WF 100 PAT

£21.99
S1F5

Respiratory
System

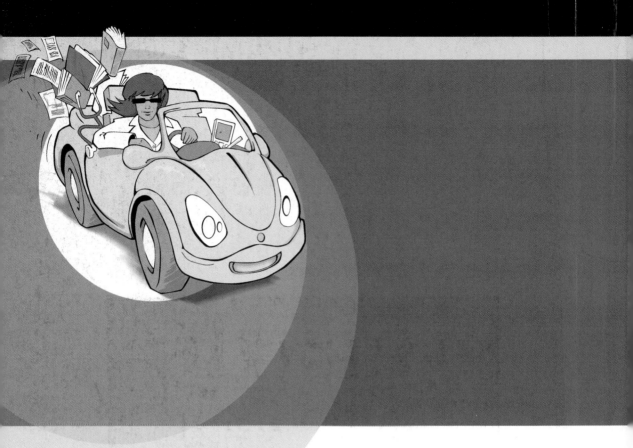

First and second edition authors:

Angus Jeffries
Andrew Turley
Pippa McGowan

CRASH COURSE

Third edition

Respiratory System

Series editor

Daniel Horton-Szar
BSC (Hons) MBBS (Hons) MRCGP

Northgate Medical Practice
Canterbury
Kent, UK

Faculty advisor

Dr Ian Adcock
PhD

National Heart and Lung Institute
Royal Brompton Hospital
Dovehouse Street
London, UK

Harish Patel

BSc (Hons)

5th Year Medical Student, Imperial College School of Medicine
South Kensington, London

Catherine Gwilt

BSc (Hons)

5th Year Medical Student, Imperial College School of Medicine
South Kensington, London

MOSBY

ELSEVIER

Edinburgh • London • New York • Oxford • Philadelphia • St Louis • Sydney • Toronto 2008

MOSBY
ELSEVIER

MOSBY An imprint of Elsevier Limited

Commissioning Editors:	**Andrew Miller, Alison Taylor**
Development Editor:	**Lulu Stader**
Project Manager:	**Jess Thompson**
Senior Designer:	**Sarah Russell**
Cover and icon illustrations:	**Stewart Larking**

First edition © 1999, Mosby International Ltd
Second edition © 2003, Elsevier Science Ltd
This edition © 2008, Elsevier Limited. All rights reserved.

First edition 1999
Second edition 2003
Third edition 2008
  Reprinted 2008

ISBN: 978-0-7234-3419-1

British Library Cataloguing in Publication Data
A catalogue record for this book is available from the British Library

Library of Congress Cataloging in Publication Data
A catalog record for this book is available from the Library of Congress

Note
Neither the publisher nor the authors assume any responsibility for any loss or injury and/or damage to persons or property arising out of or related to any use of the material contained in this book. It is the responsibility of the treating practitioner, relying on independent expertise and knowledge of the patient, to determine the best treatment and method of application for the patient.

The Publisher

ELSEVIER your source for books, journals and multimedia in the health sciences

www.elsevierhealth.com

Working together to grow
libraries in developing countries

www.elsevier.com | www.bookaid.org | www.sabre.org

ELSEVIER   BOOK AID International   Sabre Foundation

The publisher's policy is to use **paper manufactured from sustainable forests**

Printed in China

Preface

In this third edition we have tried to build a stronger bridge between the basic science and the clinical aspects of respiratory medicine. We have added lots of clinical cases and tried to make the text more clinically relevant. We have given this book a new layout, making it easier for the reader to access the information and made the text more 'digestible' as we have added plenty of summary tables and figures to reinforce key points.

We've aimed to make this book useful for the entire medical course, helping you from the first year when learning lung physiology, to the final year when you need to grasp good clinical understanding of the key respiratory topics.

We hope you enjoy using this third edition and we wish you the best of luck for your exams.

Harish Patel, Catherine Gwilt

More than a decade has now passed since work began on the first editions of the Crash Course series, and over four years since the publication of the second editions. Medicine never stands still, and the work of keeping this series relevant for today's students is an ongoing process. These third editions build upon the success of the preceding books and incorporate a great deal of new and revised material, keeping the series up to date with the latest medical research and developments in pharmacology and current best practice.

As always, we listen to feedback from the thousands of students who use Crash Course and have made further improvements to the layout and structure of the books. Each chapter now starts with a set of learning objectives, and the self-assessment sections have been enhanced and brought up to date with modern exam formats. We have also worked to integrate points of clinical relevance into the basic medical science material, which will not only add to the interest of the text but will reinforce the principles being described.

Despite fully revising the books, we hold fast to the principles on which we first developed the series: Crash Course will always bring you all the information you need to revise in compact, manageable volumes that integrate basic medical science and clinical practice. The books still maintain the balance between clarity and conciseness, and providing sufficient depth for those aiming at distinction. The authors are medical students and junior doctors who have recent experience of the exams you are now facing, and the accuracy of the material is checked by senior faculty members from across the UK.

I wish you all the best for your future careers!

Dr Dan Horton-Szar
Series Editor

Acknowledgements

We would like to thank Dan Horton-Szar and the rest of the team at Elsevier. especially Lulu Stader for all her advice and enthusiasm during the project, not to mention being so flexible with our deadlines.

A huge thanks to Professor Ian Adcock, firstly for giving us the opportunity for this task and always promptly checking our chapters even if he was half-way across the world.

Thanks also to the rest of the academic staff at the National Heart and Lung Institute who taught us during our BSc year there, for being so welcoming and giving us such a good foundation in respiratory sciences.

Finally, we would like to thank our friends and family for their continual encouragement.

Figure acknowledgements

Figs 1.1 and 1.2 adapted with permission from A Stevens and J Lowe. Human Histology, 2nd edition. Mosby, 1997

Figs 5.32, 5.33, 5.34 and 5.35 with kind permission from C J Lote. Principles of Renal Physiology, 4th edition. Kluwer Academic Publishers, 2000

Fig 7.21 adapted with permission from A Stevens and J Lowe. Pathology. Mosby, 1995

Figs 10.21, 10.23 and 10.28 adapted with permission from O Epstein, G D Perkin, D P de Bono and J Cookson. Clinical Examination, 2nd edition. Mosby, 1997

Figs 11.16, 11.17, 11.19, 11.26, 11.27 and 11.28 reproduced from D Sutton and J W R Young. Concise Textbook of Clinical Imaging, 2nd edition. Mosby, 1995

Figs 11.21, 11.22 and 11.23 reproduced from C D Forbes and W F Jackson. Color Atlas and Text of Clinical Medicine, 2nd edition. Mosby, 1997

Dedication

To my mum and dad and not forgetting my two brothers, for all the support they have given me during this project and during my medical course.

Harish Patel

To my mum, dad and sisters. Thank you for your help.

Catherine Gwilt

Contents

Contents

Glossary

Acinus Airways involved in gaseous exchange, beginning with respiratory bronchioles and ending with the alveoli.

Alveolar dead space Air reaching the alveoli that does not partake in gas exchange, for example because the alveoli are not perfused. This volume is included in physiological dead space.

Anatomical dead space Airways that do not partake in gas exchange, i.e. the nose and mouth to and including the terminal bronchioles. This volume is usually about 150 mL and included in physiological dead space.

Antitussive An intervention aiming to relieve the symptom of cough.

Asthma An airway disease with symptoms caused by reversible and intermittent airway obstruction. There is underlying inflammation characterized by eosinophilic infiltration. Often associated with other allergic diseases.

Atelectasis Collapse of part of the lung.

Bronchiectasis Permanent dilatation of the bronchi secondary to chronic infection. It is the end stage of many pulmonary diseases, including cystic fibrosis.

Bronchitis See 'Chronic bronchitis'.

Bronchoalveolar lavage A diagnostic test performed during bronchoscopy. Saline is squirted down the bronchoscope into the lungs, then sucked back up and the cells collected sent for cytology. The cellular profiles indicate different pathologies.

Bronchoscopy A diagnostic technique where a (usually fibreoptic) camera is inserted into the lungs to visualize pathology and take biopsy samples.

Chronic bronchitis A disease that is defined clinically by a persistent cough for at least 3 months of the year, for 2 consecutive years. Part of the spectrum of COPD.

Chronic obstructive pulmonary disease (COPD) A collective term for inflammatory airway diseases (emphysema, chronic bronchitis and others) occurring almost exclusively in smokers, characterized by irreversible and progressive airway obstruction. Inflammation is characterized by neutrophilic infiltration.

Conducting airways Airways not involved in gas exchange, i.e. airways proximal to respiratory bronchiole.

Continuous airways positive pressure (CPAP) A method of non-invasive ventilation whereby air is blown into the airways (positive pressure) for the whole of the respiratory cycle. CPAP is delivered by mask and is a common treatment for obstructive sleep apnoea.

Corticosteroid (glucocorticosteroid) A commonly used immunosuppressive drug that acts at a nuclear level to inhibit inflammation.

Cystic fibrosis An autosomal recessive condition causing a defect in the cystic fibrosis transmembrane receptor (CFTR), resulting in abnormally viscous lung secretions. In the lung the mutation predisposes to chronic lung infection and bronchiectasis; it also affects the pancreas and can cause male infertility.

Diffuse parenchymal lung disease See 'Interstitial lung disease'.

Emphysema Defined anatomically as destruction of the alveolar septae resulting in permanent enlargement of the air spaces distal to the terminal bronchiole. Part of the spectrum of COPD.

Haemoptysis A term to describe the symptom of coughing up blood.

Hypoxic vasoconstriction Constriction of pulmonary blood vessels in response to low alveolar oxygen tension. This mechanism acts to prevent a ventilation : perfusion mismatch.

Interstitial lung disease (ILD) A diverse group of more than 200 different lung diseases affecting the interstitium (the tissue extending from and including the alveolar epithelium to capillary endothelium). May be used interchangeably with 'diffuse parenchymal lung disease'.

Mediastinum The collective name to describe structures situated in the midline and separating the two lungs. It contains the heart, great vessels, trachea, oesophagus, lymph nodes, phrenic and vagus nerves.

Mesothelioma Cancer of the lung pleura, almost always caused by asbestos inhalation.

Obstructive lung disease Diseases which narrow the airways and increase resistance to air flow.

Physiological dead space The total amount of air in the lung that does not partake in gas exchange. Includes anatomical dead space and alveolar dead space.

Pleura An epithelial lining which covers the external surface of the lungs (visceral pleura) and then is reflected back to line the chest wall (parietal pleura).

Pleural effusion Fluid in the pleural space.

Pneumocytes The cells lining the alveoli. They are either type I, which are thin and primarily structural, or type II, which are rounded and secrete surfactant.

Pneumonia Infection of peripheral lung tissue.

Pneumothorax Air in the pleural space; the tension type is a medical emergency.

Pulmonary embolism Thrombi lodging in pulmonary vasculature causing ventilation : perfusion mismatches of varying severity. A serious complication of venous thrombosis.

Pulmonary fibrosis A restrictive lung disease where lung parenchyma is stiffened by deposition of collagen; the end-point of many different lung diseases.

Respiratory tree Another name for the airways, particularly referring to their branching pattern. Does not include alveoli.

Restrictive lung diseases Diseases which stiffen the lungs so that expansion of the lungs is compromised.

Sarcoidosis A multisystem granulomatous disorder of unknown origin that can cause a granulomatous interstitial lung disease.

Surfactant A liquid rich in phospholipids and apoproteins that lines the alveoli to reduce surface tension and defend the host against inhaled pathogens. It is secreted by type II pneumocytes.

Spirometry A diagnostic technique used to measure speed of air flow and the volume of air exhaled from the lungs.

Wheeze The musical sound heard on expiration, caused by airway narrowing.

BASIC MEDICAL SCIENCE

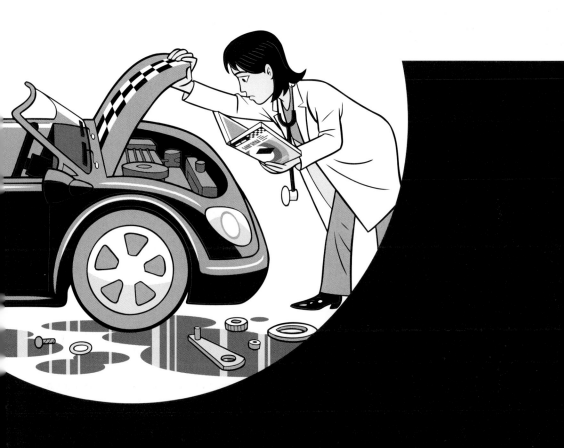

Overview of the respiratory system

Objectives

By the end of this chapter you should be able to:

- Understand why humans have developed a respiratory system.
- Describe how breathing is brought about.
- Understand the differences between the partial pressure of a gas and its concentration.
- Understand how defects in ventilation, perfusion and diffusion cause hypoxaemia.
- Understand the effect anaemia will have on P_aO_2, S_aO_2 and on the total oxygen content of the blood.
- Know which structures are involved in gas exchange.
- Show the differences between restrictive and obstructive disorders.
- Show what happens if lung disease increases the work of breathing to excessive levels.
- Describe how respiration is controlled.
- List the main functions of the respiratory system.

OVERALL STRUCTURE AND FUNCTION

Respiration

Respiration refers to the processes involved in oxygen transport from the atmosphere to the body tissues and the release and transportation of carbon dioxide produced in the tissues to the atmosphere.

This book will not discuss tissue respiration, in which oxygen is used by the cell to liberate energy; this is also known as internal respiration and is covered in *Crash Course: Metabolism and Nutrition*. The focus of this book is external respiration, or the exchange of gases between the environment and the blood.

Microorganisms rely on diffusion to and from their environment for the supply of oxygen and removal of carbon dioxide. Humans, however, are unable to rely on diffusion because:

- Their surface area : volume ratio is too small.
- The diffusion distance from the surface of the body to the cells is too large and the process would be far too slow to be compatible with life.

Remember that diffusion time increases with the square of the distance, and as a result, the human body has had to develop a specialized respiratory system to overcome these problems. This system has two components:

- A gas-exchange system that provides a large surface area for the uptake of oxygen from, and the release of carbon dioxide to, the environment. This function is performed by the lungs.
- A transport system that delivers oxygen to the tissues from the lungs and carbon dioxide to the lungs from the tissues. This function is carried out by the cardiovascular system.

Structure

The respiratory system can be neatly divided into upper respiratory tract (nasal and oral cavities, pharynx, larynx and trachea) and lower respiratory tract (main bronchi and lungs) (Fig. 1.1).

Upper respiratory tract

The upper respiratory tract has a large surface area, a rich blood supply, and its epithelium (respiratory epithelium) is covered by a mucous secretion. Within the nose, hairs are present, which act as a filter. The function of the upper respiratory tract is to warm, moisten, and filter the air so that it is in a suitable condition for gaseous exchange in the distal part of the lower respiratory tract.

Fig. 1.1 A schematic diagram of the respiratory tract.

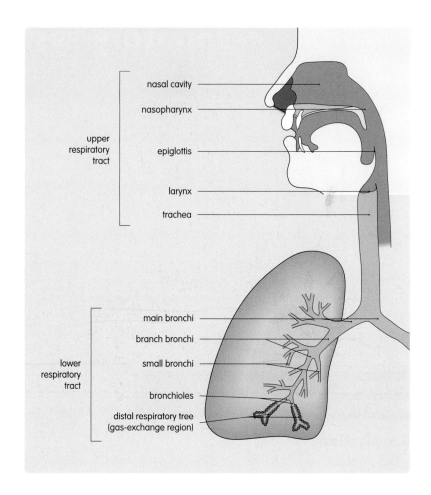

upper respiratory tract

nasal cavity

nasopharynx

epiglottis

larynx

trachea

lower respiratory tract

main bronchi

branch bronchi

small bronchi

bronchioles

distal respiratory tree (gas-exchange region)

Lower respiratory tract

The lower respiratory tract consists of the lower part of the trachea, the two primary bronchi and the lungs. These structures are contained within the thoracic cavity.

Lungs

The lungs are the organs of gas exchange and act as both a conduit for air flow (the airway) and a surface for movement of oxygen into the blood and carbon dioxide out of the blood (the alveolar capillary membrane).

The lungs consist of airways, blood vessels, nerves and lymphatics, supported by parenchymal tissue. Inside the lungs, the two main bronchi divide into smaller and smaller airways until the end respiratory unit (acinus) is reached (Fig. 1.2).

Acinus

The acinus is that part of the airway that is involved in gaseous exchange (i.e. the passage of oxygen from the lungs to the blood and carbon dioxide from the blood to the lungs). It begins with the respiratory bronchioles and includes the subsequent divisions of the airway and alveoli. The structure of the acinus is considered in detail in Chapter 3.

Conducting airways

Conducting airways allow the transport of gases to and from the acinus but are themselves unable to partake in gas exchange. They include all divisions of the bronchi proximal to, but excluding, respiratory bronchioles.

Pleurae

The lung, chest wall and mediastinum are covered by two continuous layers of epithelium known as the pleurae. The inner pleura covering the lung is the visceral pleura and the outer pleura covering the chest wall and mediastinum is the parietal pleura. These two pleurae are closely opposed and are

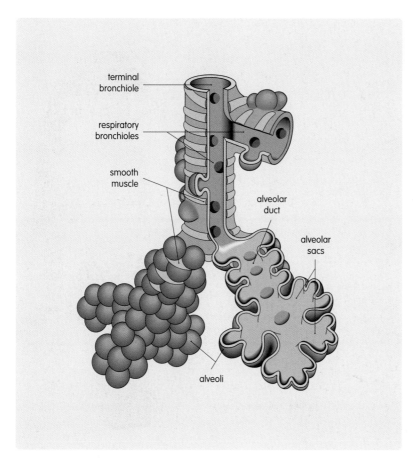

Fig. 1.2 The acinus, or respiratory unit. This part of the airway is involved in gas exchange.

terminal bronchiole

respiratory bronchioles

smooth muscle

alveolar duct

alveolar sacs

alveoli

separated by only a thin layer of liquid. The liquid acts as a lubricant and allows the two surfaces to slip over each other during breathing.

BASIC CONCEPTS IN RESPIRATION

The supply of oxygen to body tissues is essential for life; after only a brief period without oxygen, cells undergo irreversible change and eventually death. The respiratory system plays an essential role in preventing tissue hypoxia by optimizing the oxygen content of arterial blood through efficient gas exchange. The three key steps involved in gas exchange are:

- Ventilation.
- Perfusion.
- Diffusion.

Together these processes ensure that oxygen is available for transport to the body tissues and that carbon dioxide is eliminated (Fig. 1.3). If any of the three steps are compromised, for example through lung disease, then the oxygen content of the blood will fall below normal (hypoxaemia) and levels of carbon dioxide may rise (hypercapnia) (Fig. 1.4). In clinical practice, we do not directly test for tissue hypoxia but look for:

- Symptoms and signs of impaired gas exchange (e.g. breathlessness or central cyanosis).
- Abnormal results from arterial blood gas tests (see Ch. 11).

Severe hypoxaemia, with or without hypercapnia, is known as respiratory failure (see Ch. 9).

Ventilation

Ventilation is the movement of air in and out of the respiratory system. It is determined by both:

- The respiratory rate (i.e. number of breaths per minute, normally 12–20).

Fig 1.3 Key steps involved in respiration. (After Hlastala & Berger 2001, with permission of Oxford University Press.)

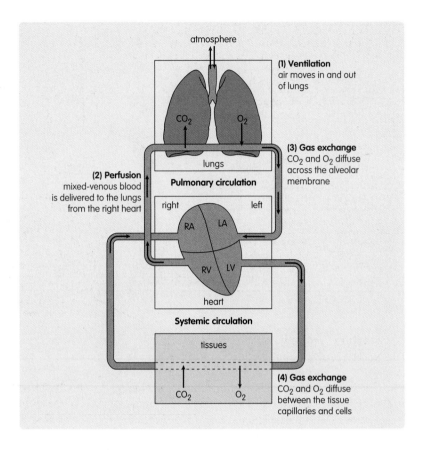

- The volume of each breath, also known as the tidal volume.

A change in ventilation, in response to the metabolic needs of the body, can therefore be brought about by either:

- Altering the number of breaths per minute.
- Adjusting the amount of air that enters the lungs with each breath.

In practice, the most common response to hypoxaemia is rapid, shallow breathing which increases the elimination of carbon dioxide and often leads to hypocapnia.

A raised respiratory rate, or tachypnoea, is not the same as hyperventilation. The term hyperventilation refers to a situation where ventilation is too great for the body's metabolic needs (see Ch. 5, p. 92).

The mechanisms of ventilation

The movement of air into and out of the lungs takes place because of pressure differences caused by changes in lung volumes. Air flows from a high-pressure area to a low-pressure area. We cannot change the local atmospheric pressure around us to a level higher than that inside our lungs; the only obvious alternative is to lower the pressure within the lungs. We achieve this pressure reduction by expanding the size of the chest.

The main muscle of inspiration is the diaphragm, upon which the two lungs sit. The diaphragm is dome-shaped; contraction flattens the dome, increasing intrathoracic volume. This is aided by the external intercostal muscles, which raise the rib cage; this results in a lowered pressure within the thoracic cavity and hence the lungs, supplying the driving force for air flow into the lungs. Inspiration is responsible for most of the work of breathing; diseases of the lungs or chest wall may increase the workload so that accessory muscles are also required to maintain adequate ventilation.

Fig. 1.4 Common respiratory terms	
Hypocapnia	Decreased carbon dioxide tension in arterial blood (P_aCO_2 <4.8kPa or 35 mmHg)
Hypercapnia	Increased carbon dioxide tension in arterial blood (P_aCO_2 >6kPa or 45 mmHg)
Hypoxaemia	Deficient oxygenation of the arterial blood
Hypoxia	Deficient oxygenation of the tissues
Hyperventilation	Ventilation that is in excess of metabolic requirements (results in hypocapnia)
Hypoventilation	Ventilation that is too low for metabolic requirements (results in hypercapnial)

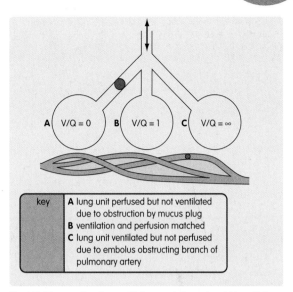

key	A lung unit perfused but not ventilated due to obstruction by mucus plug
	B ventilation and perfusion matched
	C lung unit ventilated but not perfused due to embolus obstructing branch of pulmonary artery

Fig. 1.5 Diagram showing ventilation : perfusion mismatching. (After West 2001, with permission of Lippincott, Williams & Wilkins.)

Expiration is largely passive, being a result of elastic recoil of the lung tissue. However, in forced expiration (e.g. during coughing), the abdominal muscles increase intra-abdominal pressure, forcing the contents of the abdomen against the diaphragm. In addition, the internal intercostal muscles lower the rib cage. These actions greatly increase intra-thoracic pressure and enhance expiration.

Impaired ventilation

There are two main types of disorder which impair ventilation. These are:

- Obstructive disorders:
  - Airways are narrowed and resistance to airflow is increased.
  - Mechanisms of airway narrowing include inflamed and thickened bronchial walls (e.g. asthma), airways filled with mucus (e.g. chronic bronchitis, asthma) and airway collapse (e.g. emphysema).
- Restrictive disorders:
  - Lungs are less able to expand and so the volume of gas exchanged is reduced.
  - Mechanisms include stiffening of lung tissue (e.g. pulmonary fibrosis) or inadequacy of respiratory muscles (e.g. Duchenne muscular dystrophy).

Obstructive and restrictive disorders have characteristic patterns of lung function, measured by pulmonary function tests (see Ch. 3).

Ventilatory failure occurs if the work of breathing becomes excessive and muscles fail. In this situation, or to prevent it from occurring, mechanical ventilation is required. Respiratory support is discussed in Chapter 6.

Perfusion

The walls of the alveoli contain a dense network of capillaries bringing mixed-venous blood from the right heart. The barrier separating blood in the capillaries and air in the alveoli is extremely thin. Perfusion of blood through these pulmonary capillaries allows diffusion, and therefore gas exchange, to take place.

Ventilation : perfusion inequality

To achieve efficient gaseous exchange, it is essential that the flow of gas (ventilation: $\dot{V}$) and the flow of blood (perfusion: $\dot{Q}$) are closely matched. The $\dot{V}/\dot{Q}$ ratio in a normal, healthy lung is approximately 1. Two extreme scenarios illustrate mismatching of ventilation and perfusion (Fig. 1.5). These are:

- Normal alveolar ventilation but no perfusion (e.g. due to a blood clot obstructing flow).
- Normal perfusion but no air reaching the lung unit (e.g. due to a mucus plug occluding an airway).

Make sure you grasp the concept of ventilation:perfusion matching – it makes the pathology of many lung diseases easier to understand!

Ventilation:perfusion inequality is the most common cause of hypoxaemia and underlies many respiratory diseases.

Diffusion

At the gas exchange surface, diffusion occurs across the alveolar capillary membrane.

Molecules of CO_2 and O_2 diffuse along their partial pressure gradients.

Partial pressures

Air in the atmosphere, before it is inhaled and moistened, contains 21% oxygen. This means that:

- 21% of the total molecules in air are oxygen molecules.
- Oxygen is responsible for 21% of the total air pressure; this is its partial pressure, measured in mmHg or kPa and abbreviated as PO_2 (Fig. 1.6).

Partial pressure also determines the gas content of liquids, but it is not the only factor. Gas enters the liquid as a solution, and the amount that enters depends on its solubility. The more soluble a gas the more molecules that will enter solution for a given partial pressure. The partial pressure of a gas in a liquid is sometimes referred to as its tension (i.e. arterial oxygen tension is the same as P_aO_2).

As blood perfusing the pulmonary capillaries is mixed-venous blood:

- Oxygen will diffuse from the higher PO_2 environment of the alveoli into the capillaries.
- Carbon dioxide will diffuse from the blood towards the alveoli, where PCO_2 is lower.

Blood and gas equilibrate as the partial pressures become the same in each and gas exchange then stops.

Oxygen transport

Once oxygen has diffused into the capillaries it must be transported to the body tissues. The solubility of oxygen in the blood is low and only a small percentage of the body's requirement can be carried in dissolved form. Therefore most of the oxygen is combined with haemoglobin in red blood cells. Haemoglobin has four binding sites and the amount of oxygen carried by haemoglobin in the blood depends on how many of these sites are occupied. If they are all occupied by oxygen the molecule is said to be saturated. The oxygen saturation (S_aO_2) tells us the relative percentage of the maximum possible sites that can be bound. Note that anaemia will not reduce S_aO_2; lower haemoglobin means there are fewer available sites but the relative percentage of possible sites that are saturated stays the same.

The relationship between the partial pressure of oxygen and percentage saturation of haemoglobin is represented by the oxygen dissociation curve (see Ch. 5).

Diffusion defects

If the blood–gas barrier becomes thickened through disease, then the diffusion of O_2 and CO_2 will be impaired. Any impairment is particularly noticeable during exercise, when pulmonary flow increases and blood spends an even shorter time in the capillaries, exposed to alveolar oxygen. Impaired diffusion is, however, a much less common cause of hypoxaemia than ventilation:perfusion mismatching.

Fig. 1.6 Abbreviations used in denoting partial pressures	
PO_2	Oxygen tension in blood (either arterial or venous)
P_aO_2	Arterial oxygen tension
P_vO_2	Oxygen tension in mixed-venous blood
P_AO_2	Alveolar oxygen tension
Carbon dioxide tensions follow the same format (PCO_2 etc)	

CONTROL OF RESPIRATION

Respiration must respond to the metabolic demands of the body. This is achieved by a control system within the brainstem (the respiratory centres – see Ch. 6, p. 102) which receives information from various sources in the body where sensors monitor:

It is easy to get confused about P_aO_2, S_aO_2 and oxygen content. P_aO_2 tells us the pressure of the oxygen molecules dissolved in plasma, not those bound to haemoglobin. It is not a measure of how much oxygen is in the arterial blood. S_aO_2 tells us how many of the possible haemoglobin binding sites are occupied by oxygen. To calculate the amount of oxygen you would also need to know haemoglobin levels and how much oxygen is dissolved. Oxygen content (C_aO_2) is the only value that actually tells us how much oxygen is in the blood and, unlike P_aO_2 or S_aO_2, it is given in units which denote quantity (mL O_2/dL).

- Partial pressures of oxygen and carbon dioxide in the blood.
- pH of the extracellular fluid within the brain.
- Mechanical changes in the chest wall.

On the basis of information they receive, the respiratory centres modify ventilation to ensure that oxygen supply and carbon dioxide removal from the tissues match their metabolic requirements. The actual mechanical change to ventilation is carried out by the respiratory muscles: these are known as the effectors of the control system.

Respiration can also be modified by higher centres (e.g. during speech, anxiety, emotion).

OTHER FUNCTIONS OF THE RESPIRATORY SYSTEM

Respiration is also concerned with a number of other functions, including metabolism, excretion, hormonal activity and, most importantly:

- Regulation of the pH of body fluids.
- Regulation of body temperature.

Acid–base regulation

Carbon dioxide forms carbonic acid in the blood, which dissociates to form hydrogen ions, lowering pH. By controlling the partial pressure of carbon dioxide, the respiratory system plays an important role in regulating the body's acid–base status (see Ch. 5); lung disease can therefore lead to acid–base disturbance. In acute disease it is important to test for blood pH and bicarbonate levels, and these are included in the standard arterial blood gas results.

Body temperature regulation

Body temperature is achieved mainly by insensible heat loss. Thus, by altering ventilation, body temperature may be regulated.

Metabolism

The lungs have a huge vascular supply and thus a large number of endothelial cells. Hormones such as noradrenaline (norepinephrine), prostaglandins and 5-hydroxytryptamine are taken up by these cells and destroyed. Some exogenous compounds are also taken up by the lungs and destroyed (e.g. amfetamine and imipramine).

Excretion

Carbon dioxide and some drugs (notably those administered through the lungs; e.g. general anaesthetics) are excreted by the lungs.

Hormonal activity

Hormones (e.g. steroids) act on the lungs. Insulin enhances glucose utilization and protein synthesis. Angiotensin II is formed in the lungs from angiotensin I (by angiotensin-converting enzyme). Damage to the lung tissue causes the release of prostacyclin PGI_2, which prevents platelet aggregation.

The upper respiratory tract

ORGANIZATION OF THE UPPER RESPIRATORY TRACT

Structure of the upper respiratory tract

Nose

The nose consists of an external part (the external nose) and an internal part (the nasal cavities, including the nasal septum). These structures are adapted to the main functions of the nose which are olfaction (smelling) and breathing. This book will focus on the internal nose and its function in breathing.

Nasal cavities and paranasal sinuses

The lateral wall of the nasal cavity consists of bony ridges called conchae or turbinates (Figs 2.1 and 2.2). These provide a large surface area covered in highly vascularized mucous membrane which warms and humidifies inspired air.

Under each turbinate there is a groove or meatus. The paranasal air sinuses (frontal, sphenoid, ethmoid and maxillary) drain into these meatuses via small ostia, or openings. The drainage sites of each of the sinuses are shown in Figure 2.2.

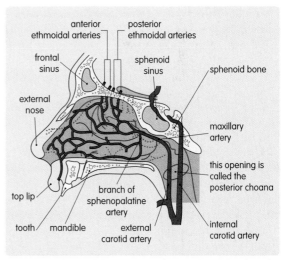

Fig. 2.1 Lateral view of the nasal cavity showing the rich blood supply.

The important role of the nasal cavities in warming and humidifying air is illustrated by patients who have had tracheostomies or endotracheal intubation for long periods. Without nose breathing, the mucosa of the trachea can become dry and crusted.

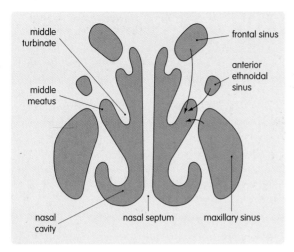

Fig. 2.2 Frontal view of the nasal cavity drainage sites of the paranasal sinuses.

Muscle tone of the pharynx, particularly at the level of the soft palate, is important in maintaining airway patency. During sleep, the upper airway dilating muscles relax and in some individuals the airway may be partially or completely occluded. This leads to recurrent episodes of sleep apnoea (p. 18).

Mr Wells had been suffering from a cold for the last 10 days and now complained of right-sided unilateral face pain (worse on chewing), fever, headache and purulent nasal discharge. On examining him, the GP noted tenderness over the right maxillary sinus, and suspected sinusitis as a complication of a common cold. The ostia of the sinuses had become blocked by mucosal inflammation and the stagnant mucus led to increased pressure and infection The GP prescribed amoxicillin and Mr Wells made a full recovery.

Blood and nerve supply and lymphatic drainage

The terminal branches of the internal and external carotid arteries provide the rich blood supply for the internal nose. The sphenopalatine artery (from the maxillary artery) and the anterior ethmoidal artery (from the ophthalmic) are the two most important branches. Sensation to the area is provided mainly by the maxillary branch of the trigeminal nerve. Lymphatic vessels drain into the submandibular node, then drain into deep cervical nodes.

Pharynx

The pharynx extends from the base of the skull to the inferior border of the cricoid cartilage where it is continuous anteriorly with the trachea and posteriorly with the oesophagus. It is described as being divided into three parts: the nasopharynx, oropharynx and the laryngopharynx, which open anteriorly into the nose, the mouth and the larynx, respectively (Fig. 2.3).

The nasopharynx is situated above the soft palate and opens anteriorly into the nasal cavities at the choanae (posterior nares). During swallowing, the nasopharynx is cut off from the oropharynx by the soft palate. The nasopharynx contains the opening of the eustachian canal (pharyngotympanic or auditory tube) and the adenoids, which lie beneath the epithelium of its posterior wall.

Detailed discussion of the oropharynx and laryngopharynx is beyond the scope of this book.

Musculature, blood and nerve supply and lymphatic drainage

Three muscles surround the fascial tube of the pharynx: the superior, middle and inferior constrictor muscles (Fig. 2.4).

The arterial blood supply of the pharynx is from the external carotid through the superior thyroid, ascending pharyngeal, facial and lingual arteries. Venous drainage is by a plexus of veins on the outer surface of the pharynx to the internal jugular vein.

Both sensory and motor nerve supplies are from the pharyngeal plexus (cranial nerves IX and X); the maxillary nerve (cranial nerve V) supplies the nasopharynx with sensory fibres.

Lymphatic vessels drain directly into the deep cervical lymph nodes.

Larynx

At its inferior end, the larynx is continuous with the trachea. At its superior end, it is attached to the U-shaped hyoid bone and lies below the epiglottis of the tongue. The larynx is made up of a cartilaginous skeleton linked by a number of membranes. This cartilaginous skeleton consists of the epiglottis, thyroid, arytenoid and cricoid cartilages. Figure 2.5

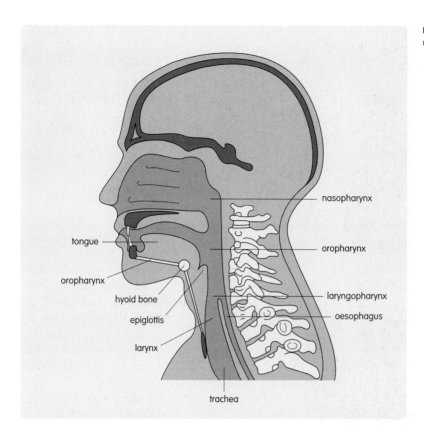

Fig. 2.3 Schematic diagram showing midline structures of the head and neck.

nasopharynx

tongue

oropharynx

oropharynx

hyoid bone

laryngopharynx

epiglottis

oesophagus

larynx

trachea

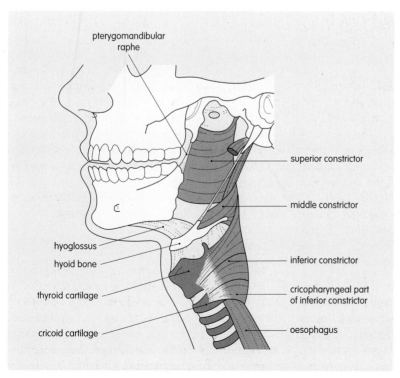

Fig. 2.4 The pharynx, showing the superior, middle and inferior constrictors.

pterygomandibular raphe

superior constrictor

middle constrictor

hyoglossus

hyoid bone

inferior constrictor

thyroid cartilage

cricopharyngeal part of inferior constrictor

cricoid cartilage

oesophagus

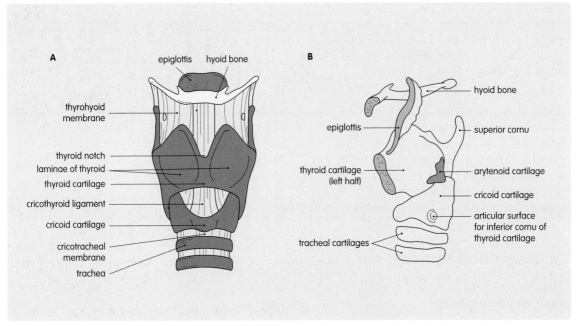

Fig. 2.5 The larynx. (A) External view – anterior aspect. (B) Median section through the larynx, hyoid bone and trachea.

shows an external view and a median section through the larynx.

The larynx has three main functions:

- As an open valve, to allow air to pass when breathing.
- Protection of the trachea and bronchi during swallowing. The vocal cords close, the epiglottis folds back covering the opening to the larynx, and the larynx is pulled upwards and forwards beneath the tongue.
- Speech production (phonation).

Musculature

The muscles of the larynx are split into external and internal muscles. There is only one external muscle of the larynx (cricothyroid), although many other muscles attach to the thyroid membrane and cartilage. Cricothyroid has its origin at the arch of the cricoid and attaches to the lower border of the thyroid cartilage. The internal muscles may change the shape of the larynx: they protect the lungs by a sphincter action and adjust the vocal cords in phonation.

Blood and nerve supply and lymphatic drainage

The blood supply of the larynx is from superior and inferior laryngeal arteries, which are accompanied by the superior and recurrent laryngeal branches of the vagus nerve (cranial nerve X). The internal

Mr Rogers, a heavy smoker, presented to his GP with a 'bovine' cough and hoarseness. Investigations revealed a left-sided lung cancer that had caused Mr Rogers's symptoms by compression of the left recurrent laryngeal nerve. The left recurrent laryngeal nerve is susceptible to compression by neoplasms since it has a long course through the thorax from the aortic arch, where it leaves the vagus, to the larynx.

branch of the superior laryngeal nerve supplies the mucosa of the larynx above the vocal cords, the external branch supplies the cricothyroid muscle. The recurrent laryngeal nerve supplies the mucosa below the vocal cords and all the intrinsic muscles apart from the cricothyroid.

Lymph vessels above the vocal cords drain into the upper deep cervical lymph nodes; below the vocal cords, lymphatic vessels drain into the lower cervical lymph nodes.

Trachea

The trachea is a cartilaginous and membranous tube of about 10 cm in length. It extends from the larynx to its bifurcation at the carina (at the level of the fourth or fifth thoracic vertebra). The trachea is approximately 2.5 cm in diameter and is supported by C-shaped rings of hyaline cartilage. The rings are completed posteriorly by the trachealis muscle. Important relations of the trachea within the neck are:

- The thyroid gland, which straddles the trachea, its two lobes sitting laterally, and its isthmus anteriorly with the inferior thyroid veins.
- The common carotid arteries, which lie lateral to the trachea.
- The oesophagus, which lies directly behind the trachea, and the recurrent laryngeal nerve, which lies between these two structures.

Tissues of the upper respiratory tract

Nose and nasopharynx

The upper one-third of the nasal cavity is the olfactory area and is covered in yellowish olfactory epithelium. The lower two-thirds of the nasal cavity, the nasal sinuses and the nasopharynx comprise the respiratory area, which is adapted to its main functions of filtering, warming and humidifying inspired air. These areas are lined with pseudostratified ciliated columnar epithelium (Fig. 2.6), also known as respiratory epithelium. With the exception of a few areas, this pattern of epithelium lines the whole of the respiratory tract down to the terminal bronchioles. Throughout these cells are numerous mucus-secreting goblet cells with microvilli on their luminal surface. Coordinated beating of the cilia propels mucus and entrapped particles to the pharynx where it is swallowed.

> The cilia play an important role in preventing microorganisms from causing infection. Abnormal ciliary motility, as seen in Kartagener's syndrome (p. 18), leads to sinusitis and bronchiectasis.

Adenoids

The nasopharyngeal tonsil is a collection of mucosa-associated lymphoid tissue (MALT) that lies behind the epithelium of the roof and the posterior surface of the nasopharynx. Together with the palatine tonsils and the lymphoid tissue on the dorsum of the tongue, these form Waldeyer's ring.

Oropharynx and laryngopharynx

The oropharynyx and laryngopharynx have two functions as parts of both the respiratory and alimentary tracts. They are lined with non-keratinized stratified squamous (NKSS) epithelium several layers thick and are kept moist by numerous salivary glands.

Larynx and trachea

The epithelium of the larynx is made up of two types: NKSS epithelium and respiratory epithelium. NKSS epithelium covers the vocal folds, vestibular fold and larynx above this level. Below the level of the vestibular fold (with the exception of the vocal folds, which are lined with keratinized stratified squamous epithelium), the larynx and trachea are covered with respiratory epithelium.

DEVELOPMENT OF THE UPPER RESPIRATORY TRACT

Branchial arches and pharyngeal pouches

During week 4 of development, the branchial arches are formed; these are gill-like pairs of folds at the cranial (head) end of the embryo. Eventually, six pairs of branchial arches are formed, which are numbered craniocaudally (head to tail) from first to sixth arches. Not all arches are present at once; the

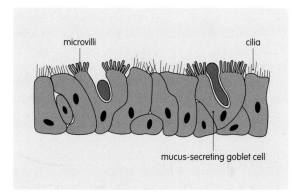

microvilli   cilia

mucus-secreting goblet cell

Fig. 2.6 Respiratory epithelium.

first two branchial arches degenerate before the sixth arch is formed. The branchial arches form the major part of the branchial apparatus, which consists of:

- Branchial arches.
- Pharyngeal pouches: evaginations of endodermal tissue, situated inside the primitive pharynx.
- Branchial grooves: located between the branchial arches.
- Branchial membrane: bilaminar layer of ectodermal and endodermal tissue between the branchial arches.

The branchial arches form the skeletal and muscular components of the head and neck. Mesenchymal cells group together within the arches to form clusters called branchial arch cartilages, which form skeletal structures. Mesenchymal cells also form myoblasts (primitive muscle cells), which migrate to form the musculature of the head and neck.

The nerve supply of the branchial arches is derived from the cranial nerves. The first and second branchial arches receive sensory fibres from cranial nerve V and motor fibres from cranial nerve VII. The nerve supply to the third branchial arch is from cranial nerve IX, which also supplies the stylopharyngeus. The fourth and sixth branchial arches are supplied by two branches of the vagus nerve (cranial nerve X): the superior laryngeal and recurrent laryngeal nerves.

Primitive mouth, nasal and oral cavities

The primitive mouth is formed by a depression in the ectoderm at the cranial end of the embryo, called the stomodeum, initially separated from the primitive pharynx by a bilaminar membrane called the oropharyngeal membrane. This membrane ruptures at about day 24–26, by which time the ectoderm of the cranial end of the embryo has already invaginated, forming the nasal and oral cavities.

Respiratory tract: larynx and trachea

The respiratory tract starts as a groove in the median plane of the primitive pharynx, the laryngotracheal groove. This groove deepens to form the laryngotracheal diverticulum and continues caudally (towards the tail) into the splanchnic mesenchyme, its distal end forming the lung bud. The cartilage and smooth muscle of the larynx are formed from the mesenchyme surrounding the diverticulum (Fig. 2.7). The foregut is separated from the diverticulum by the tracheo-oesophageal septum; when the diverticulum lengthens this is called the laryngotracheal tube. Defects in development may result in a tracheo-oesophageal fistula.

The connective tissue, cartilages and smooth muscle of the trachea develop from the splanchnic mesenchyme, the glandular tissue developing from the endoderm.

DISORDERS OF THE NOSE

Inflammatory conditions

Infectious rhinitis (acute coryza or common cold)

'Rhinitis' is inflammation of the mucosal membrane lining the nose. Inflammation seen in the common cold is caused by a number of viral infections:

- Rhinovirus (commonest cause).
- Coronavirus.
- Adenovirus.
- Parainfluenza virus.
- Respiratory syncytial virus.

The common cold is a highly contagious self-limiting condition, with the highest incidence in children. Symptoms are nasal obstruction, rhinorrhoea (runny nose) and sneezing. Complications include sinusitis, otitis media and lower respiratory tract infections such as bronchitis.

Pathology
There is acute inflammation with oedema, glandular hypersecretion and loss of surface epithelium.

Treatment
Treat symptomatically with decongestants and analgesics. Unless bacterial complications ensue, antibiotics are useless because of viral aetiology.

Chronic rhinitis

Chronic rhinitis may follow an acute inflammatory episode. Predisposing factors include inadequate drainage of sinuses, nasal obstruction caused by polyps, and enlargement of the adenoids.

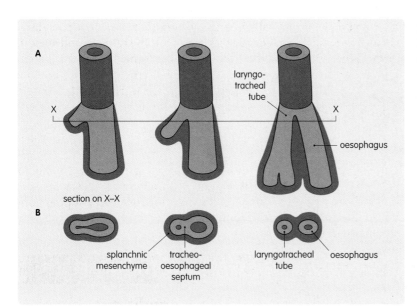

Fig. 2.7 Formation of the trachea and larynx: (A) lateral view; (B) cross-section on X–X. Note how defects in formation of the septum can lead to a fistula between trachea and oesophagus.

Allergic rhinitis

Allergic rhinitis is a common condition, affecting up to 30% of the western population. It is classified as either seasonal rhinitis (hay fever) or perennial rhinitis.

Seasonal rhinitis

Seasonal rhinitis has a maximum prevalence in patients aged 10–20 years. It occurs during summer months. Approximately 20% of patients with allergic rhinitis also suffer from asthma.

Perennial rhinitis

The incidence of perennial rhinitis decreases with age. It is most common in patients aged 10–30 years.

There is no seasonal variation in symptoms, which are mainly caused by Der p1 allergen in faecal particles of the house dust mite. Proteins from the urine and saliva of domestic pets, especially cats, also cause problems.

In some cases the pathology of perennial rhinitis is non-allergic and is due to abnormalities of the autonomic nervous system; this is termed vasomotor, or intrinsic, rhinitis. Nasal polyps may also present with perennial rhinitis secondary to nasal obstruction.

Aetiology

Rhinitis is caused by hypersensitivity to allergens; commonest allergens are highly soluble proteins or glycoproteins (e.g. from pollens, moulds, cat dander and dust mite).

Pathology

Symptoms are caused by a type I IgE-mediated hypersensitivity reaction. IgE fixes onto mast cells in nasal mucous membranes. Upon re-exposure to allergen, cross-linking of the IgE receptor occurs on the surface of the mast cells leading to mast cell degranulation and release of histamine and leukotrienes.

Investigations

Diagnosis of rhinitis is clinical. Skin prick tests, nasal smears and provocation tests can be used. Blood tests are:

- PRIST (plasma radioimmunosorbent test) – measures total plasma IgE levels.
- RAST (radioallergosorbent test) – measures specific serum IgE antibody.

Treatment

Treatment is by allergen avoidance and drug treatment with antihistamines, anti-inflammatory drugs (e.g. nasal corticosteroids) and sodium cromoglicate (mast cell stabilizers).

Acute sinusitis

Sinusitis is an inflammatory process involving the lining of paranasal sinuses. The maxillary sinus is most commonly clinically infected. The majority of infections are rhinogenic in origin and are classified as either acute or chronic.

Aetiology

The causes of acute sinusitis are:

- Secondary bacterial infection (by *Streptococcus pneumoniae* or *Haemophilus influenzae*), often after upper respiratory tract viral infection.
- Dental extraction or infection.
- Swimming and diving.
- Fractures involving sinuses.

Clinical features

Symptoms occur over several days with yellow–green nasal discharge, malaise, sinus tenderness and disturbed sense of smell. There may be fullness and pain over the cheeks, maxillary toothache or a frontal headache. Pain is classically worse on leaning forward. Postnasal discharge may lead to cough.

Pathology

Hyperaemia and oedema of the mucosa occurs. Blockage of sinus ostia and mucus production increases. Cilia stop beating; therefore, stasis of secretions leads to secondary infection.

Investigations

The investigations are:

- Blood – white cell count and erythrocyte sedimentation rate (may be raised but are often normal).
- Culture of pus from nose.
- Radiology of paranasal sinuses.

Treatment

Medical treatment is by analgesia, broad-acting antibiotic for 7 days, and a decongestant (e.g. xylomethazoline). Anti-inflammatory nasal sprays such as fluticasone propionate or budesonide (topical corticosteroids) can be used to relieve symptoms. Discourage smoking and alcohol consumption. If no response to two regimens of antibiotics, refer to ear, nose and throat (ENT) specialist.

Chronic sinusitis

Chronic sinusitis is an inflammation of the sinuses which has been present for more than 4 weeks. It usually occurs after recurrent acute sinusitis and is common in patients who are heavy smokers and work in dusty environments.

Clinical features

Clinical features are similar to those of acute sinusitis but are typically less severe.

Pathology

Prolonged infection leads to irreversible changes in the sinus cavity, including:

- An increase in vascular permeability.
- Oedema and hypertrophy of the mucosa.
- Goblet-cell hyperplasia.
- Chronic cellular infiltrate.
- Ulceration of the epithelium, resulting in granulated tissue formation.

Investigations

The investigations are through sinus radiographs, high-definition coronal section CT and diagnostic endoscopy.

Treatment

This condition is difficult to treat. Treatments are:

- Medical – broad-acting antibiotics and decongestant.
- Surgical – antral lavage, inferior meatal intranasal antrostomy and functional endoscopic sinus surgery.

Rarely, recurrent sinusitis may be caused by Kartagener's syndrome, a congenital mucociliary disorder due to the absence of the ciliary protein dynein (Fig. 2.8). It is characterized by sinusitis, bronchiectasis, otitis media, dextrocardia and infertility.

DISORDERS OF THE PHARYNX

Sleep apnoea

Sleep apnoea is the cessation of breathing during sleep. There are two types: obstructive sleep apnoea and central sleep apnoea.

It is thought that the defect in the cilia in Kartagener's syndrome affects cell motility during embryogenesis, resulting in situs inversus, e.g. dextrocardia, left-sided liver and right-sided spleen. Although the condition is rare, examiners love inviting these patients for OSCEs for cardiovascular and abdominal examinations.

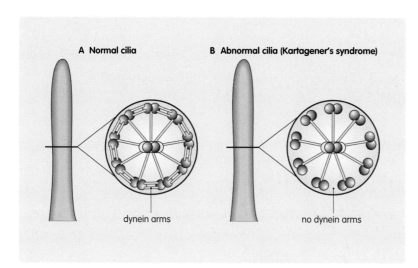

Fig. 2.8 Cross-section of: (A) normal cilium; (B) cilium in Kartagener's syndrome.

Obstructive sleep apnoea results from occlusion of the upper airway and is common in overweight, middle-aged men. In inspiration upper airway pressure becomes negative, but airway patency is maintained by upper airway muscle (e.g. genioglossus) tone. During sleep these muscles relax, causing narrowing of the upper airways even in normal subjects. However, if the airway is already narrowed, for example by the weight of adipose tissue in obese patients or a small jaw (micrognathia), the airway collapses and obstructive sleep apnoea results. Other risk factors include:

- Down's syndrome.
- Adenotonsillar hypertrophy.
- Macroglossia – 'enlarged tongue' (seen in hypothyroidism, acromegaly and amyloidosis).
- Nasal obstruction (as in rhinitis).
- Alcohol (which has been shown to reduce muscle tone and reduces the arousal response). A cycle is generated during sleep in which:
- The upper airway dilating muscles lose tone (usually accompanied by loud snoring).
- The airway is occluded.
- The patient wakes.
- The airway reopens.

As a consequence of this cycle, sleep is unrefreshing and daytime sleepiness is common, particularly during monotonous situations such as motorway driving. Each arousal also causes a transient rise in blood pressure, which may lead to sustained hypertension, pulmonary hypertension and cor pulmonale, ischaemic heart disease and stroke.

Conversely, in central sleep apnoea, the airway remains patent but there is no efferent output from the respiratory centres in the brain. There is no respiratory effort by the respiratory muscles, causing P_aCO_2 levels to rise. The high P_aCO_2 arouses the patient who then rebreathes to normalize the P_aCO_2 and then falls asleep again. This cycle can be repeated many times during the night and leads to a disruptive sleep pattern. Central sleep apnoea is rarer than obstructive sleep apnoea but is more common in patients with congestive heart failure and patients with neurological diseases (e.g. strokes). It can also be seen in people with no abnormalities, such as those that live at high altitude.

Investigations and treatment

Patients are referred to a sleep or respiratory specialist for overnight sleep study, polysomnography (Fig. 2.9): 15 apnoeas/hypoapnoeas (of 10 seconds or longer) per hour of sleep is diagnostic.

Some patients can be managed conservatively and are advised to lose weight and avoid alcohol and

> Sleep apnoea can markedly reduce a patient's quality of life. It is also a public health problem – patients with sleep apnoea are at an increased risk of road accidents as they have difficulty concentrating when driving and may even fall asleep at the wheel.

Fig. 2.9 Example results of polysomnographs showing the two types of sleep apnoea. Sleep apnoea can be detected by reduced airflow and a delayed desaturation following the apnoea. Normally the thorax and abdomen move in the same direction as each other; however, in obstructive sleep apnoea the thorax and abdomen move in opposite directions to each other – an abnormal pattern called paradoxical breathing. Conversely, in central sleep apnoea there is neither thoracic nor abdominal movement because the respiratory centre in the brain has stopped instructing the respiratory muscles to move.

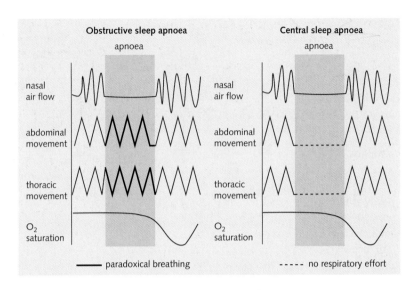

sedatives as these relax the upper airway dilating muscles. However, for most patients nightly continuous positive airway pressure (CPAP) is recommended (see p. 174). Some success has been obtained with medications which have a stimulator effect on the respiratory system, such as theophylline.

Neoplasms

Nasopharyngeal carcinoma

Nasopharyngeal carcinoma is commonly a poorly differentiated squamous cell carcinoma. Men are more likely to suffer from the disease, which usually presents in patients aged 50–70 years. The disease is common in South East Asia, and is associated with the Epstein–Barr virus and salted preserved fish. Nasopharyngeal carcinoma presents with epistaxis, nasal obstruction or a neck lump: 70% of patients have metastatic lymph node involvement at presentation. The overall 5-year survival rate is 35%. Treatment is by radiotherapy.

Nasopharyngeal angiofibroma

Nasopharyngeal angiofibroma is a benign neoplasm occurring in childhood, affecting boys more than girls. It arises unilaterally and frequently coincides with a pubertal growth spurt. The disease presents with epistaxis and nasal obstruction.

Pathology

An enlarging vascular tumour is present, which contains a fibrous component. The disease can cause bone erosion and destruction by pressure atrophy. The sphenopalatine foramen is always involved.

Investigations and treatment

Investigate by MR imaging or CT scanning. Surgical treatment is possible, but vascularity may be a problem. Radiotherapy is used only in unresectable cases.

DISORDERS OF THE LARYNX

Inflammatory conditions

Acute laryngitis

Acute laryngitis is a common condition, usually caused by viral infection, although secondary infection with streptococci or staphylococci can occur. Patients typically present with a hoarse voice and feel unwell. Rarely, dysphagia and pain on phonation occur.

Acute laryngitis is usually a self-limiting condition. If symptoms persist, refer to an ENT specialist.

Chronic laryngitis

Chronic laryngitis is inflammation of the larynx and trachea associated with excessive smoking, continued vocal abuse and excessive alcohol.

The mucous glands are swollen and the epithelium hypertrophied. Heavy smoking leads to squamous metaplasia of the larynx. Biopsy is mandatory to rule out malignancy. Management is directed at avoidance of aetiological factors.

Laryngotracheobronchitis (croup) and acute epiglottitis

The features of laryngotracheobronchitis (croup) and acute epiglottitis are described in Figure 2.10. The incidence of epiglottitis has dramatically fallen due to the introduction of the Hib (*Haemophilus influenzae* type B) vaccine.

Pathology

In laryngotracheobronchitis, there is necrosis of epithelium and formation of an extensive fibrous membrane on the trachea and main bronchi. Oedema of the subglottic area occurs, with subsequent danger of laryngeal obstruction.

In acute epiglottitis, there is an acute inflammatory oedema and infiltration by neutrophil polymorphs. No mucosal ulceration occurs. Acute epiglottitis may also occur in adults, although it is much more common in children (see Fig. 2.10).

Treatment

To treat laryngotracheobronchitis, keep the patient calm and hydrated. Nurse in a warm room in an upright position. Drug treatment, if required, includes steroids, oxygen and nebulized adrenaline (epinephrine).

Acute epiglottitis is a medical emergency. Call for anaesthetist, ENT surgeon and, if appropriate, the

Lucy, a 2-year-old girl, came into A&E with a cough, difficulty breathing and a sore throat. Her mother said that she had had a cold for the past week. Closer examination revealed that Lucy had a hoarse voice and a cough that sounded like a bark. There was some sternal recession and discomfort when lying down. Lucy was diagnosed as having croup.

She had moderate to severe croup and was treated with 100% oxygen, nebulized adrenaline (epinephrine) and budesonide as well as having oral dexamethasone.

paediatric team. Never attempt to visualize the epiglottis. Keep calm and reassure the patient. Never leave the patient alone. As with other serious *Haemophilus influenzae* infections, prophylactic treatment with rifampicin is offered to the close contacts.

Reactive nodules

Reactive nodules are common, small, inflammatory polyps usually measuring less than 10 mm in diameter. They are also known as singer's nodules. They present in patients aged 40–50 years and are more common in men. Reactive nodules are caused by excessive untrained use of vocal cords. Patients present with hoarseness of the voice.

Pathology

Keratosis develops at the junction of the anterior and middle thirds of the vocal cord on each side. Oedematous myxoid connective tissue is covered by squamous epithelium. The reactive nodules may become painful because of ulceration.

Neoplasms

Squamous papilloma

Squamous papilloma is the commonest benign tumour of larynx; it usually occurs in children aged 0–5 years, but can also affect adults.

Aetiology

The disease is caused by infection of the epithelial cells with human papillomavirus (HPV) types 6 and 11, and can be acquired at birth from maternal genital warts.

Fig. 2.10 Laryngotracheobronchitis (croup) and acute epiglottitis

	Croup	Epiglottitis
Aetiology	Viral	Bacterial
Organism	Parainfluenza, respiratory syncytial virus	Group B haemophilus influenza
Age range	6 months to 3 years	3–7 years
Onset	Gradual over days	Sudden over hours
Cough	Severe barking	Minimal
Temperature	Pyrexia <38.5°C	Pyrexia >38.5°C
Stridor	Harsh	Soft
Drooling	No	Yes
Voice	Hoarse	Reluctant to speak
Able to drink	Yes	No
Active	Yes	No, completely still
Mortality	Low	High

Clinical features

Clinical features include hoarseness of the voice and an abnormal cry (Fig. 2.11).

Pathology

Tumours may be sessile or pedunculated. They can occur anywhere on the vocal cords. Lesions are commoner at points of airway constriction (Fig. 2.12A and B).

Investigations and treatment

Investigations include endoscopy, followed by histological confirmation.

Surgical treatment is by removal with a carbon dioxide laser. Medical treatment is with alpha interferon.

Squamous cell carcinoma

Squamous cell carcinoma is the commonest malignant tumour of the larynx, affecting men and women in the ratio of 5 : 1. The disease accounts for 1% of all male malignancies. Incidence increases with age, with peak incidence occurring in those aged 60–70 years. Patients present with hoarseness, although dyspnoea and stridor are late signs.

Predisposing factors include alcohol and tobacco smoke (the condition is very rare in non-smokers).

Pathology

Carcinoma of vocal cord appears first, and subsequently ulcerates. Carcinoma of the larynx infiltrates and destroys surrounding tissue. Infection may follow ulceration.

Investigations and treatment

Investigations include chest radiography, full blood count, serum analysis (liver function tests for metastatic disease), direct laryngoscopy under general anaesthesia, and full paraendoscopy and bronchoscopy. Treatment is by radiotherapy and surgery.

Prognosis

Prognosis is poor if the tumour involves the upper part of the larynx or subglottic region.

Fig. 2.11 Features of squamous papilloma	Adult	Child
Incidence	Rare	Common
Number of lesions	Single mass	Multiple masses
Outcome	Surgical removal	Regress spontaneously at puberty

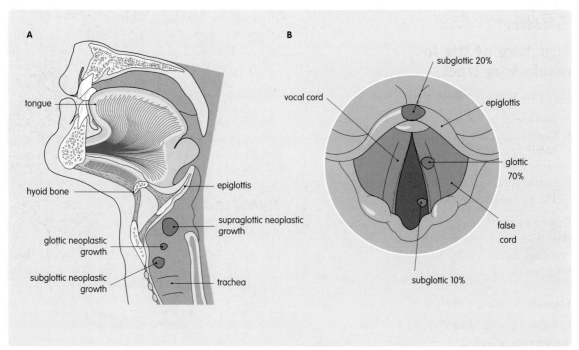

Fig. 2.12 Position of laryngeal carcinoma (A) and as seen on mirror examination (B).

The lower respiratory tract

3

Objectives

By the end of this chapter you should be able to:

- Describe the anatomy and function of the pleurae.
- List the medial relations of the lungs and the contents of the hilum.
- Describe the structure of the tracheobronchial tree and define the differences between conducting and respiratory zones.
- List the differences between bronchi and bronchioles.
- Describe the ultrastructure of the airways.
- Describe the differences in function between the pulmonary and bronchial circulations.
- Outline the fetal circulation.
- Know how the circulation changes at birth.
- Describe the mechanisms available to the lung to prevent entry of particulate matter.
- Describe the key functions of the alveolar macrophage.
- List the metabolic functions of the lung.
- Describe, with the use of a diagram, the activation of angiotensin.
- Outline, with the aid of a diagram, arachidonic acid metabolism.

ORGANIZATION OF THE LOWER RESPIRATORY TRACT

Structure of the lower respiratory tract

The lower respiratory tract consists of:

- The lower part of the trachea.
- The two main bronchi.
- Lobar bronchi, segmental bronchi and smaller bronchi.
- Bronchioles and terminal bronchioles.
- The end respiratory unit.

These structures make up the tracheobronchial tree (Fig. 3.1). The structures distal to the two main bronchi are contained within a tissue known as the lung parenchyma.

Thorax

The cone-shaped thoracic cavity is bounded superiorly by the first rib and inferiorly by the diaphragm. The thorax is narrow at the top (thoracic inlet) and wide at its base (thoracic outlet).

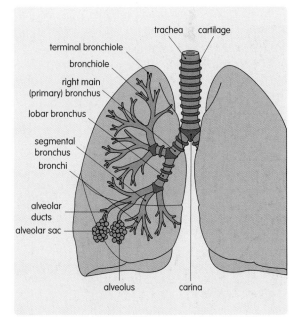

Fig. 3.1 Tracheobronchial tree. Schematic showing the divisions of the airway down to the end respiratory unit (acinus).

The thoracic wall is supported and protected by the bony thoracic cage consisting of:

- Thoracic vertebrae.
- Manubrium.
- Sternum.
- Twelve pairs of ribs with associated costal cartilages (Fig. 3.2A).

Each rib makes an acute angle with the spine and:

- Articulates with the body and transverse process of its equivalent thoracic vertebra.
- Articulates with the body of the vertebra above.

The upper seven ribs (true ribs) articulate anteriorly through their costal cartilages with the sternum. The eighth, ninth, and tenth ribs (false ribs) articulate with the costal cartilages of the next rib above. The eleventh and twelfth ribs (floating ribs) are smaller and their tips are covered with a cap of cartilage.

The space between ribs is known as the intercostal space. Lying obliquely between adjacent ribs are the internal and external intercostal muscles. The intercostal muscles support the thoracic cage; their other functions include:

- External intercostal muscles – raise the rib cage and increase intrathoracic volume.
- Internal intercostal muscles – lower the rib cage and reduce intrathoracic volume.

Deep to the intercostal muscles and under cover of the costal groove lies a neurovascular bundle of vein, artery and nerve (see Fig. 3.2B). This anatomy is important during some procedures (e.g. when inserting a chest drain into a pneumothorax, the drain is inserted through the intercostal space just above the rib to avoid hitting the subcostal vessels).

The thorax contains:

- Lungs, heart and major vessels.
- Oesophagus, lower part of the trachea and main bronchi.

Mediastinum

The mediastinum is situated in the midline and lies between the two lungs. It contains the:

- Heart and great vessels.
- Trachea and oesophagus.
- Phrenic and vagus nerves.
- Lymph nodes.

Pleurae and pleural cavities

The pleurae consist of a continuous serous membrane, which covers the external surface of the lung and is then reflected to cover the inner surface of the thoracic cavity (Fig. 3.3).

The differences between the visceral and parietal pleurae are:

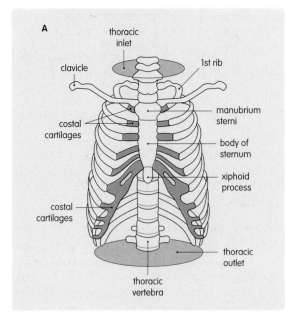

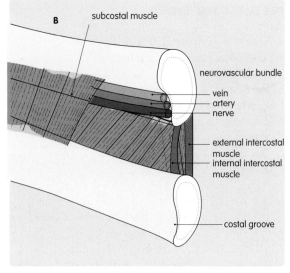

Fig. 3.2 The thoracic cage (A) and details of the subcostal neurovascular bundle (B).

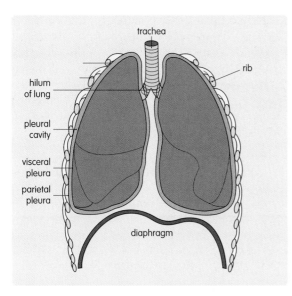

hilum of lung

pleural cavity

visceral pleura

parietal pleura

trachea

rib

diaphragm

Fig. 3.3 The two pleurae form a potential space called the pleural cavity (shown in light blue).

- The visceral pleura lines the surface of the lungs.
- The parietal pleura lines the thoracic wall and the diaphragm.

The pleurae form a double layer, creating a potential space known as the pleural cavity. The visceral and parietal pleurae are so closely apposed that only a thin film of fluid is contained within the pleural cavity. This allows the pleurae to slip over each other during breathing, thus reducing friction. Normally, no cavity is actually present, although in pathological states this potential space may expand.

Where the pleura is reflected off the diaphragm onto the thoracic wall, a small space is created which is not filled by the lung tissue; this space is known as the costodiaphragmatic recess. At the root of the lung (the hilum), the pleurae become continuous and form a double layer known as the pulmonary ligament.

The parietal pleura has a blood supply from intercostal arteries and branches of the internal thoracic artery. Venous and lymph drainage follow a return course similar to that of the arterial supply. Nerve supply is from the phrenic nerve; thus, if the pleura becomes inflamed this may cause ipsilateral (on the same side of the body) shoulder-tip pain.

The visceral pleura has a blood supply from bronchial arteries. Venous drainage is through the bronchial veins to the azygous and hemiazygous veins. Lymph vessels drain through the superficial plexus over the surface of the lung to bronchopulmonary nodes at the hilum. The visceral pleura has an autonomic nerve supply and therefore does not give rise to the sensation of pain.

Inflammation of the pleurae can cause an increase in fluid between the parietal and visceral pleurae. This inflammation may give rise to a pleural rub on auscultation, which is said to mimic the sound of a foot crunching through fresh snow. Excess liquid or air may be present within the pleural cavity, caused by:

- Pneumothorax.
- Haemothorax.
- Pleurisy and pneumonia.
- Malignancy.
- Chylothorax.

Lungs

The two lungs are situated within the thoracic cavity and lie on either side of the mediastinum. During life, they appear pink and spongy, although carbon deposits give patchy discolouration. The lungs contain:

- Airways: bronchi, bronchioles, respiratory bronchioles, alveolar ducts, alveolar sacs and alveoli.
- Vessels: pulmonary artery and vein and bronchial artery and vein.
- Lymphatics and lymph nodes.
- Nerves.
- Supportive connective tissue (lung parenchyma), which has elastic qualities.

Figures 3.4 and 3.5 show the lateral and medial surfaces of the lung.

Hilum of the lung

The hilum or root of the lung (Fig. 3.6) consists of:

- Bronchi.
- Vessels: pulmonary artery and vein.
- Nerves.
- Lymph nodes and lymphatic vessels.
- Pulmonary ligament.

Bronchopulmonary segments

The trachea divides to form the left and right primary bronchi, which in turn divide to form lobar bronchi, supplying air to the lobes of each lung. The lobar bronchi divide again to give segmental bronchi, which supply air to regions of lung known as bronchopulmonary segments. The bronchopulmonary segment is both anatomically and functionally distinct. This is important because it means that a segment of diseased lung can be removed surgically (e.g. in tuberculosis).

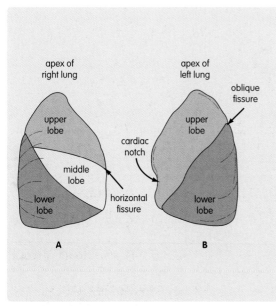

Fig. 3.4 Lateral aspect of the lungs. The outer surfaces show impression of the ribs. (A) Left lung; (B) right lung.

Surface anatomy

The surface anatomy of the lungs is shown in Figure 3.7.

Airways and the blood–air interface

Airways (respiratory tree)

Inside the thorax, the trachea divides into the left and right primary bronchi. The right main bronchus is shorter and more vertical than the left; for this reason, inhaled foreign bodies are more likely to pass into the right lung.

The primary bronchi within each lung divide into secondary or lobar bronchi. The lobar bronchi divide again into tertiary or segmental bronchi. The airways continue to divide, always splitting into two daughter airways of progressively smaller calibre until eventually forming bronchioles.

Figure 3.1 outlines the structure of the respiratory tree. Each branch of the tracheobronchial tree can be classified by its number of divisions (called the generation number); the trachea is generation number 0. The trachea and bronchi contain cartilage in their walls for support and to prevent collapse of the airway. At about generation 10 or 11, the airways contain no cartilage in their walls and are

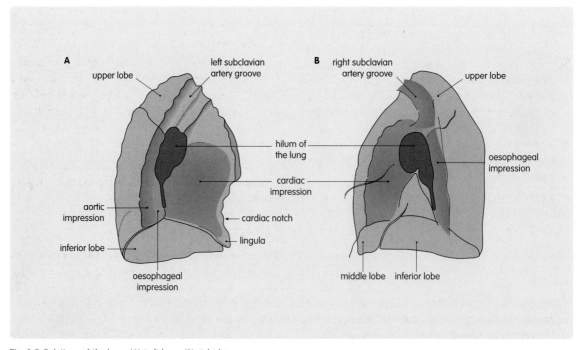

Fig. 3.5 Relations of the lung. (A) Left lung; (B) right lung.

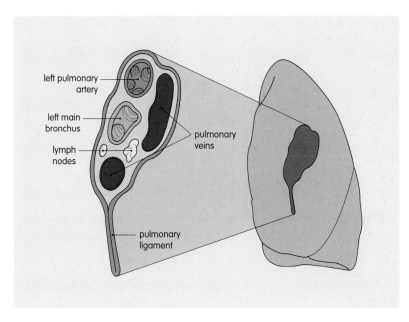

Fig. 3.6 Contents of the hilum.

left pulmonary
artery

left main
bronchus

lymph
nodes

pulmonary
veins

pulmonary
ligament

known as bronchioles. Airways distal to the bronchi that contain no cartilage rely on lung parenchymal tissue for their support and are kept open by sub-atmospheric intrapleural pressure (radial traction).

Bronchioles continue dividing for up to 20 or more generations before reaching the terminal bronchiole. Terminal bronchioles are those bronchioles which supply the end respiratory unit (the acinus).

The tracheobronchial tree can be classified into two zones:

- The conducting zone (airways proximal to the respiratory bronchioles), involved in air movement by bulk flow to the end respiratory units.
- The respiratory zone (airways distal to the terminal bronchiole), involved in gaseous exchange.

As the conducting zone does not take part in gaseous exchange, it can be seen as an area of 'wasted' ventilation and is described as anatomical dead space.

Acinus

The acinus is that part of the airway that is involved in gaseous exchange (i.e. the passage of oxygen from the lungs to the blood and carbon dioxide from the blood to the lungs). The acinus consists of:

- Respiratory bronchioles, leading to the alveolar ducts.
- Alveolar ducts, opening into two or three alveolar sacs, which in turn open into several alveoli (see Fig. 1.2 on p. 5).
- Alveoli also open directly into alveolar ducts and a few open directly into the respiratory bronchiole.

Lung lobules

Lung lobules (Fig. 3.8) are areas of lung containing groups of between three and five acini surrounded by parenchymal tissue. Each lobule is separated from a neighbouring lobule by an interlobular septum.

Structure of the airways

The structure of the airways changes as the tracheobronchial tree descends; these differences are outlined in Figure 3.9.

The blood–air interface

The blood–air interface is a term that describes the site at which gaseous exchange takes place within the lung (Fig. 3.10).

The alveoli are microscopic blind-ending air pouches, of which there are 150–400 million in each normal lung. The alveoli open into alveolar sacs and then into alveolar ducts (see Fig. 1.2, p. 5).

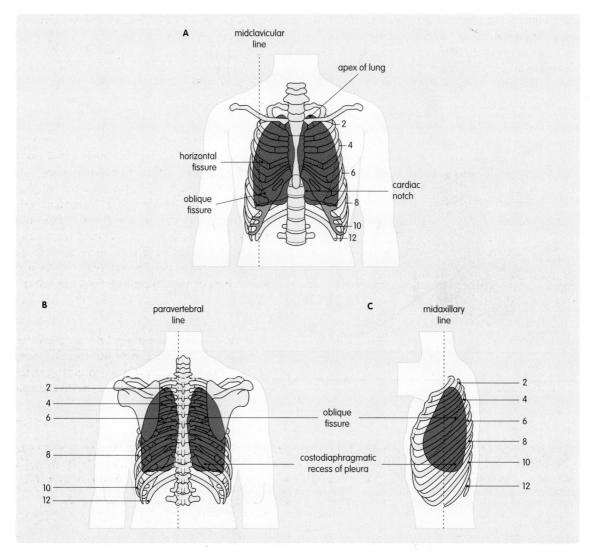

Fig. 3.7 Surface anatomy of the lungs and pleura (shaded area). (A) Anterior aspect; (B) posterior aspect; (C) lateral aspect.

The walls of the alveoli are extremely thin and the alveoli are lined by a single layer of pneumocytes (types I and II) lying on a basement membrane.

The alveolar surface is covered with alveolar lining fluid. The walls of the alveoli also contain capillaries. It should be noted that:

- Average surface area of the alveolar–capillary membrane = $50–100\,\text{m}^2$ (about the same size as two tennis courts).
- Average thickness of alveolar–capillary membrane = $0.4\,\mu\text{m}$.

This allows an enormous area for gaseous exchange and a very short diffusion distance.

A common short-answer question in exams is: 'Name the differences in structure between the bronchi and the bronchioles'. It is a good idea to memorize the information in Figure 3.9.

Tissues of the lower respiratory tract

The basic structural components of the walls of the airways are shown in Figure 3.11. The proportions of these components vary in different regions of the tracheobronchial tree. The absence of cartilage in the bronchioles and distal airways means that these airways must be kept open by radial traction (see Ch. 4). The walls of the airways are composed of:

- Respiratory epithelium (ciliated columnar type).
- Basement membrane.
- Lamina propria.
- Elastic fibres.
- Smooth muscle.
- Cartilage.

Trachea

The respiratory epithelium of the trachea is tall and sits on a particularly thick basement membrane separating it from the lamina propria. The lamina propria of the trachea is loose and highly vascular, with a fibromuscular band of elastic tissue. Under the lamina propria lies a loose submucosa containing numerous glands that secrete mucinous and serous fluid. The C-shaped cartilage found within the trachea is hyaline in type and merges with the submucosa.

Bronchi

The respiratory epithelium of the bronchi is shorter than the epithelium of the trachea and contains fewer goblet cells. The lamina propria is denser with more elastic fibres and it is separated from the submucosa

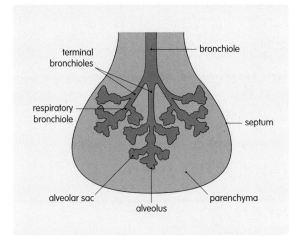

Fig. 3.8 The lung lobule.

Fig. 3.9 Differences in structure of the airways

Airway	Generation No.	Lining	Wall structure	Diameter	Function	Contractile
trachea	0	respiratory epithelium	membranous tube supported by C-shaped rings of cartilage, loose submucosa and glands	25 mm	Con	No
bronchus	1–11	respiratory epithelium	fibromuscular tubes containing smooth muscle are reinforced by incomplete rings of cartilage and express β-receptors	1–10 mm	Con	Yes
bronchiole	12–16	simple ciliated cuboidal epithelium and Clara cells	membranous and smooth muscle in the wall; no submucosal glands and no cartilage	1.0 mm	Con	Yes
respiratory bronchiole	18+	simple ciliated cuboidal epithelium and Clara cells	merging of cuboidal epithelium with flattened epithelial lining of alveolar ducts; membranous wall	0.5 mm	Con/Gas	Yes
alveolar duct	20–23	flat non-ciliated epithelium; no glands	outer lining of spiral smooth muscle; walls of ducts contain many openings laterally into alveolar sacs	0.5 mm	Gas	Yes
alveolus	24	pneumocytes types I and II	types I and II pneumocytes lie on an alveolar basement membrane; capillaries lie on the outer surface of the wall and form the blood–air interface	75–300 mm	Gas	No

Fig. 3.10 Blood–air interface.

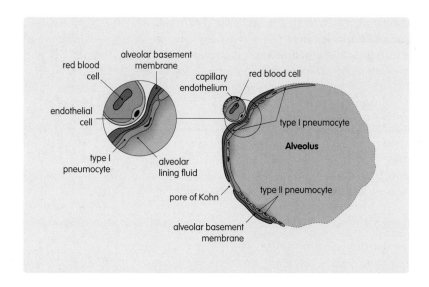

Fig. 3.11 Structure of the airways: (A) bronchial structure; (B) bronchiolar structure. *Note there are no submucosal glands or cartilage in the bronchiole.* (From Widdecombe & Davies 1991, with permission of Arnold.)

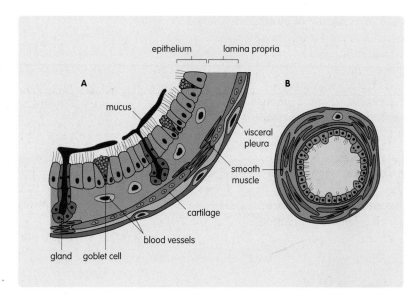

by a discontinuous layer of smooth muscle. The lamina propria also contains mast cells.

The cartilage of the bronchi forms discontinuous flat plates and there are no C-shaped rings.

Tertiary bronchi

The epithelium in the tertiary bronchi is similar to that in the bronchi. The lamina propria of the tertiary bronchi is thin and elastic, being completely encompassed by smooth muscle. Submucosal glands are sparse and the submucosa merges with surrounding adventitia. Mucosa-associated lymphoid tissue (MALT) is present (see p. 31).

Bronchioles

The epithelium of a bronchiole is ciliated cuboidal and contains Clara cells, which are non-ciliated and secrete proteinaceous fluid. Bronchioles contain no cartilage and no glands in the submucosa. The smooth muscle layer is prominent. Adjusting the tone of the smooth muscle layer alters airway diameter, enabling resistance to air flow to be effectively controlled.

Respiratory bronchioles

The respiratory bronchioles are lined by ciliated cuboidal epithelium, which is surrounded by smooth muscle. Clara cells are present within the walls of the respiratory bronchioles. Goblet cells are absent but there are a few alveoli in the walls; thus, the respiratory bronchiole is a site for gaseous exchange.

Alveolar ducts

Alveolar ducts consist of rings of smooth muscle, collagen and elastic fibres. They open into two or three alveolar sacs, which in turn open into several alveoli. There are alveoli present in the walls and this is a site for gaseous exchange.

Alveoli

An alveolus is a blind-ending terminal sac of respiratory tract (Fig. 3.12). Most gaseous exchange occurs in the alveoli. Because alveoli are so numerous, they provide the majority of lung volume and surface area. The majority of alveoli open into the alveolar sacs. Communication between adjacent alveoli is possible through perforations in the alveolar wall called pores of Kohn. The alveoli are lined with type I and type II pneumocytes, which sit on a basement membrane. Type I pneumocytes are structural, whereas type II pneumocytes produce surfactant (see Ch. 4).

Type I pneumocytes

To aid gaseous diffusion, type I pneumocytes are very thin; they contain flattened nuclei and few mitochondria. Type I pneumocytes make up 40% of the alveolar cell population and 90% of the surface

> Layers through which gas exchange occurs are:
> - Alveolar lining fluid.
> - Pneumocytes.
> - Alveolar basement membrane.
> - Capillary endothelium.

lining of the alveolar wall. Cells are joined by tight junctions.

Type II pneumocytes

Type II pneumocytes are rounded cells containing rounded nuclei; their cytoplasm is rich in mitochondria and endoplasmic reticulum, and microvilli exist on their exposed surface. Type II pneumocytes make up 60% of the alveolar cell population and 5–10% of the surface lining of the alveolar wall. They produce surfactant.

Alveolar macrophages

Alveolar macrophages are derived from circulating blood monocytes. They lie on an alveolar surface lining or on alveolar septal tissue. The alveolar macrophages phagocytose foreign material and bacteria; they are transported up the respiratory tract by mucociliary clearance. They are discussed further under the lung defences (see p. 36).

Mucosa-associated lymphoid tissue (MALT)

The immune system has a major role in the defence of the respiratory tract against pathogens (see below). To aid this key role, lymphoid cells concentrate in the mucosal surfaces of the body to provide immunological protection. This specialized local system of lymphoid tissue is known as mucosa-associated lymphoid tissue (MALT).

MALT is non-capsulated lymphoid tissue located in the walls of the gastrointestinal, respiratory and urogenital tracts, providing immunological protection. These tissues are also a main site of lymphocyte activation and activated lymphocytes will specifically return to respiratory mucosa.

Examples of MALT were mentioned among the tissues of the upper respiratory tract (e.g. the adenoids and the tonsils). MALT in the lung is termed BALT (bronchus-associated lymphoid tissue). BALT

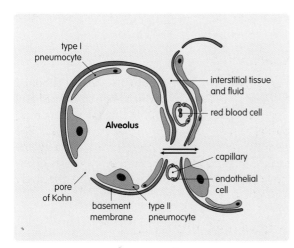

Fig. 3.12 The alveolus. *Note communication between alveoli through pores of Kohn.*

is located beneath the mucosa of the bronchi and is covered by M cells, specialized epithelial cells that sample and transport antigen to the lymphoid tissue.

The lymphoid tissue of the respiratory tract is similar to that in the gut; aggregates are a diffuse distribution of mostly B lymphocytes within the lamina propria, covered by similar antigen-targeting and antigen-transporting cells (M cells). The lymphatic vessels associated with MALT are all efferent lymphatics, which drain to regional (hilar) lymph nodes. Large aggregations function in a similar manner to lymph nodes, containing T-cell and B-cell zones.

DEVELOPMENT OF THE LOWER RESPIRATORY TRACT

Development of the bronchi and the lungs

Bronchi and lung development is divided into five stages: embryonic, pseudoglandular, canalicular, terminal sac and alveolar periods.

Stage 1 – embryonic period (3–7 weeks)

The laryngotracheal diverticulum develops into the lung bud, which divides into two bronchial buds by the end of week 4 (Fig. 3.13). As the bronchial bud enlarges, it forms two primary bronchi: the right and left primary bronchi (occurring in week 5). The right main bronchus is slightly larger and more vertical than the left. By the end of week 5, the secondary bronchi start to form.

By week 8, the segmental bronchi develop and together with the splanchnic mesenchyme form the bronchopulmonary segment. The splanchnic mesenchyme forms:

- Visceral pleura (mesoderm).
- Pulmonary capillaries and vasculature.
- Bronchial smooth muscle.
- Pulmonary connective tissue.

Stage 2 – pseudoglandular period (7–16 weeks)

During the pseudoglandular period, the conducting airways up to the terminal bronchioles are present. The large airways are lined with ciliated cells, goblet cells and Clara cells. Breathing movements occur at 10 weeks although the fetal lungs themselves are not able to perform gaseous exchange. Babies born at this stage do not survive.

Stage 3 – canalicular period (16–28 weeks)

During the canalicular period, there are increases in the diameter of airways, bronchi and terminal bronchioles. The squamous epithelium (type I pneumocytes) develops at about week 24, whereas secretory cells (type II pneumocytes) develop at around weeks 24–28. The lung vasculature develops, and primitive end respiratory units are formed: respiratory bronchiole, alveolar duct and terminal sac (primitive alveolus). Some gaseous exchange is possible, and there is a very small chance of survival if born after week 22 (although intensive care is required).

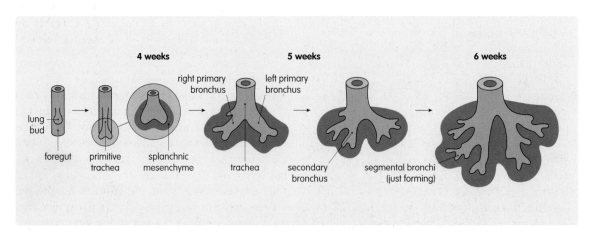

Fig. 3.13 Development of primary bronchi and the formation of the secondary and segmental bronchi.

Stage 4 – terminal sac period (28–36 weeks)

During the terminal sac period, numerous terminal sacs develop; there is thinning of the epithelial lining of terminal sacs. Type II pneumocytes produce surfactant, reducing surface tension within the liquid film within an alveolus and thus preventing alveolar collapse. After week 32, sufficient surfactant has been produced to allow the neonate to inflate its own lungs and allow the alveoli to continue to develop.

Stage 5 – alveolar period (36 weeks – 3 years postnatal)

During the alveolar period, clusters of primitive alveoli are formed. Breathing occurs in utero by aspiration of amniotic fluid. The lungs are half full of liquid at birth; fluid is emptied through the mouth and also absorbed into the blood and lymph. The alveoli mature after birth: for the first 3 years after birth, alveoli increase only in number, not size; between the ages of 3 and 8 years, alveoli increase in both size and number.

The first breath

After delivery, the baby's external environment suddenly changes. The placental blood supply is cut off and the baby must begin to use its lungs. A reduction in temperature and, more likely, hypercapnia may trigger the baby's first breath. The fetal lungs are

Babies born via caesarean section do not experience the physical and chemical stimulation of a normal vaginal delivery. Hence lung fluid will not be rapidly absorbed and the baby may experience respiratory distress (transient tachypnoea of the newborn). Therefore, these babies may need respiratory assistance and oxygen.

filled with fluid. During labour, fetal catecholamine levels rise and trigger the movement of fluid from the air spaces into the interstitium, via epithelial sodium channels, from where it drains into the lymph. The process of delivery itself exerts pressure on the baby's thorax and can assist with fluid drainage.

THE PULMONARY CIRCULATION

Blood vessels

The lungs have a dual blood supply from the pulmonary and bronchial circulations. The bronchial circulation is part of the systemic circulation.

Pulmonary circulation

Function
The primary function of the pulmonary circulation is to allow the exchange of oxygen and carbon dioxide between the blood in the pulmonary capillaries and air in the alveoli. Oxygen is taken up into the blood while carbon dioxide is released from the blood into alveolar air.

Anatomy
Mixed-venous blood is pumped from the right ventricle through the pulmonary arteries and thence through the pulmonary capillary network, which is in contact with the respiratory surface (Fig. 3.14). Gaseous exchange occurs (carbon dioxide given up by the blood, oxygen taken up by the blood) and the oxygenated blood returns through the pulmonary venules and veins to the left atrium. The pulmonary capillary network offers a huge gas exchange area of approximately 50–100 m^2.

Sam, a male infant born at 26 weeks' gestation, was observed to have an increased respiratory rate, chest wall recession, expiratory grunting and cyanosis. Infant respiratory distress syndrome (IRDS) was diagnosed. Since Sam was born before 28 weeks' gestation he had not developed surfactant-producing type II pneumocytes, and surfactant deficiency was causing respiratory distress. In addition, his adrenal glands had not fully developed. Hence, lack of cortisol to stimulate surfactant production.

Sam was treated with exogenous surfactant directly sprayed into his lungs via the endotracheal tube. Alternatively, if Sam's mother had been given antenatal glucocorticoids, fetal lung maturation and production of surfactant would have been stimulated and decreased Sam's chance of developing IRDS.

Fig. 3.14 Pulmonary circulation. The pulmonary capillaries lie within the lungs, situated in the alveolar walls. They are in contact with alveolar gas and this is the site where gaseous exchange takes place.

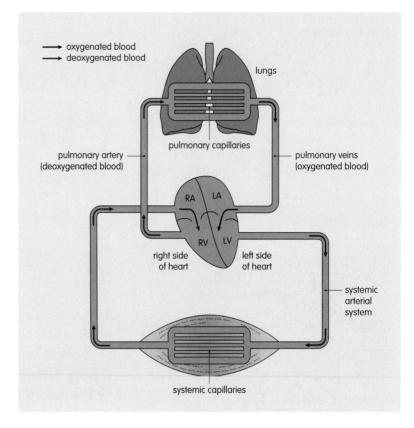

Bronchial circulation

The bronchial circulation is part of the systemic circulation; bronchial arteries are branches of the descending aorta.

Function

The function of the bronchial circulation is to supply oxygen, water and nutrients to:

- Lung parenchyma.
- Airways – smooth muscle, mucosa and glands.
- Pulmonary arteries and veins.
- Pleurae.

An additional function of the bronchial circulation is in the conditioning (warming) of inspired air. The airways distal to the terminal bronchiole are supplied only by alveolar wall capillaries. For this reason, a pulmonary embolus may result in infarction of the tissues supplied by the alveolar wall capillaries, shown as a wedge-shaped opacity on the lung periphery of a chest X-ray.

Development of the pulmonary circulation

The primitive heart is divided into four chambers during weeks 4 and 5. This involves:

- Formation of endocardial cushions.
- Division of the primitive atrium.

During week 6, the six primitive aortic arches are transformed into the adult arterial layout. However, the ductus arteriosus is still patent. For further information on development of the heart see *Crash Course: Cardiovascular System*.

Fetal circulation

The main difference between adult and fetal circulation (Fig. 3.15) is that oxygenation of the fetal blood is by the maternal placental circulation. Consequently, the pulmonary circulation is largely bypassed through:

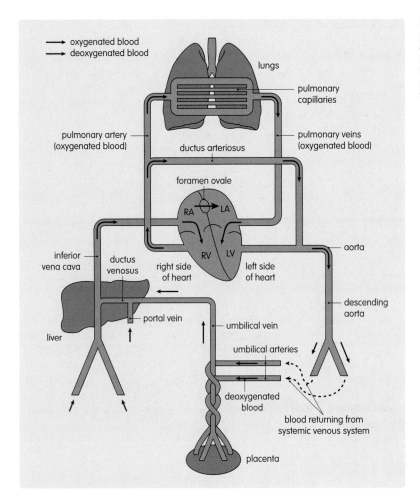

- The foramen ovale – which connects the right atrium to the left atrium.
- The ductus arteriosus – which connects the pulmonary artery to the aorta.

Deoxygenated fetal blood flows through the two umbilical arteries (branches of the common iliacs) to the placenta (Fig. 3.15). Oxygen and nutrients are taken up from the maternal blood by the fetal circulation. Waste products of metabolism and carbon dioxide are passed from fetal blood to the maternal circulation. Oxygenated blood returns to the fetal heart through the umbilical vein, ductus venosus and inferior vena cava. The oxygenated blood from the umbilical vein mixes with deoxygenated blood from the portal circulation and lower limbs and is returned to the right side of the heart. The majority of the fetal blood bypasses the pulmonary circulation, passing through the foramen ovale into the left atrium (see large arrow in Fig. 3.15).

In fetal life, the pressure in the pulmonary circulation is greater than in the systemic circulation, and less than one-third of the right ventricular output passes through the lungs; the remainder flows from the pulmonary artery through the ductus arteriosus into the aorta.

Changes of circulation after birth

At birth, blood flow through the umbilical vessels stops. When blood flow through the umbilical vein ceases, the ductus venosus, a thick-walled vessel with a muscular sphincter, closes. As the neonate takes its first breath, the lungs fill with air and pulmonary vascular resistance falls to 10% of its value before lung expansion. Left atrial pressure is raised above that in the inferior vena cava by three methods:

- Decreased pulmonary vascular resistance leading to a large increase in blood flow through the lungs to the left atrium.

- Decreased blood flow to the right atrium caused by occlusion of the umbilical vein.
- Increased resistance to the left ventricular output produced by occlusion of the umbilical arteries.

The reversal of pressure gradient between the atria closes the valve over the foramen ovale. Fusion of the septal leaflets occurs over a period of several days.

The fall in pulmonary arterial pressure reverses the flow through the ductus arteriosus, but within a few moments of birth the ductus arteriosus begins to constrict, producing a turbulent flow heard as a murmur in the newborn child. The constriction is progressive and usually complete within 1–2 days after birth.

The exact mechanism for closure of the ductus arteriosus is not entirely clear, although it is thought to involve bradykinin, prostaglandins (because indometacin can delay closure), adenosine and endothelin-1.

The following factors have been suggested as causes of closure of the ductus arteriosus:

- Cutting of the umbilical cord.
- Exposure to cold air.
- Increase in arterial partial pressure of oxygen.
- Pressure difference between pulmonary and systemic circulations.

At birth, the walls of the left and right ventricles are the same thickness. After birth, the thickness of the right ventricular wall diminishes whereas that of the left ventricle increases.

Patent ductus arteriosus

Patent ductus arteriosus (PDA) is a common congenital heart defect, especially in girls. It is associated with maternal rubella (togavirus infection) in early pregnancy. As discussed above, the ductus arteriosus normally closes within 24 hours of birth. If closure fails to occur, blood flows from the aorta through the patent ductus and into the pulmonary artery (a left-to-right shunt). This increases pulmonary artery pressure (hydrodynamic pulmonary hypertension). The defect is classified as either small ductus or large ductus. The murmur heard has a machine-like quality and extends throughout the cardiac cycle. The treatment of choice is surgical ligation of the ductus. If the defect is large, the infant may require medical treatment with indometacin, a prostaglandin E inhibitor, to alleviate heart failure.

Atrial septal defect

Atrial septal defect (ASD) is a defect in the atrial septum around the area of the fossa ovalis, caused by a defect in the ostium secundum. Blood flows from the left atrium to the right atrium and then into the right ventricle (a left-to-right shunt), increasing the pulmonary blood flow, causing hydrodynamic pulmonary hypertension. Symptoms do not usually occur until about 30–40 years of age, when patients present with heart failure; at presentation, a soft heart murmur is usually heard, and a fixed splitting of the second heart sound.

DEFENCE MECHANISMS OF THE LUNGS

Overview

The lungs have a very large surface area for gaseous exchange and present a small barrier to diffusion between air and the blood flowing through the lungs. In fact, they possess the largest surface area of the body in contact with the environment and, therefore, are extremely susceptible to damage by foreign material and provide an excellent gateway for infection. The lungs are exposed to many foreign materials:

- Dust particles.
- Pollen.
- Fungal spores.
- Bacteria.
- Viruses.
- Airborne pollutants.

Therefore, it is necessary for defence mechanisms to prevent infection and reduce the risk of damage

The following fetal vessels lose their function and become ligaments at birth:
- Ductus arteriosus – becomes the ligamentum arteriosum.
- Ductus venosus – becomes the ligamentum venosum.
- Umbilical arteries – become the medial umbilical ligaments.
- Umbilical veins – become the ligamentum teres.

by inhalation of foreign material (Fig. 3.16). There are three main mechanisms of defence:

- Physical.
- Humoral.
- Cellular.

Physical defences are particularly important in the upper respiratory tract, whilst at the level of the alveoli other defences, such as alveolar macrophages, predominate.

Physical defences

Preventing entry to distal lower respiratory tract

Entry is restricted by the following three mechanisms:

- Filtering at the nasopharynx – hairs within the nose act as a coarse filter for inhaled particles; sticky mucus lying on the surface of the respiratory epithelium traps particles, which are then transported by the wafting of cilia to the nasopharynx; the particles are then swallowed into the gastrointestinal tract.
- Swallowing – during swallowing, the epiglottis folds back, the laryngeal muscles constrict the opening to the larynx, and the larynx itself is lifted; this prevents aspiration of food particles.
- Irritant C-fibres – stimulation of receptors within the bronchi by inhalation of chemicals, particles, or infective material produces a reflex contraction of bronchial smooth muscle; this reduces the diameter of airways and increases mucus secretion, thus limiting the penetration of the offending material.

Airway clearance

Cough reflex

Inhaled material and material brought up the bronchopulmonary tree to the trachea and larynx by mucociliary clearance can trigger a cough reflex (see Ch. 9). This is achieved by a reflex deep inspiration, increasing intrathoracic pressure while the larynx is closed. The larynx is suddenly opened, producing a

Fig. 3.16 Summary of defences of the respiratory system.

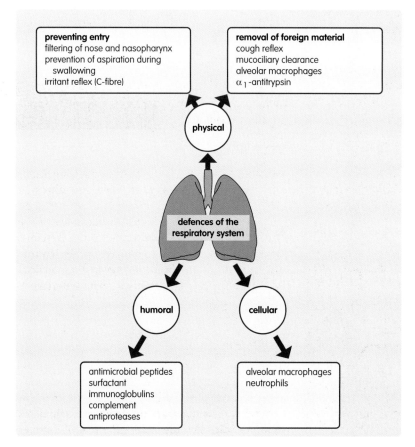

high-velocity jet of air, which ejects unwanted material at high speed through the mouth.

Mucociliary clearance

Mucociliary clearance deals with a lot of the large particles trapped in the bronchi and bronchioles and debris brought up by alveolar macrophages. Respiratory epithelium is covered by a layer of mucus secreted by goblet cells and submucosal glands. Approximately 10–100 mL of mucus is secreted by the lung daily. The mucus film is divided into two layers:

- Periciliary fluid layer about 6 μm deep, immediately adjacent to the surface of the epithelium. The mucus here is hydrated by epithelial cells. This reduces its viscosity and allows movement of the cilia.
- Superficial gel layer about 5–10 μm deep. This is a relatively viscous layer forming a sticky blanket, which traps particles.

The cilia beat synchronously at 1000–1500 strokes per minute. Coordinated movement causes the superficial gel layer, together with trapped particles, to be continually transported towards the mouth at 1–3 cm/min. The mucus and particles reach the trachea and larynx where they are swallowed or expectorated (coughed up).

Mucociliary clearance is inhibited by:

- Tobacco smoke.
- Cold air.
- Many drugs (e.g. general anaesthetics).
- Sulphur oxides.
- Nitrogen oxides.

The importance of mucociliary clearance is illustrated by cystic fibrosis, in which a defect in chloride channels throughout the body leads to hyperviscous secretions. In the lung, inadequate hydration causes excessive stickiness of the mucus lining the airways, preventing the action of the cilia

It is possible to measure the efficiency of the cilia with a simple clinical test. The saccharin screening test establishes the amount of time it takes for saccharin placed in the anterior nares to taste sweet.

Smaller inhaled particles will travel further down the respiratory tract. The method that is used to deal with inhaled particles depends upon which area of the respiratory tract the particle finally reaches (e.g. large particles may be filtered out by the nasopharynx).

in effecting mucociliary clearance. Failure to remove bacteria leads to repeated severe respiratory infections, which progressively damage the lungs. Impaired mucociliary clearance is the major cause of morbidity and mortality in cystic fibrosis.

Humoral defences

Lung secretions contain a wide range of proteins which defend the lungs by various different mechanisms.

Humoral and cellular aspects of the immune system are considered only briefly here; for more information see *Crash Course: Immunology and Haematology*.

Antimicrobial peptides

A number of proteins in lung fluid have antibacterial properties. These are generally low-molecular-weight proteins such as:

- Defensins.
- Lysozyme.
- Lactoferrin.

Surfactant

The alveoli are bathed in surfactant and this reduces surface tension and prevents the lungs from collapsing (see p. 58). Surfactant also contains proteins which play an important role in defending the host. Surfactant protein A (Sp-A) is the most abundant of these proteins and is hydrophilic. Sp-A has been shown to have similar properties to those of mannose binding proteins and acts as an opsonin – enhancing the phagocytosis of microorganisms by alveolar macrophages. Sp-D, which is also hydrophilic, has a similar role to Sp-A with regards to immune defence.

Sp-B and Sp-C, which are hydrophobic in nature, have a more structural role in that they are involved in maintaining the surfactant monolayer and further reducing the surface tension.

Immunoglobulins

Effector B lymphocytes (plasma cells) in the submucosa produce immunoglobulins. All classes of antibody are produced, but IgA production predominates. The immunoglobulins are contained within the mucous secretions in the respiratory tract and are directed against specific antigens.

Complement

Complement proteins are found in lung secretions in particularly high concentrations during inflammation and they play an important role in propagating the inflammatory response. Complement components can be secreted by alveolar macrophages (see below) and act as chemoattractants for the migration of cells such as neutrophils to the site of injury.

Antiproteases

Lung secretions contain a number of enzymes (antiproteases) that break down the destructive proteases released from dead bacteria, macrophages and neutrophils. One of the most important of these antiproteases is α_1-antitrypsin.

Cigarette smoke increases the number of pulmonary macrophages; these release a chemical that attracts leucocytes to the lung. The leucocytes in turn release proteases, including elastase, that attack elastic tissue in the lungs. This process is usually inhibited by α_1-antitrypsin, but this itself is inhibited by oxygen radicals released by leucocytes. The result is a protease–antiprotease imbalance that leads to the destruction of lung tissue and the development of emphysema.

A deficiency in α_1-antitrypsin (inherited as an autosomal dominant condition) leads to a reduction in the breakdown of proteolytic enzymes, such as elastase, released from neutrophils during acute inflammation. This results in increased destruction of the alveolar wall and lung parenchymal tissue. Thus, any insult to the lungs (e.g. smoking) will lead to increased destruction of tissue and emphysema. It should be noted, however, that only 2% of individuals who have emphysema have α_1-antitrypsin

Inherited defects in any of these humoral mechanisms can lead to lung disease. Patients with deficiencies in IgA or complement (C3) are prone to recurrent respiratory tract infections.

deficiency; the vast majority of cases of emphysema are related to smoking alone.

Cellular defences

Alveolar macrophages

Alveolar macrophages are differentiated monocytes, and are both phagocytic and mobile. They normally reside in the lining of the alveoli where they ingest bacteria and debris, before transporting it to the bronchioles where it can be removed from the lungs by mucociliary clearance. Alveolar macrophages can also initiate and amplify the inflammatory response by secreting proteins that recruit other cells. These proteins include:

- Complement components.
- Cytokines (e.g. IL-1, IL-6) and chemokines.
- Growth factors.

Neutrophils

Neutrophils are the predominant cell recruited in the acute inflammatory response. Neutrophils emigrate from the intravascular space to the alveolar lumen where intracellular killing of bacteria takes place by two mechanisms:

- Oxidative – via reactive oxygen species.
- Non-oxidative – via proteases.

In some cases, defence mechanisms can cause injury to lung tissue. Uncontrolled degranulation of neutrophils releases large amounts of elastase, damaging the lung parenchyma in diseases such as emphysema.

METABOLIC FUNCTIONS OF THE LUNGS

Overview

The lungs, in addition to their role as gas-exchange organs, have some important metabolic functions, notably:

- Conversion of angiotensin I to angiotensin II.
- Deactivation of vasoactive substances.
- Arachidonic acid metabolism.
- Phospholipid synthesis.
- Protein synthesis.

Angiotensin-converting enzyme

Renin released from the juxtaglomerular cells of the kidney enters the bloodstream where it acts on a plasma protein, angiotensinogen, to produce angiotensin I (Fig. 3.17). Angiotensin I is further converted by angiotensin-converting enzyme (ACE) to angiotensin II, which stimulates aldosterone secretion and acts as a potent vasoconstrictor. ACE is produced by the vascular endothelial cells of the lungs.

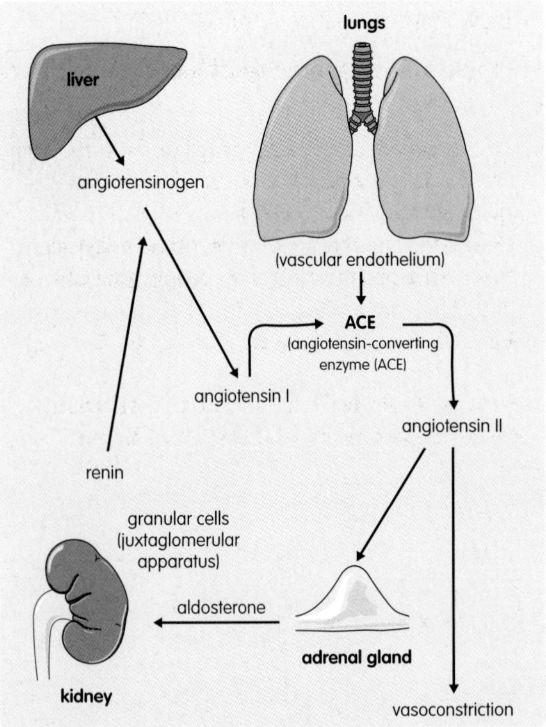

Deactivation of vasoactive substances

Many different vasoactive substances are deactivated as they pass through the lungs. An example of this is the degradation of bradykinin (a potent vasodilator) to inactive peptides by ACE (Fig. 3.18).

The administration of an ACE inhibitor (such as captopril) inhibits both the production of angiotensin II and the breakdown of bradykinin.

Arachidonic acid metabolism

The lungs are capable of both production and removal of arachidonic acid metabolites. The following metabolites are removed by the lung:

- Prostaglandin E_2.
- Prostaglandin $F_{2\alpha}$.
- Leukotrienes.

Arachidonic acid synthesis

Arachidonic acid is released from membrane phospholipids by the action of phospholipase A_2 (Fig. 3.19). Arachidonic acid is converted into endoperoxides (e.g. prostaglandins) by the action of cyclo-oxygenase or into leukotrienes by the action of lipoxygenase.

Leukotrienes (LTB_4, LTC_4, LTD_4) are implicated as a cause of bronchoconstriction in asthma (Chs 6 and 7). Thromboxane A_2 increases platelet aggregation and vasoconstriction, whereas prostacyclin has opposite effects. The prostaglandins produced have vasodilatory and vasoconstrictory effects.

Fig. 3.17 The renin–angiotensin system. Conversion of angiotensin I to angiotensin II by angiotensin-converting enzyme (ACE) occurs mainly in the pulmonary vascular endothelium.

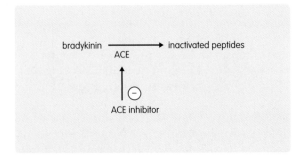

Fig. 3.18 Bradykinin degradation.

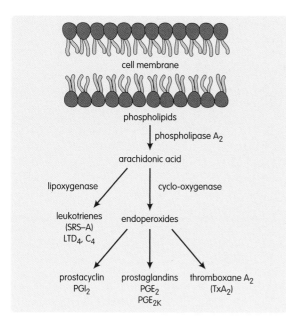

Fig. 3.19 Arachidonic acid metabolism. The production of endoperoxides and leukotrienes.

Phospholipid synthesis

Type II pneumocytes produce surfactant which contains an important phospholipid (dipalmitoyl phosphatidylcholine, DPC). As noted above, surfactant has the property of reducing surface tension in proportion to its surface concentration and plays an important role in defence.

Phospholipids are produced from fatty acids in association with smooth endoplasmic reticular membrane. Synthesis occurs at the interface between cytosol and the endoplasmic reticular membrane. The synthesized phospholipids are transported to vesicles by 'membrane budding' (endoplasmic reticular membrane fuses with the vesicle).

The surfactant mixture is extruded into the alveolus and lowers the surface tension. The synthesis is rapid and allows quick turnover of surfactant.

Protein synthesis

Structural proteins, collagen, and elastin form the parenchyma of the lung; their synthesis and breakdown are important to the normal functioning of the lung. An increase in their breakdown is associated with increased protease activity (as seen in α_1-antitrypsin deficiency) and leads to emphysema.

THE EFFECT OF SMOKING ON THE LOWER RESPIRATORY TRACT

Smoking is associated with increased morbidity and mortality in many different diseases, e.g. ischaemic heart disease, peripheral vascular disease and carcinoma of the oesophagus and bladder. Focusing on the respiratory system, smoking increases the number of deaths from laryngeal cancer and is strongly associated with the following lower respiratory tract diseases:

- Lung cancer (see p. 151).
- Chronic obstructive pulmonary disease (COPD) (see p. 124).
- Cor pulmonale.
- Treatment-insensitive asthma.

The main mechanisms by which smoking causes harm include:

- The direct effect of toxic compounds in tobacco smoke (e.g. hydrocarbons, reactive oxygen species and nitrosamines).
- Increasing the release of proteolytic enzymes from neutrophils and macrophages (see above, p. 39).
- Reduction in endogenous nitric oxide production.
- Increased permeability of blood vessel walls. Smoking cessation is discussed in Chapter 6.

Ventilation and gas exchange

4

Objectives

By the end of this chapter you should be able to:

- Define minute ventilation and alveolar ventilation.
- Define anatomical dead space, quoting its normal value, and describe two methods of measuring anatomical dead space.
- Define all lung volumes and capacities, giving normal values, and state the significance of each volume and capacity.
- Name four methods for measuring lung volume.
- Outline the regional variations in ventilation of the lung and how these might be measured.
- Explain why intrapleural pressure is negative and describe its variation during breathing.
- Describe how breathing is brought about, naming the muscles involved and their actions.
- Define lung compliance and explain what is meant by static and dynamic lung compliance, including a description of the pressure–volume curve.
- Describe the role of surfactant.
- Define airway resistance and viscous tissue resistance.
- List the factors determining airway resistance.
- Describe how airway resistance is altered in asthma.
- Explain what is meant by dynamic compression of the airways.
- Summarize the mechanisms that impair ventilation in COPD.
- Describe factors affecting the rate of diffusion across the blood–air interface.
- Give the normal values of the partial pressures of carbon dioxide and oxygen within the respiratory system.
- Explain the terms 'partial pressure of a gas' and 'vapour pressure'.
- Name three conditions that lower the transfer of oxygen to the blood and describe how they affect diffusion.
- Using examples, define perfusion limitation and diffusion limitation.
- Define diffusing capacity and describe its measurement.

OVERVIEW

Ventilation is the flow of air in and out of the respiratory system (breathing); it is defined physiologically as the amount of air breathed in and out in a given time. The function of ventilation is to maintain blood gases at their optimum level, by delivering air to the alveoli where gas exchange can take place. The movement of air in and out of the lungs occurs due to pressure differences brought about by changes in lung volume. The respiratory muscles bring about these changes, but other factors are also involved, namely the physical properties of the lungs, including their elasticity and the resistance of the airways. Lung diseases that affect these physical properties therefore impair gas exchange by reducing the delivery of fresh gas to the lungs, ultimately leading to a mismatch in ventilation : perfusion.

VENTILATION

Anatomical dead space

Not all of the air entering the respiratory system actually reaches the alveoli and takes part in gas exchange. Chapter 3 introduced the concept of anatomical dead space, or those areas of the airway not involved in gaseous exchange (i.e. the conducting zone). Included in this space are:

- Nose and mouth.
- Pharynx.
- Larynx.
- Trachea.
- Bronchi and bronchioles, down to and including the terminal bronchioles.

Inspired air held within these areas is referred to as dead air. The volume of the anatomical dead space (V_D) is usually about 150 mL (or 2 mL/kg of bodyweight). Anatomical dead space varies with the size of the subject and also increases with increased inspiration because greater expansion of the lungs lengthens and widens the conducting airways.

Anatomical dead space can be measured using Fowler's method, which is based on the single-breath nitrogen test. This test is described in Chapter 11.

Physiological dead space

Anatomical dead space is not the only cause of 'wasted' ventilation, even in the healthy lung. The total dead space is known as physiological dead space and includes gas in the alveoli that does not participate in gas exchange.

Physiological dead space = anatomical dead space + alveolar dead space

Alveolar dead space comes about because gas exchange is less than optimal in some parts of the lung. If each acinus (or end respiratory unit) were perfect, the amount of air received by each alveolus would be matched by the flow of blood through the pulmonary capillaries. In reality:

- Some areas receive less ventilation than others.
- Some areas receive less blood flow than others.

In a normal, healthy person, anatomical and physiological dead space are almost equal, alveolar dead space being very small (< 5 mL). However, when lung disease alters ventilation : perfusion

Respiratory physiology involves a number of equations and you may find this aspect difficult. Memorizing these equations is less important than understanding the underlying concepts and being able to relate them to clinical practice. For this reason, in most cases we have separated the equations from the main body of the text; if you want more detail or need to memorize them for your exams, you will find the equations and brief explanations in the figures.

A component balance works on the basis of conservation of mass (i.e. what goes into a system must equal what comes out). Several tests in respiratory medicine (e.g. helium dilution, nitrogen washout) are based on this principle.

relationships, the volume of alveolar dead space increases.

Measurement of physiological dead space

Physiological dead space is measured using the Bohr equation (Fig. 4.1).

The method requires a sample of arterial blood and involves the analysis of carbon dioxide in expired air. Knowing that carbon dioxide is not blown off from end respiratory units that are not perfused, and that carbon dioxide in air is almost zero, it is possible to carry out a component balance for carbon dioxide to establish the volume of physiological dead space.

Minute ventilation

Minute ventilation ($\dot{V}_E$) is the volume of gas moved in and out of the lungs in 1 minute (Fig. 4.2).

In order to calculate $\dot{V}_E$ you need to know:

- The number of breaths per minute.
- The volume of air moved in and out with each breath (the tidal volume: V_T).

Alveolar ventilation

We have already noted that not all the air inspired reaches the alveoli; some stays within the trachea or other conducting airways.

Therefore, two values of minute ventilation need to be considered:

- Minute ventilation ($\dot{V}_E$), as described above.
- Minute alveolar ventilation ($\dot{V}_A$), which is the amount of air that reaches the alveoli in 1 minute.

From our understanding of anatomical dead space, we can say that for one breath:

$$V_A = V_T - V_D$$

where V_A = the volume reaching the alveolus in one breath, and V_D = the volume of dead space. Hence, in 1 minute:

$$\dot{V}_A = (V_T - V_D)f$$

Variation in ventilation within the lung

Not all regions of the lungs are ventilated equally. Ventilation per unit volume can be measured by inhalation of a radioactive isotope of xenon (^{133}Xe). If radiation counters are placed at different levels of the lungs, the volume of inhaled radioactive xenon in various areas of the lung can be measured.

It has been shown that the lower zones of the lungs are ventilated better than the upper zones. The causes of regional differences in ventilation will be discussed in the next section.

Lung volumes

The gas held by the lungs can be thought of in terms of subdivisions, or specific lung volumes. Some of these volumes can be measured using spirometry, a technique which is described in Chapter 11. A trace from a spirometer, showing key lung volumes, is reproduced in Figure 4.3. Note that one of the

---

Fig. 4.1 The Bohr equation

The Bohr equation is used in measuring physiological dead space

$V_D/V_T = (P_ACO_2 - P_ECO_2)/P_ACO_2$
V_D = Volume of dead space
V_T = Tidal volume
P_ACO_2 = Partial pressure of carbon dioxide in alveolar air
P_ECO_2 = Partial pressure of carbon dioxide in mixed expired air

Normally, the partial pressures of carbon dioxide in alveolar gas and arterial blood are the same.

The equation can therefore be shown as:
$V_D/V_T = (P_aCO_2 - P_ECO_2)/P_aCO_2$

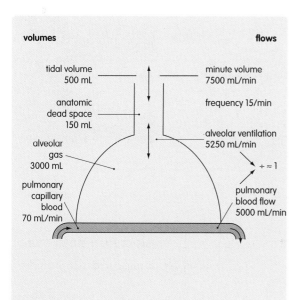

Fig. 4.2 Ventilation in the simplified lung. (From Criner & D'Alonzo 1999, with permission of Fence Creek Publishing.)

The normal frequency of breathing varies between 12 and 20 breaths per minute. Normal tidal volume is approximately 500 mL in quiet breathing. If a subject with a tidal volume of 500 mL took 12 breaths a minute, it would seem obvious that the volume exhaled per minute (minute ventilation) would be $500 \times 12 = 6000$ mL/min. Or, more generally:

$$\dot{V}_E = V_Tf$$

where $\dot{V}_E$ = minute ventilation, V_T = tidal volume, and f = the respiratory rate (breaths/minute).

Note that at this stage we are still considering the healthy lung. In clinical practice, disease has a much greater effect on variation of ventilation.

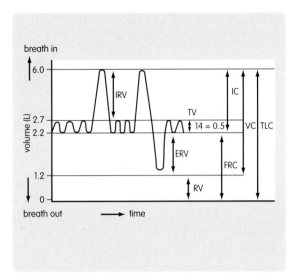

Fig. 4.3 Typical spirometer trace. Note that functional residual capacity (FRC) and residual volume (RV) cannot be measured using a spirometer; thus, neither can total lung capacity (TLC). ERV = expiratory reserve volume; IRV = inspiratory reserve volume; TV = tidal volume; IC = inspiratory capacity; VC = vital capacity.

subdivisions shown here, tidal volume, has already been introduced above under the concept of minute ventilation. Definitions of all the lung volumes and capacities (combinations of two or more volumes) are given in Figure 4.4.

Measuring lung volumes

There are four main methods of measuring lung volumes:

- Spirometry.
- Nitrogen washout.
- Helium dilution.
- Plethysmography.

These techniques are considered in detail in Chapter 11.

Effect of disease on lung volumes

Understanding lung volumes is important because they can be affected by disease. Two particular volumes are important in common diseases such as

Fig. 4.4 Descriptions of lung volumes and capacities	
Air in lungs is divided into 4 volumes	
tidal volume (TV)	volume of air breathed in and out in a single breath: 0.5 L
inspiratory reserve volume (IRV)	volume of air breathed in by a maximum inspiration at the end of a normal inspiration: 3.3 L
expiratory reserve volume (ERV)	volume of air that can be expelled by a maximum effort at the end of a normal expiration: 1.0 L
residual volume (RV)	volume of air remaining in lungs at end of a maximum expiration: 1.2 L
Pulmonary capacities are combinations of 2 or more volumes	
inspiratory capacity (IC) = TV + IRV	volume of air breathed in by a maximum inspiration at the end of a normal expiration: 3.8 L
functional residual capacity (FRC) = ERV + RV	volume of air remaining in lungs at the end of a normal expiration. Acts as buffer against extreme changes in alveolar gas levels with each breath: 2.2 L
vital capacity (VC) = IRV + TV + ERV	volume of air that can be breathed in by a maximum inspiration following a maximum expiration: 4.8 L
total lung capacity (TLC) = VC + RV	only a fraction of TLC is used in normal breathing: 6.0 L
Most of these volumes can be measures with a spirometer (see Fig. 4.3)	

asthma and COPD and are considered in more detail below. These are residual volume (RV) and functional residual capacity (FRC).

Residual volume and functional residual capacity

After breathing out, the lungs are not completely emptied of air. A completely deflated lung would require a much greater amount of energy to inflate it than one in which the alveoli have not collapsed (see Fig. 4.17). Even a maximum respiratory effort (forced expiration) fails to expel all the air from the lungs. When the expiratory muscles contract, all the structures in the lungs (not only the alveoli but also the airways) are compressed by the positive intrapleural pressure. During forced expiration, the smaller airways collapse before the alveoli empty completely. Thus, some air remains within the lungs; this is known as the residual volume (Fig. 4.3).

During normal breathing (quiet breathing), the lung volume oscillates between inhalation and exhalation. In quiet breathing, after the tidal volume has been expired:

- Pressure outside the chest is equal to pressure inside the alveoli (i.e. atmospheric pressure).
- Elastic forces tending to collapse the lung are balanced by the elastic recoil trying to expand the chest (Fig. 4.5).

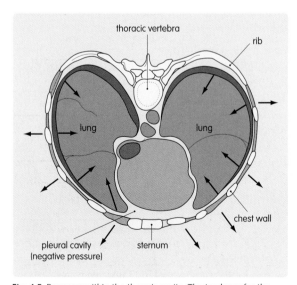

Fig. 4.5 Pressures within the thoracic cavity. The tendency for the lungs to collapse (elastic recoil) and the opposing forces' tendency to expand the chest wall create a subatmospheric (negative) pressure in the intrapleural space.

thoracic vertebra
rib
lung
lung
chest wall
pleural cavity (negative pressure)
sternum

- This creates a subatmospheric (negative) pressure in the intrapleural space.

The lung volume at this point is known as functional residual capacity. RV and FRC can be measured using nitrogen washout, helium dilution and plethysmography (see Ch. 11).

Patterns of lung function

Disease affects lung volumes in specific patterns, depending on the pathological processes. Diseases can be classified as obstructive, restrictive or mixed, with each showing characteristic changes in lung volumes. Figures 4.6 and 4.7 summarize the common patterns seen.

Obstructive disorders

This group of disorders is characterized by obstruction of normal air flow due to airway narrowing (see p. 124), which, in general, leads to hyperinflation of the lungs as air is trapped behind closed airways. RV is increased as gas that is trapped cannot leave the lung, and the RV:TLC ratio increases also. In patients with severe obstruction, air trapping is so extensive that vital capacity is decreased.

Restrictive disorders

Restrictive disorders (see p. 145) result in stiffer lungs which cannot expand to normal volumes. All the subdivisions of volume are decreased and the RV:TLC ratio will be normal, or where VC decreases more quickly than RV, increased.

MECHANICS OF BREATHING

In order to understand ventilation we must also understand the mechanism by which it takes place: breathing. This section reviews the mechanics of breathing including:

- The pressure differences that generate air flow.
- The respiratory muscles that effect these pressure differences.
- Tissue properties that influence how easily the lungs expand.

Flow of air into the lungs

To achieve air flow into the lungs, we require a driving pressure (remember air flows from high

Fig. 4.6 Lung volumes in health, and in obstructive and restrictive disease. See Figure 4.4 for abbreviations. Note that in obstructive diseases TLC and FRC are increased. VC may be entirely normal or reduced. In restrictive diseases all lung volumes are reduced. (From Criner & D'Alonzo 1999, with permission of Fence Creek Publishing.)

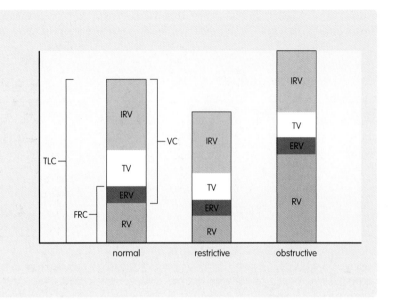

Fig. 4.7 Patterns of lung function			
	Obstructive	Restrictive	Mixed
FEV$_1$	↓	↓	↓
FVC	N or ↓	↓	↓
FEV$_1$/FVC ratio	↓	N	↓
TLC	N or ↓	↓	↓
VC	N or ↓	↓	↓
RV	↑	N or ↓	N or ↑
RV/TLC ratio	↑	N or ↑	↑?

pressure to low pressure). Pressure at the entrance to the respiratory tract (i.e. at the nose and mouth) is atmospheric (P_{atm}). Pressure inside the lungs is alveolar pressure (P_A).

Therefore:

- If $P_A = P_{atm}$, no air flow occurs (e.g. at functional residual capacity).
- If $P_A < P_{atm}$, air flows into the lungs.
- If $P_A > P_{atm}$, air flows out of the lungs.

Because we cannot change atmospheric pressure, alveolar pressure must be altered to achieve air flow. Thus, if the volume inside the lungs is changed, Boyle's law predicts that pressure inside the lungs will also change. How can this be achieved? (Fig. 4.8).

- The lungs contain no muscle that can actively expand or contract.
- Therefore the chest must be expanded, which lowers intrapleural pressure, expanding the lungs.
- The majority of chest expansion in quiet breathing is caused by contraction of the diaphragm.
- Relaxation of the muscles of the chest wall allows the elastic recoil of the lungs to cause contraction of the lungs and expulsion of gas.

Intrapleural pressure

In the previous section, we saw that at FRC elastic recoil of the lungs is exactly balanced by the elastic recoil of the chest wall trying to expand the chest. These two opposing forces create a subatmospheric (negative) pressure within the intrapleural space; as the alveoli communicate with the atmosphere, the intrapleural pressure is also less than the pressure inside the lungs (Fig. 4.9). The intrapleural pressure fluctuates during breathing (Fig. 4.10) but is about 0.5 kPa at the end of quiet expiration. In summary, there is a gradient between the pressure on the inside and the outside of the lungs, or across the lung walls; this is known as the transmural pressure. It is transmural pressure (caused by the negative pressure in the pleural space) that ensures that the lungs are held partially expanded in the thorax. It effectively links the lungs (which are like suspended balloons) with the chest wall.

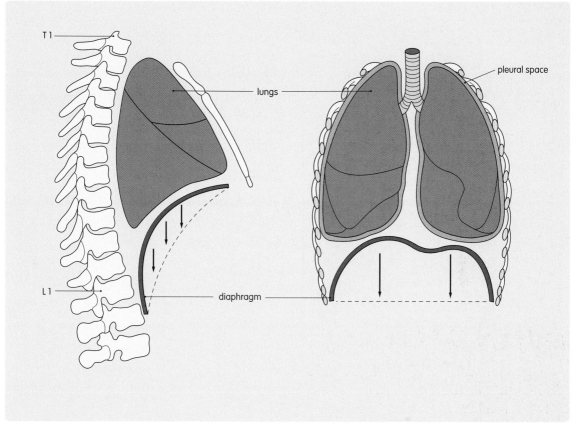

Fig. 4.8 Expanding the lungs to draw in air. Flattening the diaphragm increases the thoracic volume, lowering the intrapleural pressure and expanding the lungs.

On inspiration, intrathoracic volume is increased; this lowers intrapleural pressure making it more negative, causing the lungs to expand and air to enter. On expiration, the muscles of the chest wall relax and the lungs return to their original size by elastic recoil, with the expulsion of air.

It should be noted that during quiet breathing, intrapleural pressure is always negative. In forced expiration, however, the intrapleural pressure becomes positive, forcing a reduction in lung volume with the expulsion of air.

Puncture wounds through the thorax can mean that the intrapleural space is open to the atmosphere – a pneumothorax. The pressures equilibrate and the lungs are no longer held expanded, leading to collapse.

Differences in intrapleural pressure between apex and base

The lungs are not rigid and therefore not self-supportive. As we pass vertically down the lung, each layer of lung hangs down from the layer of lung above and sits on the layer of lung below. Thus, at the apex, there is a larger weight of lung pulling away from the chest wall causing the intrapleural pressure to be more negative at the apex than at the base. For an upright subject at functional residual capacity (before inspiration) the intrapleural pressure at the apex is –0.8 kPa, and at the base about –0.2 kPa. The lung base is compressed compared with the apex.

It should be noted that:

- Alveolar volumes at the base and the apex of the lung are of different values before inspiration.
- However, intrapleural pressure changes at lung base and apex during breathing are of equal magnitude.

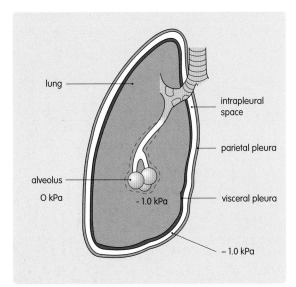

Fig. 4.9 Transmural pressure and inflation pressure. The transmural pressure is the difference in pressure across the walls of the airways. There is a slight difference in pressure between the intrapleural space and the outside of the airway, but this has been ignored in this example and the inflation pressure can be considered as the pressure difference between the intrapleural pressure and the pressure inside the alveoli (−1.0 kPa).

These two factors will be important later when we look at why ventilation varies from lung base to apex.

Muscles of respiration

We have seen that the chest must be expanded in order to reduce intrapleural pressure and drive air into the lungs. This section describes the muscles of respiration that bring about this change in volume.

Thoracic wall

The thoracic wall is made up of (from superficial to deep):

- Skin and subcutaneous tissue.
- Ribs, thoracic vertebrae, sternum and manubrium.
- Intercostal muscles: external, internal and thoracis transversus.
- Parietal pleura.

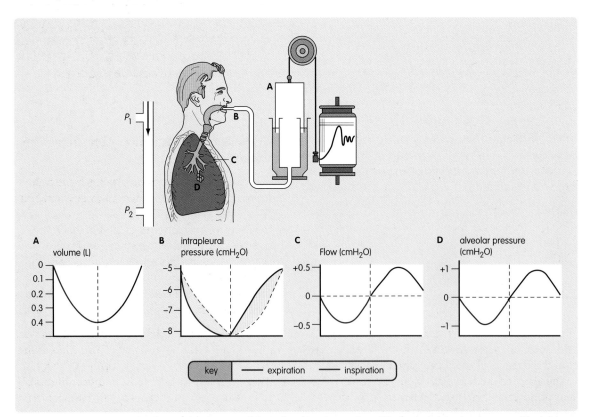

Fig. 4.10 Negative pressure within the intrapleural space and during breathing. Lung volume (A); change in intrapleural pressure (B); air flow (C); and alveolar pressure (D). All measurements are relative to inspiration and expiration. *Note that intrapleural pressure becomes more negative during inspiration as intrathoracic volume increases.*

Situated at the thoracic outlet is the diaphragm, which attaches to the costal margin, xyphoid process and lumbar vertebrae.

Intercostal muscles

The action of the intercostal muscles is to pull the ribs closer together. There are therefore two main actions:

- If the first rib is fixed by scalene muscle, the external intercostal muscles pull the ribs upwards.
- If the last rib is fixed by quadratus lumborum, the internal intercostal muscles pull the ribs downwards.

Their action during respiration is discussed in 'function of the muscles of respiration'.

External intercostal muscles
External intercostal muscles span the space between adjacent ribs, originating from the inferior border of the upper rib, and attaching to the superior border of the rib below. The muscle attaches along the length of the rib, from the tubercle to the costal-chondral junction, and its fibres run forward and downward (Fig. 4.11A).

Internal intercostal muscles
Internal intercostal muscles span the space between adjacent ribs, originating from the subcostal groove of the rib above, and attaching to the superior border of the rib below. The muscle attaches along the length of the rib from the angle of the rib to the sternum, and its fibres run downward and backward (Fig. 4.11B).

Thoracis transversus
Thoracis transversus muscle is incomplete and has the parietal pleura and neurovascular bundle as its relations.

Diaphragm

The diaphragm is the main muscle of respiration (Fig. 4.12). The central region of the diaphragm is tendinous; the outer margin is muscular, originating from the borders of the thoracic outlet.

The diaphragm has right and left domes. The right dome is higher than the left to accommodate the liver below. There is a central tendon that sits below the two domes, attaching to the xiphisternum anteriorly and the lumbar vertebrae posteriorly.

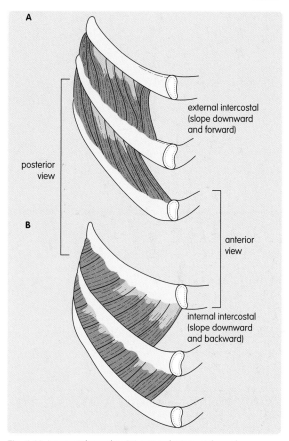

Fig. 4.11 Intercostal muscles. (A) External intercostal muscles; (B) internal intercostal muscles.

Several important structures pass through the diaphragm:

- The inferior vena cava passes through the right dome at the level of the eighth thoracic vertebra (T8).
- The oesophagus passes through a sling of muscular fibres from the right crus of the diaphragm at the level of the tenth thoracic vertebra (T10).
- The aorta pierces the diaphragm anterior to the twelfth thoracic vertebra (T12).

The diaphragm attaches to the costal margin anteriorly and laterally. Posteriorly, it attaches to the lumbar vertebrae by the crura (left crus at L1 and L2, right crus at L1, L2 and L3). In addition, the position of the diaphragm changes relative to posture: it is lower when standing than sitting.

The motor and sensory nerve supply of the diaphragm is from the phrenic nerve. Blood supply of the

Fig. 4.12 The diaphragm. Many structures pass through the diaphragm, notably the inferior vena cava, the aorta and the oesophagus.

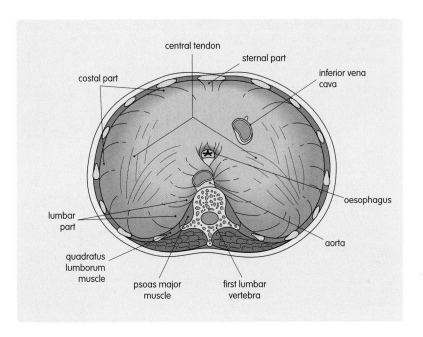

The phrenic nerve supplies the diaphragm (60% motor, 40% sensory). Remember, 'nerve roots 3, 4 and 5 keep the diaphragm alive'. Thus, if you break your neck at C3, you die.

A chest X-ray of a 66-year-old smoker complaining of shortness of breath and reduced exercise capacity shows a flattened diaphragm. Flattening of the diaphragm suggests air trapping and an obstructive lung disease, which in light of the history is likely to be COPD.

diaphragm is from pericardiophrenic and musculophrenic branches of the internal thoracic artery.

Function of the muscles of respiration

Breathing can be classified into inspiration and expiration, quiet or forced.

Quiet inspiration

In quiet inspiration, contraction of the diaphragm flattens its domes. This action increases the length of the thorax and thus its volume. This lowers intrapleural pressure and draws air into the lungs. At the same time, the abdominal wall must relax to allow the abdominal contents to be displaced as the diaphragm moves down.

The main muscle in quiet breathing is the diaphragm, but the intercostal muscles are involved. With the first rib fixed, the intercostal muscles can expand the rib cage by two movements:

- Forward movement of the lower end of the sternum – pump-handle action (Fig. 4.13A).
- Upward and outward – bucket-handle action (Fig. 4.13B).

During quiet inspiration, these actions are small and the intercostal muscles mainly prevent deformation of the tissue between the ribs, which would otherwise lower the volume of the thoracic cage (Fig. 4.14). The internal intercostal muscles carry out this role.

Quiet expiration

Quiet expiration is passive and there is no direct muscle action. During inspiration, the lungs are expanded against their elastic recoil. This recoil is sufficient to drive air out of the lungs in expiration. Thus, quiet expiration involves the controlled relaxation of the intercostal muscles and the diaphragm.

Forced inspiration

In addition to the action of the diaphragm:

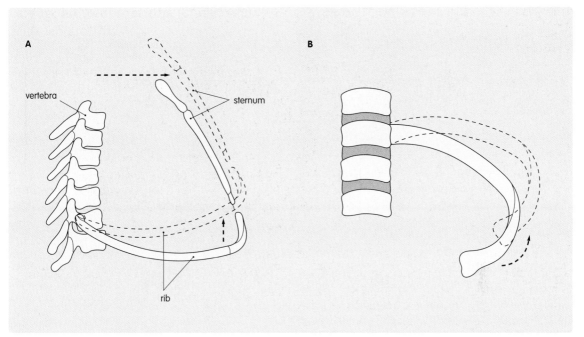

Fig. 4.13 Posterior (A) and lateral (B) expansion of the chest. Note the expansion of the chest (A) in a forward and upward movement (pump-handle action) and (B) an outward and upward movement (bucket-handle action).

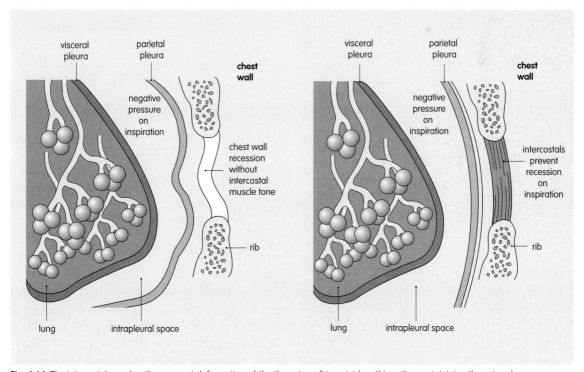

Fig. 4.14 The intercostal muscles: they prevent deformation of the thoracic wall in quiet breathing, thus maintaining thoracic volume.

The change in intrathoracic volume is mainly caused by the movement of the diaphragm downwards. Contraction of the diaphragm comprises 75% of the energy expenditure during quiet breathing.

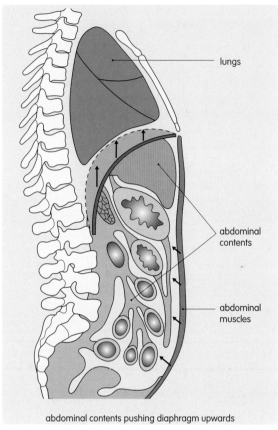

- Scalene muscles and sternocleidomastoids raise the ribs anteroposteriorly, producing movement at the manubriosternal joint.
- Intercostal muscles are much more active and raise the ribs to a much greater extent than in quiet inspiration.
- The twelfth rib, which is attached to quadratus lumborum, allows forcible downward movement of the diaphragm.
- Arching the back using erector spinae also increases thoracic volume.

During respiratory distress, the scapulae are fixed by trapezius muscles, rhomboid muscles and levator scapulae; pectoralis minor and serratus anterior raise the ribs; the arms can be fixed (e.g. by holding the back of a chair), allowing the use of pectoralis major.

Fig. 4.15 Forced expiration. *Note the abdominal contents pushing the diaphragm upwards.*

Forced expiration

Elastic recoil of the lungs is reinforced by contraction of the muscles of the abdominal wall. These force the abdominal contents against the diaphragm, pushing it up (Fig. 4.15).

In addition, quadratus lumborum pulls the ribs down, thus adding to the force of the abdominal contents against the diaphragm. Intercostal muscles prevent outward deformation of the tissue between the ribs. Latissimus dorsi and serratus posterior inferior also may play some role.

You are called to assess a patient in casualty complaining of shortness of breath. The patient is using his accessory muscles of respiration and has fixed his torso by leaning forward and holding onto his knees. In your assessment of the patient's condition, these signs suggest that the patient is in respiratory distress and urgent action is required.

Elastic properties of the lung

In order for ventilation to take place, the respiratory muscles described above must overcome the mechanical properties of the lungs and thorax, specifically their tendency to elastic recoil.

The elastic properties of the lung are caused by:

- Elastic fibres and collagen in the tissues in the lung.
- Surface tension forces in the lung caused by the alveolar–liquid interface.

When we discuss the elastic properties of the lung, we often focus not on recoil but on stretch; the capacity of the lung to stretch is known as compliance and is discussed below.

Compliance

Compliance describes the distensibility or ease of stretch of a material when an external force is applied to it. Elasticity (E) is the resistance to that stretch. Therefore:

$$C = 1/E$$

In respiratory physiology, we deal with:

- Compliance of the lung (C_L).
- Compliance of the chest wall (C_W).
- Total compliance (C_{TOT}) of the chest wall and lung together.

Lung compliance

Lung compliance is the ease with which the lungs expand under pressure. The pressure to inflate comes from the transmural pressure (i.e. the difference between the intrapleural pressure and the intrapulmonary pressure); this is plotted against the change in volume on a pressure–volume curve (Fig. 4.16). Compliance represents the slope of the curve ($\Delta V : \Delta P$).

> Lung mechanics are often categorized as static or dynamic. This can sometimes be confusing. As the name implies, static qualities do not change with time; lung statics help us to explore certain qualities of the lungs in isolation. Obviously, in real life, air in the respiratory tree flows (i.e. it changes with time). Therefore lung dynamics give us a fuller picture of what actually happens during respiration.

Lung compliance can be looked at in two ways:

- Static lung compliance.
- Dynamic lung compliance.

Dynamic lung compliance is a measure of the change in volume of the lung during breathing, and will thus include the work required to overcome airway resistance. This will be discussed later.

Static lung compliance involves the inflation of the lungs in steps of various inflating pressures and recording the volume at the new inflation pressure. The lungs are expanded from complete collapse to total lung capacity, and measurements are also taken in deflation (see dotted line in Fig. 4.17A). This is carried out in vitro because, in life, we cannot completely deflate the lungs. The difference between inflation and deflation curves is called hysteresis and will be explained later.

Figure 4.17B also shows the pressure–volume curve for inflation of the lungs from functional residual capacity to total lung capacity. The curve still shows hysteresis, but not to the extent of the pressure–volume curve from complete lung collapse to total lung capacity. The slope of the curve (i.e. compliance) varies with lung volume. It can be seen that compliance is greatest at the lower lung volumes and is smallest at higher lung volumes. For these reasons, lung compliance is sometimes quoted as specific lung compliance (sp.C_L).

$$sp.C_L = C_L/V_L$$

This change in lung compliance helps explain the difference in ventilation of the lung between apex and base.

The lung volume in the base is less (because it is compressed) relative to the apex (see p. 49). Thus, the base of the lung has greater initial compliance than that of the apex. Because both base and apex are subject to intrapleural pressure changes of the same magnitude during inspiration, the base of the

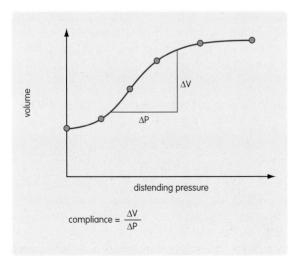

compliance = $\dfrac{\Delta V}{\Delta P}$

Fig. 4.16 The pressure–volume curve.

> You can see from the pressure–volume curve that expanding the lung is like blowing up a balloon. At first, high pressure is required for a small increase in volume. Then the slope becomes steeper before flattening out again.

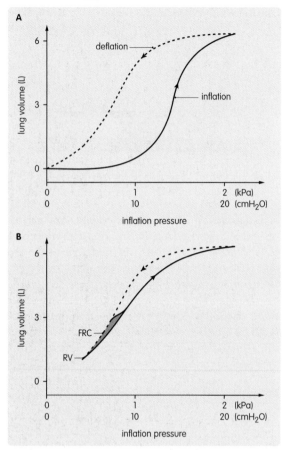

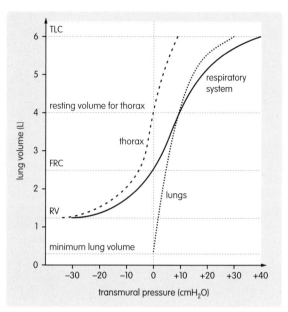

Fig. 4.18 Pressure–volume curve of the entire respiratory system. Only at functional residual capacity does the passively inflated lung–thorax system (respiratory system) have no pressure difference between the alveoli and the body surface.

Fig. 4.17 Pressure–volume curves for inflation of the lungs: (A) in vitro; (B) in life, from residual volume to total lung capacity. *Note the curve still shows hysteresis but to a lesser extent.*

lung will therefore expand to a greater extent than the apex. This explains in part the regional difference of ventilation.

Chest wall compliance

As we have discussed before, the chest wall has elastic properties; at functional residual capacity, these are equal and opposite to those in the lung (i.e. tending to expand the chest). If the sternum were cut (e.g. in surgery) or if air were introduced into the intrapleural space then this would cause the chest wall to spring open.

As we breathe in, elastic forces (tending to expand the chest wall) aid inflation; however, at about two-thirds of total lung capacity, the chest wall has reached its resting position and any expansion beyond this point requires a positive pressure to stretch the chest wall.

Below this resting position, the chest wall is being compressed by the pressure difference between atmospheric pressure and intrapleural pressure. Thus, if we plot inflation pressure against volume of the chest wall, the inflation pressure is negative below two-thirds of total lung capacity (the dashed line in Fig. 4.18). However, compliance (the slope of the pressure–volume curve for the chest wall) remains positive, because we are looking at the change in volume caused by a change in inflation pressure. Above the resting position the inflation pressure required to expand the chest is positive. Compliance of the lung is also plotted (dotted line in Fig. 4.18). Total compliance is plotted on the same graph and is derived from:

$$1/C_{TOT} = 1/C_L + 1/C_W$$

Effect of disease on compliance

Structural change in the thorax (e.g. kyphoscoliosis) may alter compliance of the chest wall; however, in practice, disease more often has an effect on compliance of the lung. Emphysema and pulmonary fibrosis (Fig. 4.19) represent two extremes of lung compliance in disease. In emphysema the compliance of the lung is increased, that is it becomes more easily distended. This is due to the destruction

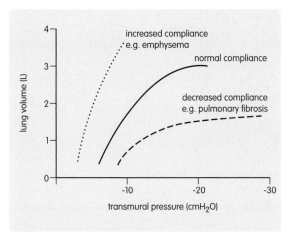

Fig. 4.19 Pressure–volume curves in disease.

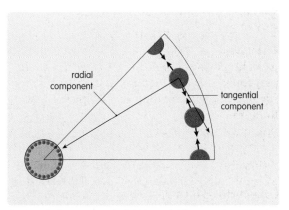

Fig. 4.20 Surface tension. (After Berne & Levy 1993, with permission of Mosby.)

of the normal lung architecture, including the elastic fibres and collagen. Impaired elastic recoil means that the lungs do not deflate as easily, contributing to air trapping.

In diseases that cause fibrosis, scar tissue replaces normal interstitial tissue. As a result, the lungs become stiffer and compliance decreases.

Surface tension and surfactant

As noted above, the elasticity, and therefore compliance of the lungs, is dependent on two factors. The first is the elastic fibres in lung tissue. The second is the surface tension of the alveolar lining. This lining is a thin film of liquid, the main component of which is surfactant.

Surface tension

Surface tension is a physical property of liquids and arises because fluid molecules have a stronger attraction to each other than to air molecules (Fig. 4.20). Molecules on the surface of a liquid in contact with air are therefore pulled close together and act like a skin.

When molecules of a liquid lie on a curved surface (e.g. in a bubble), surface tension acts to pull that surface inwards. If the bubble is to be prevented from collapsing there must be an equal and opposite force tending to expand it. This is provided by positive pressure within the bubble.

The alveoli are lined with liquid and are in contact with air. They can therefore be considered similar to tiny bubbles. Laplace's law (Fig. 4.21) tells us that the smaller a bubble, the greater the internal pressure needed to keep it inflated (Fig. 4.22). If a bubble of

> **Fig. 4.21** Laplace's law
>
> Laplace's law: states that 'The pressure within a bubble is equal to twice the surface tension divided by the radius'
>
> $$P = \frac{2T}{r}$$
>
> P=pressure within bubble
> T=surface tension
> r=radius
>
> The smaller a bubble (i.e. the more curved the surface) the larger the radial component.
> The larger the radial component the greater the tendency to collapse.
> Smaller bubbles must have a greater internal pressure to keep them inflated.

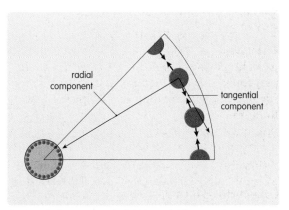

Fig. 4.22 Surface tension of a bubble. Radial forces tend to collapse the bubble and there must be a positive pressure inside the bubble to prevent it from collapsing. The smaller the bubble, the greater the internal pressure.

about the same size as an alveolus was made of interstitial fluid and filled with air it would require an internal pressure in the order of 3 kPa to prevent it from collapsing. The lungs would have a very low compliance and the forces involved in breathing would be extremely large. This would seem to argue against the lungs having a liquid lining.

This problem was investigated by von Neergaard, who measured the compliance of excised lungs, first using air to inflate them and then using saline (Fig. 4.23). He noticed that:

- Lungs were much easier to inflate (i.e. more compliant) with saline than with air.
- When he used air, the pressure required was greater during inflation than during deflation.

This phenomenon is called hysteresis.

Since there was no surface tension when saline was used, the alveoli did seem to have a liquid lining; surface tension was contributing to the elastic recoil of the lungs making them harder to inflate. However, the pressure needed to inflate the lungs was actually much lower than if the fluid were water or interstitial fluid. Something in the fluid lining the lungs reduces surface tension, making the lungs more compliant and therefore easier to expand.

This leads us to three questions:

- How is this low surface tension achieved?
- Laplace's law says that small bubbles have higher internal pressure than larger ones. If two bubbles of different sizes were connected, air would flow from the small bubble to the large,

causing the small bubble to collapse (Fig. 4.24). Why does this not happen to alveoli?
- How does the phenomenon of hysteresis of the pressure–volume curve occur?

The answers to all these questions are linked to surfactant.

Surfactant

Surfactant is manufactured by type II pneumocytes. It is first stored intracellularly as lamellar bodies and then released as tubular myelin, the storage form of active surfactant. Once in the alveolar air space, tubular myelin unravels to form a thin layer of surfactant over type I and type II pneumocytes. Surfactant is 90% lipid (mostly a phospholipid called dipalmitoyl phosphatidylcholine) and 10% protein. The three mechanical functions of surfactant are:

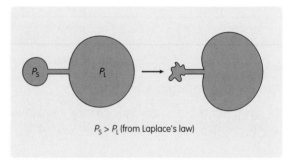

$P_S > P_L$ (from Laplace's law)

Fig. 4.24 The pressure in the smaller bubble (P_S) from Laplace's law. The smaller bubble collapses, emptying into the larger, lower-pressure bubble.

Fig. 4.23 Note the marked difference between the pressure–volume curves of air-filled and saline-filled lungs. It is much easier to inflate the lung without air. (After Berne & Levy 1993, with permission of Mosby.)

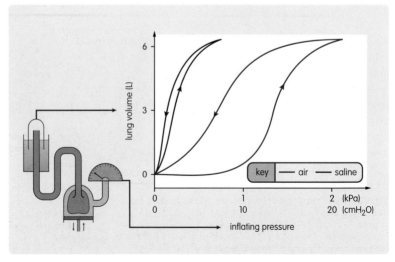

- Prevention of alveolar collapse (gives alveolar stability).
- Increase in lung compliance by reducing surface tension of alveolar lining fluid.
- Prevention of transudation of fluid into alveoli.

Immunological functions of surfactant are discussed in Chapter 3.

Prevention of alveolar collapse

Because of two factors, alveoli of different sizes do not collapse:

- Surface tension of the alveolar lining fluid varies with surface area. This is because surfactant reduces surface tension in proportion to its surface concentration. Surfactant is insoluble in water and floats on the surface of the alveolar lining fluid. In larger alveoli the surfactant is more spread out (dilute) and the surface tension is higher (Fig. 4.25).
- There is interaction between adjacent groups of alveoli. Therefore, collapsing alveoli pull on adjacent alveoli preventing further collapse. This is termed alveolar interdependence.

Prevention of transudation of fluid into alveoli

Surfactant reduces the surface tension in the alveolar lining fluid, which reduces the tendency for the alveolus to collapse. If the alveoli were lined with interstitial fluid, their collapse would cause a more negative pressure in the interstitial space. This would lead to an increase in hydrostatic pressure difference between the pulmonary capillary and the interstitial space, leading to transudation of fluid.

Hysteresis

Hysteresis of the pressure–volume curve is explained by a property of surfactant. The surface tension of surfactant shows different values when being expanded (e.g. during inspiration) or compressed (e.g. during expiration) (Fig. 4.26). Because lung compliance is dependent upon surface tension, this explains why hysteresis of the pressure–volume curve occurs.

Respiratory distress syndrome

Respiratory distress syndrome (RDS) occurs in premature babies of less than 32 weeks' gestation; it is caused by a deficiency of surfactant production by type II pneumocytes. Difficulty in breathing occurs; breathing is rapid and laboured, often with an expiratory grunt. There is diffuse damage to alveoli with hyaline membrane formation. Treatment is with high-concentration oxygen therapy, which reverses the hypoxaemia.

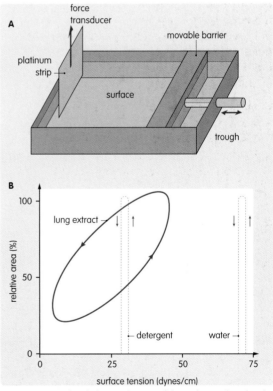

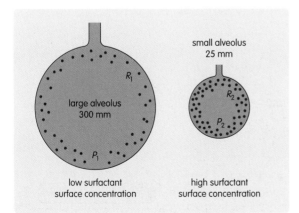

Fig. 4.25 The surface tension (T_1) within the larger alveolus (with radius R_1) is greater than the surface tension (T_2) within the smaller alveolus (with radius R_2). This is because the surfactant is more spread out in the larger alveolus. Thus, the T : R ratio remains constant and the same pressure is required to inflate alveoli of all sizes ($P_1 = P_2$).

Fig. 4.26 (A) Surface balance. The area of the surface is altered and the surface tension is measured from the force exerted on a platinum strip dipped into the surface. (B) Plots of surface tension and area obtained with a surface balance. *Note that lung washings show a change in surface tension with area and that the minimum tension is very small.* (After West 1995, with permission of Lippincott, Williams & Wilkins.)

DYNAMICS OF VENTILATION

The previous section discusses the elastic properties of the lungs (i.e. those caused by surface tension and tissue elasticity). These were looked at under static conditions; however, if we inflate the lungs, dynamic conditions exist. So, in addition to overcoming the elastic properties of the lung during breathing, we must also overcome the dynamic resistance to inflation of the lungs.

The total pressure difference (P_{TOT}) required to inflate the lungs is the sum of the pressure to overcome lung compliance and the pressure to overcome dynamic resistance:

$$P_{TOT} = P_{COM} + P_{DYN}$$

where P_{COM} = pressure to overcome lung compliance and P_{DYN} = pressure to overcome the dynamic resistance.

Dynamic resistance itself comprises:

- Resistance presented by the airways to flow of air into the lungs – airway resistance.
- Resistance to tissues as they slide over each other – viscous tissue resistance.

$$P_{DYN} = P_{AR} + P_{VTR}$$

where P_{AR} = pressure to overcome airways resistance and P_{VTR} = pressure to overcome viscous tissue resistance.

Viscous tissue resistance comprises approximately 20% of the total dynamic resistance, i.e. the vast majority of the total resistance is provided by the airways.

Dynamic lung compliance

Now that we have introduced dynamic conditions, in which airway resistance is a factor, we need to review our measurements of lung compliance. If a pressure–volume curve is plotted under dynamic conditions, the pressure–volume loop is widened when compared with the curve under static conditions (Fig. 4.27). Dynamic lung compliance is the slope of this curve at any one point. Dynamic lung compliance is less than static lung compliance.

Airway resistance

Airway resistance is an important concept because it is increased in common diseases such as asthma

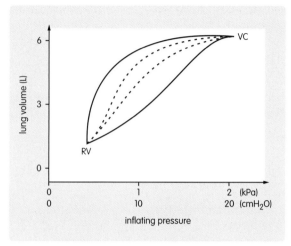

Fig. 4.27 Difference in pressure–volume relationships in lungs inflated and deflated (measurements made under static conditions with no air flowing: dotted lines; dynamic conditions with air flowing continuously into or out of the lung: solid lines).

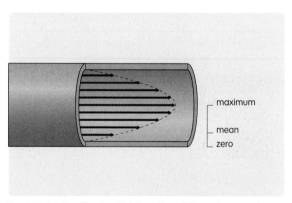

Fig. 4.28 Laminar flow in which the coloured filament remained central. The flow occurs in streamlines, or laminae. The greatest velocity of flow is centrally and the velocity profile is parabolic. (After Berne & Levy 1993, with permission of Mosby.)

and COPD. It is defined as the resistance to flow of gas within the airways of the lung.

Before we discuss airway resistance, it is important to outline pattern of flow.

Pattern of flow

The pattern of fluid flowing through a tube (e.g. an airway or blood vessel) varies with the velocity and physical properties of the fluid. This was established by a French engineer, Reynolds, who injected a coloured dye into the centre of a clear pipe of water flowing at various velocities. He discovered two phenomena, which he described as laminar flow (which appeared at low flow rates; Fig. 4.28) and turbulent flow (which appeared at high flow rates; Fig. 4.29).

Figure 4.30 describes some of the differences between laminar and turbulent flow. Both types of flow are seen in the respiratory system.

Turbulent flow

Turbulent flow is much more likely to occur with:

- High velocities (e.g. within the airways during exercise).
- Larger-diameter airways.
- Low-viscosity, high-density fluids.

Branching or irregular surfaces can also initiate turbulence.

Laminar flow

Laminar flow is described by Poiseuille's law (Fig. 4.31). In basic terms, Poiseuille's law means that the wider the tube, the lower the resistance to air flow. Importantly, the change in width is not directly proportional to the change in resistance: for a given reduction in the radius there is a 16-fold increase in resistance. Narrower or longer pipes or a higher fluid viscosity have a higher resistance to flow and so flow rate is reduced.

Sites of airway resistance

Considering the whole respiratory system, approximately one-half of the resistance to air flow occurs in the upper respiratory tract when breathing through the nose. This is significantly reduced when mouth breathing. Thus, approximately one-half of the resistance lies within the lower respiratory tract.

Assuming laminar air flow, Poiseuille's law would predict that the major resistance to air flow would

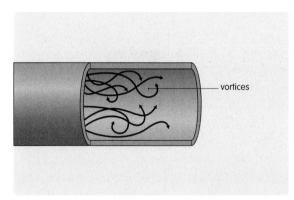

Fig. 4.29 Turbulent flow in which the coloured filament broke up into eddies. (After Berne & Levy 1993, with permission of Mosby.)

Remembering Poiseuille's law isn't drastically important, but understanding it is! So, remember that in laminar flow: A small change in radius significantly affects either flow rate or pressure drop required to achieve the same flow. An example of this is bronchoconstriction in asthma.
- Flow varies directly with pressure drop.
- Flow varies inversely with viscosity (e.g. during scuba diving).

Fig. 4.30 Differences between laminar and turbulent flow	
Laminar	**Turbulent**
fluid moves parallel to walls only	flow has some movement at right angles
no mixing between fluid other than by diffusion	well-mixed flow eddies and diffusion
non-erosive flow regime	flow regime can be erosive
flow is quiet	may account for murmurs heard clinically
poor flow for arterial thrombi but venous stasis may lead to thrombi	arterial thrombi more likely to form
resistance to flow is independent of surface roughness	resistance to flow is dependent on surface roughness
flow is proportional to the radius to the power 4	flow is proportional to diameter to the power 5

Fig. 4.31 Poiseuille's law

Poiseuille's law: states that for a fluid under laminar flow conditions, the flow rate is directly related to the pressure drop between the two ends of a tube and the fourth power of the radius but inversely related to viscosity and length of pipe:

$$F = \frac{P\pi r^4}{8\eta L}$$

(F) = flow rate
(P) = pressure drop
(r) = radius
(η) = viscosity
(L) = length of pipe

Remember, Poiseuille's law applies to laminar, not turbulent, flow

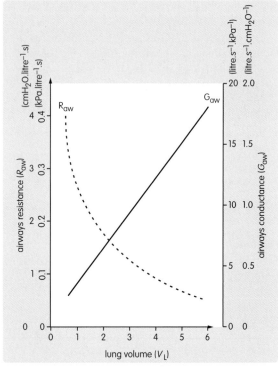

Fig. 4.32 The relationship between lung volume (V_L) and airway resistance (R_{aw}) and conductance (G_{aw}). *Note that at low lung volumes, R_{aw} is high and G_{aw} is low.* (After Widdicombe & Davies 1991, with permission of Edward Arnold.)

occur in the airways with a smaller radius. This is not the case because although the individual diameter of each airway is small, the total cross-sectional area for flow increases (large number of small airways) as we go down the tracheobronchial tree.

In exercise, the airway resistance may increase significantly due to high air flows inducing turbulence. It is normal under these conditions to switch to mouth breathing to reduce airway resistance.

It is important to note that resistance of the smaller airways is difficult to measure. Thus, these small airways may be damaged by disease and it may be some time before this damage is detectable, thus representing a 'silent' zone.

Factors determining airway resistance

Factors affecting airway resistance are:

- Lung volume.
- Bronchial smooth muscle tone.
- Altered airway calibre.
- Change in density and viscosity of inspired gas.

Lung volume

Airways are supported by radial traction of lung parenchyma and thus their diameter and resistance to flow are affected by lung volume (Fig. 4.32):

- Low lung volumes tend to collapse and compress the airways, reducing their diameter and thus increasing resistance to flow.
- High lung volumes tend to increase radial traction, increasing the length and diameter of airways.

- The increase in diameter reduces airway resistance. The increase in length has a much smaller effect of increasing resistance, which is explained by Poiseuille's law.

Bronchial smooth muscle tone

Motor innervation of the smooth muscle of the airways is via the vagus nerve. The muscle has resting tone determined by the autonomic nervous system. This tone can be affected by a number of factors (Fig. 4.33).

Things to remember:
- The major site of airway resistance is medium-sized bronchi.
- 80% of the resistance of the lower respiratory tract is presented by the trachea and bronchi.
- Less than 20% of airway resistance is caused by airways less than 2 mm in diameter.

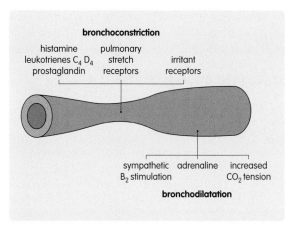

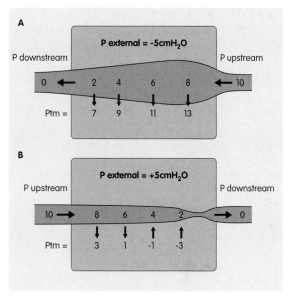

Fig. 4.33 Factors affecting bronchial motor tone. (After Berne & Levy 1993, with permission of Mosby.)

Fig. 4.34 Transmural pressure: (A) during inspiration; (B) during expiration. Ptm = transmural pressure.

Factors acting to decrease the airway diameter include:

- Irritant and cough receptors, C-fibre reflex – reflex and bronchoconstriction act to close the airway.
- Pulmonary stretch receptors.
- Mediator release – inflammatory mediators (histamine, leukotrienes, etc.) cause bronchoconstriction.

Factors acting to increase the airway diameter include:

- Carbon dioxide.
- Catecholamine release.
- Other nerves – non-adrenergic, non-cholinergic (NANC) nerves cause bronchodilatation.

Reduced airway calibre can be caused either by disease or by an inhaled foreign body. A change in density and viscosity of gas occurs in scuba diving (Ch. 6).

Effect of transmural pressure on airway resistance

Remember that the airways are not rigid tubes; they are affected by the pressures around them. The pressure difference between the gas in the airway and the pressure outside the airway is known as the transmural pressure difference. The pressure outside the airway reflects the intrapleural pressure (Fig. 4.34).

During inspiration
The pressure within the pleural cavity is always negative and the alveolar pressure is greater than intrapleural pressure. The transmural pressure difference is always positive, thus the airway is distended (radial traction).

During expiration
The pressure within the alveolus is positive with respect to the intrapleural pressure; hence, the alveolus stays open. The transmural pressure difference, however, is dependent upon expiratory flow rate and intrapleural pressure.

During forced expiration, the positive intrapleural pressure is transmitted through the lungs to the external wall of the airways. In addition, there is a dynamic pressure drop from the alveolus to the airway caused by airway resistance. This is greater at high expiratory flow rates. Thus, the pressure in the lumen of the airway may be lower than the external wall pressure (negative transmural pressure), leading to collapse of the airways.

Thus, the harder the subject tries to exhale forcibly, the more the airways are compressed, so the rate of expiration does not rise as the increased

Increased smooth muscle tone is very important in asthma. Inflammatory mediators act to narrow the airways and increase resistance to air flow.

pressure gradient (from alveoli to atmospheric pressure) is offset by the reduced calibre of the airways. This phenomenon is known as the dynamic compression of airways.

Dynamic compression of airways is greater at lower lung volumes because the effect of radial traction holding the airways open is less. Thus it can be seen that for a specific lung volume there is a maximum expiratory flow rate caused by dynamic compression of the airways (Fig. 4.35). Any rate of expiration below this flow rate is dependent on how much effort is made to expel the air from the lungs and the flow is said to be effort dependent. At maximum expiratory flow rate, any additional effort does not alter the expiratory flow rate (because of dynamic compression of airways) and the flow is said to be effort independent.

Dynamic compression in disease

In patients with COPD, dynamic compression limits expiratory flow even in tidal breathing. The main reasons for this are:

- Loss of radial traction (due to destruction of the lung architecture) means the airways are more readily compressed.
- Increased lung compliance, leading to lower alveolar pressure and less force driving air out of the lungs.

The clinical consequences are airway collapse on expiration and air trapping in the alveoli. Patients

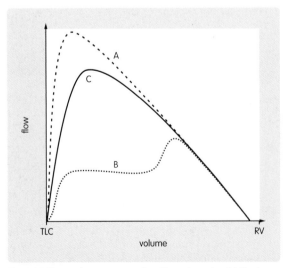

Fig. 4.35 Flow–volume curves made with a spirometer. (A) Maximum inspiration and forced expiration. (B) Slow expiration initially then forced. (C) Expiratory flow almost to maximum effort. *Note that the three descending curves are almost superimposed.*

sometimes demonstrate pursed lip breathing as they attempt to increase pressure on expiration and reduce the amount of air trapped.

Measuring airway resistance

Airway resistance can be measured by plethysmography. In practice, estimates of airway resistance are made every day using simpler methods which rely on the relationship between resistance and air flow. Peak expiratory flow rate (PEFR) measures the maximum air flow achieved in a rapid, forced expiration. Spirometry measures the volume exhaled in a specified time (e.g. the forced expired volume in 1 second or FEV_1). These investigations are described in Chapter 11.

The work of breathing

The work of breathing is the work done by the respiratory muscles to overcome the forces described above, i.e. resistance to air flow and the elastic recoil of the lungs.

The work done (W) to change a volume (ΔV) of gas at constant pressure (P) is shown by the relationship below:

$$W = P \bullet \Delta V$$

Work done is measured in joules; a volume change of 10 L at a pressure of $1\,cmH_2O = 1\,J$ of energy.

Respiration normally represents just a small fraction of the total cost of metabolism (approximately 2%). However, the work required to inflate the lungs, along with this percentage, will rise if:

- Lungs are inflated to a larger volume (e.g. COPD and chronic severe asthma).
- Lung compliance decreases (e.g. fibrotic lungs).
- Airway resistance increases (e.g. COPD and asthma).
- Turbulence is induced in the airways (e.g. in high flow rates experienced during strenuous exercise).

In contrast, the work of breathing is reduced by bronchodilators, which act to decrease airway resistance.

The increased work requirement can be dramatic in patients with severe COPD; a great deal of energy is required just in order to breathe. This can also be understood in terms of the efficiency of ventilation (i.e. the amount of work done divided by energy expenditure). Efficiency of normal quiet breathing is low (about 10%) even in health. In COPD, efficiency decreases, and the work done increases, so much that all the oxygen supplied from increasing ventilation is consumed by the respiratory muscles.

The work of breathing can be illustrated by volume–pressure curves (Fig. 4.36). Figure 4.37 shows

Try to relate these concepts to respiratory failure. A patient with lung disease may be able to respond to impaired gas exchange by raising the ventilatory rate, leading to rapid, shallow breaths. This increases the work of breathing. If lung disease is severe, the work of breathing may become unsustainable. Respiratory muscles tire, ventilatory failure ensues and the patient must be mechanically ventilated, to reduce the work of breathing.

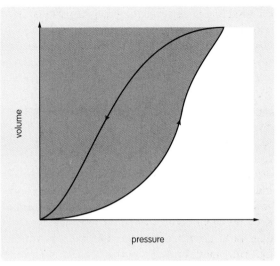

Fig. 4.36 Graph of normal lung volume against trans-lung pressure. The shaded area is the inspiratory work of breathing. (After Widdicombe & Davies 1991, with permission of Edward Arnold.)

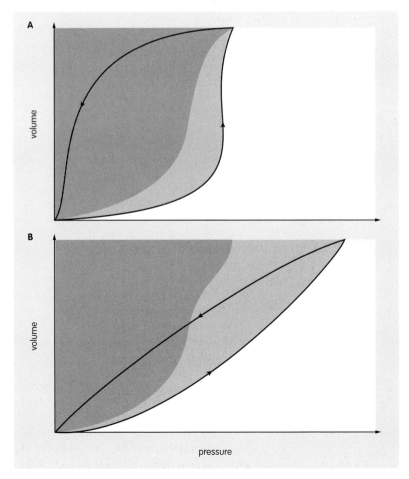

Fig. 4.37 Changes to breathing work during diseased states. Paler shading denotes disease state; dark shading shows the normal work prefills from Figure 4.36. (A) Increased airway resistance (e.g. in asthma); (B) decreased compliance (e.g. in fibrotic lung disease). (After Widdicombe & Davies 1991, with permission of Edward Arnold.)

the effect of disease on these curves. Figure 4.38 shows the effect of the pattern of breathing on work; there is an optimal balance between volume and rate of breathing at which the work of breathing is minimal.

GASEOUS EXCHANGE IN THE LUNGS

This section discusses how gas is transferred from the alveoli to the bloodstream and from the bloodstream to the alveoli. A brief outline of how the laws of diffusion apply to the diffusion of gas from the airways to the circulation is given below. Time for diffusion and diffusion–perfusion limitations are also discussed.

Diffusion

Gas exchange between alveolar air and blood in the pulmonary capillaries takes place by diffusion.

Diffusion is the process in which molecules move due to their random motion (Brownian motion). The process of diffusion is seen to be a net movement of particles:

- Diffusion occurs from an area of high concentration to an area of low concentration. Thus, the driving force for diffusion is concentration difference (ΔC).
- Diffusion will occur until the concentration in the two areas is equalized (i.e. net movement has ceased). Random movement of particles continues to occur and this is known as dynamic equilibrium.

Fig. 4.38 The work done in breathing is altered by the pattern of breathing. (A) Optimal pattern; (B) increased frequency and decreased volume; (C) decreased frequency and increased volume. *Note that the work of breathing is highest when frequency decreases and volume increases.* (After Widdicombe & Davies 1991, with permission of Edward Arnold.)

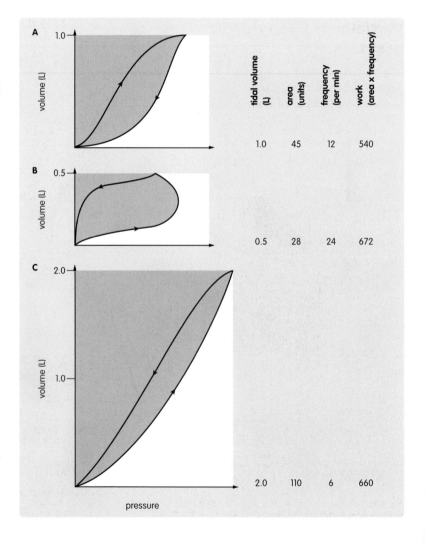

tidal volume (L)	area (units)	frequency (per min)	work (area x frequency)
1.0	45	12	540
0.5	28	24	672
2.0	110	6	660

Diffusion in the lungs occurs across a membrane and is therefore governed by Fick's law (Fig. 4.39). Fick's law tells us that the rate of diffusion of a gas increases:

- As the surface area of the membrane increases.
- The thinner the membrane.
- The greater the partial pressure gradient across the membrane.
- The more soluble the gas.

It is clear that the blood–gas interface with its large surface area of 50–100 m^2 and average thickness of 0.4 μm permits the high rate of diffusion required by the body.

We can also see that the rate of diffusion across the alveoli is directly dependent upon the difference in partial pressures between a gas in the alveoli (P_A) and in arterial blood (P_a).

Partial pressures of respiratory gases

The partial pressure of a gas can be calculated by Dalton's law. Dalton's law states that 'The pressure exerted by a mixture of non-reacting gases is equal to the sum of the partial pressures of the separate components.' In other words, each gas in a mixture of gases exerts the same pressure as it would if it were present alone in the volume occupied by the mixture (Fig. 4.40).

From Dalton's law we see that:

- The total pressure of a gas is the sum of all the partial pressures of its constituents.
- The partial pressure of a gas can be calculated from its fractional concentration.

If we consider the total barometric pressure of air (P_{atm}, about 760 mmHg at sea level), this is composed of the sum of all the partial pressures of its constituent gases:

$$P_{atm} = PO_2 + PN_2 + PCO_2 + PH_2O$$

> Henry's law states that at equilibrium, the amount of gas dissolved in a given volume of liquid at a given temperature (C) is proportional to the partial pressure (P) of the gas in the gas phase and its solubility in the liquid (S).
>
> $$C = S \bullet P$$

> The following will increase the rate of oxygen diffusion into the blood:
> - Increased surface area of the alveolus.
> - Decreased thickness of the alveolar wall.
> - Increased alveolar partial pressure of oxygen (oxygen therapy).

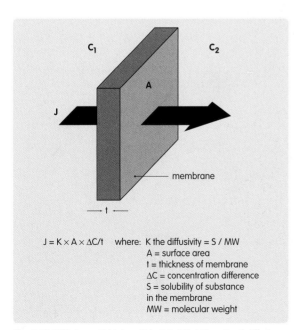

$J = K \times A \times \Delta C / t$ where: K the diffusivity = S / MW
A = surface area
t = thickness of membrane
ΔC = concentration difference
S = solubility of substance in the membrane
MW = molecular weight

Fig. 4.39 Diffusion – Fick's law. Fick stated that the rate of diffusion (J) of a gas through a membrane was: $J = K \times A \times \Delta C / t$

Fig. 4.40 Partial pressures of respiratory gases

Gas	PO_2 (kPa)	PCO_2 (kPa)	PH_2O (kPa)
atmosphere	21	0	variable
trachea (inspiration)	20	0	6.3[*]
alveolar gas	13.5	5.3	6.3
exhaled breath	16	3.5	variable

*note inspired air is fully saturated with water vapour before it enters the lungs

Secondly, taking one of the constituent gases, we can multiply the fractional concentration of that gas by the total pressure to find the partial pressure that the gas exerts, or its tension:

$$PO_2 = FO_2 \times P_{atm}$$

where FO_2 is the fractional concentration of oxygen.

Dry air has a fractional concentration of oxygen of 21%; inserting this value into the equation above gives us an oxygen tension at sea level of 159 mmHg.

We specified sea level because the partial pressure of a gas in a system will alter with total pressure. If atmospheric pressure is reduced (e.g. when climbing Mount Everest), so is the partial pressure of oxygen.

Water vapour pressure

Dry gas pressures are, however, of little relevance in respiratory medicine. On inspiration, air is warmed and humidified. Therefore water vapour also exerts a pressure, which reduces the pressure available to the partial pressures of the gases.

The water vapour pressure (WVP) of a gas depends on:

- Saturation of the gas (quoted as % saturation).
- Temperature of the gas (WVP increases as temperature rises).

It is important to know that for fully (100%) saturated air, the water vapour pressure at 37°C is 47 mmHg. Using this value we can calculate the partial pressure of oxygen in inspired (or 'tracheal') air.

$$PO_2 = 0.21 \times (760 - 47) = 150\,mmHg$$

Perfusion and diffusion limitation

At the gas-exchange surface, gas transfer occurs through a membrane into a flowing liquid. There are two processes (Fig. 4.41) occurring:

- Diffusion across the alveolar capillary membrane.
- Perfusion of blood through pulmonary capillaries.

Uptake of a gas into the blood is dependent on its solubility and the chemical combination (e.g. with haemoglobin: Hb). If the chemical combination is strong, the gas is taken up by the blood with little rise in arterial partial pressure.

The solubility of nitrous oxide (N_2O) in the blood is low, and it does not undergo chemical combination with any component of the blood. Thus, rate of transfer of gas into the liquid phase is slow and partial pressure of the gas in the blood rises rapidly (Fig. 4.42). This reduces the partial pressure difference between alveolar gas and the blood and hence the driving force for diffusion. Nitrous oxide is, therefore, an example of a gas that is said to be perfusion limited. Thus, the amount of nitrous oxide taken up by the blood is dependent almost solely upon the rate of blood flow through the pulmonary capillaries.

In the case of carbon monoxide (CO), the gas is taken up rapidly and bound tightly by haemoglobin; the arterial partial pressure rises slowly (Fig. 4.42). Thus, there is always a driving force (partial pressure difference) for diffusion (even at low perfusion rates), and the overall rate of transfer will be dependent on the rate of diffusion. This type of transfer is said to be diffusion limited. Thus, the amount of

The following will decrease the rate of oxygen diffusion into the blood:
- Reduction in the overall alveolar surface area (e.g. emphysema).
- Increased distance for diffusion (e.g. emphysema).
- Increased thickness of the alveolar wall (e.g. fibrosing alveolitis).
- Reduction in the alveolar partial pressure of oxygen (e.g. altitude).

Partial pressures are also expressed in kPa. 1 kPa is 7.5 mmHg.

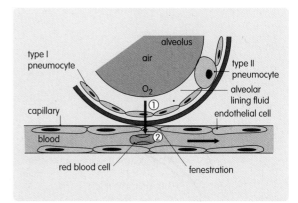

Fig. 4.41 Gas transfer across alveolar capillary membrane. (1) Diffusion across membrane; (2) perfusion of blood through pulmonary capillaries.

carbon monoxide taken up by the blood is dependent on the rate of diffusion of carbon monoxide from the alveoli to the blood.

The transfer of oxygen is normally perfusion limited because the arterial partial pressure of oxygen (P_aO_2) reaches equilibrium with the alveolar gas (P_AO_2) by about one-third of the way along the pulmonary capillary (Fig. 4.42); there is, therefore, no driving force for diffusion after this point. However, if the diffusion is slow because of emphysematous changes to the lung, then P_aO_2 may not reach equilibrium with the alveolar gas before the blood reaches the end of the capillary. Under these conditions, the transfer of oxygen is diffusion limited.

Oxygen uptake in the capillary network

The time taken for the partial pressure of oxygen to reach its plateau is approximately 0.25 seconds. The pulmonary capillary volume under resting conditions is about 75 mL, which is approximately the same size as the stroke volume of the right ventricle. Pulmonary capillary blood is therefore replaced with every heart beat, approximately every 0.75 seconds. This far exceeds the time for transfer of oxygen into the bloodstream.

During exercise, however, the cardiac output increases and the flow rate through the pulmonary capillaries also increases. Because the lungs have the ability to recruit new capillaries and distend already open capillaries (see Ch. 5), the effect of increased blood flow rate on the time allowed for diffusion is not as great as one might expect. In strenuous exercise, the pulmonary capillary network volume may increase by up to 200 mL. This helps maintain the time allowed for diffusion, although it cannot keep it to the same value as at rest (Fig. 4.43).

Carbon dioxide transfer

Fick's is not the only law that describes the diffusion of gases in the lung. Graham's law tells us that gases with greater molecular weights diffuse more slowly than those that are lighter.

However, we are also concerned with the diffusion rates of gas in blood. Diffusion in liquids is directly dependent upon the solubility of the gas, but inversely proportional to the square root of its molecular weight. Carbon monoxide diffuses 20 times more rapidly than oxygen, but has a similar molecular weight. Thus, the difference in rates of

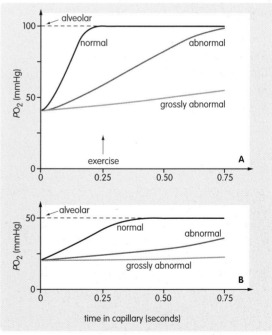

Fig. 4.43 Pulmonary capillary partial pressure of oxygen vs. time in the pulmonary capillary network: (A) alveolar PO_2 normal; (B) low alveolar PO_2. Curves are for normal blood–gas interface and abnormal in diseased state. *Note that the difference between the normal and abnormal lungs increases at low alveolar PO_2.* (After West 1995, with permission of Lippincott, Williams & Wilkins.)

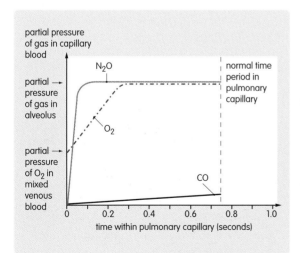

Fig. 4.42 Graph of partial pressure of respiratory gases against time within the pulmonary capillary bed. Transfer of N_2O is perfusion limited, transfer of CO is diffusion limited. Transfer of O_2 is usually perfusion limited but may change with diseased states.

diffusion is caused by the much higher solubility of carbon dioxide.

Under normal conditions, the transfer of carbon dioxide is not diffusion limited (Fig. 4.44).

Measuring diffusion

As we have already seen (p. 67), gas transfer (J) can be calculated using Fick's law:

$$J = K \times A \times (P_A - P_a)/t.$$

It is not possible to measure the area and thickness of a complex structure like the blood–gas barrier, so the equation is rewritten:

$$J = D_L(P_A \times P_a)$$

where D_L is the diffusing capacity of the lung, defined as the ease of diffusion of gas into the blood (the rate of uptake of a gas divided by the partial pressure difference between alveoli and blood).

$$D_L = J/(P_A - P_a)$$

Carbon monoxide is the gas most commonly used to study diffusing capacity. Because carbon monoxide is taken up into the liquid phase very quickly, the rate of perfusion of pulmonary capillaries does not significantly affect the partial pressure difference between alveolar gas and the bloodstream. In addition, carbon monoxide binds irreversibly to haemoglobin and is not taken up by the tissues.

In contrast, oxygen is not a good candidate for calculating diffusing capacity because it binds reversibly to haemoglobin; thus, mixed-venous

The terms diffusing capacity (D_LCO) and transfer factor (T_LCO) are interchangeable.

partial pressure may not be the same as that of blood entering the pulmonary capillary bed. In addition, because oxygen is taken up less quickly than CO, perfusion has more of an effect.

We therefore use the diffusing capacity of carbon monoxide (D_LCO) as a general measure of the diffusion properties of the lung.

The partial pressure of carbon monoxide in the blood (P_aCO) is negligible, so the equation can be rewritten:

$$D_L CO = JCO/P_A CO$$

One of the methods used to measure diffusion across the blood–gas interface is the single-breath method. A single breath of a mixture of carbon monoxide and air is taken. The breath is then held for approximately 10 seconds. The difference between inspiratory and expiratory concentrations of carbon monoxide is measured and therefore the amount of carbon monoxide taken up by the blood in 10 seconds is known. If the lung volume is also measured by the helium dilution method, it is possible to determine the transfer coefficient (KCO) or diffusion rate per unit of lung volume. This is a more useful measure of diffusion where lung volume has been lost, for example after surgery or in pleural effusion. Because there can be many causes of a reduction in diffusing capacity, it is not a specific test for lung disease. It is, however, a sensitive test; it is able to demonstrate minor impediments to gas diffusion.

Factors that decrease the rate of diffusion include:

- Thickening of the alveolar capillary membrane (e.g. in fibrosing alveolitis).
- Oedema of the alveolar capillary walls.
- Increased lining fluid within the alveoli.
- Increased distance for gaseous diffusion (e.g. in emphysema).
- Reduced area of alveolar capillary membrane (e.g. in emphysema).
- Reduced flow of fresh air to the alveoli from terminal bronchioles.
- Hypoventilation.

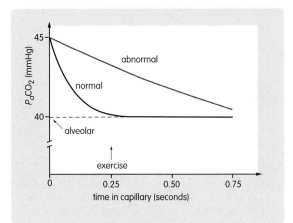

Fig. 4.44 Change in $P_a CO_2$. Calculated when alveolar capillary membrane is normal or abnormal. (After West 1995, with permission of Lippincott, Williams & Wilkins.)

Perfusion and gas transport

Objectives

By the end of this chapter you should be able to:

- State the normal diastolic and systolic pressures in the pulmonary circulation.
- Describe recruitment and distension and how they affect pulmonary vascular resistance.
- Outline the factors that affect pulmonary blood flow and resistance of the pulmonary vasculature.
- Describe the pattern of blood flow through the lungs in terms of three zones.
- Explain the term hypoxic vasoconstriction and its importance.
- Describe what is meant by the ventilation : perfusion ratio.
- Describe with the aid of a diagram how disease might affect the ventilation : perfusion ratio distribution.
- Describe the structure of haemoglobin and its ability to bind oxygen.
- Draw and explain the oxygen dissociation curve for haemoglobin and explain what factors affect the curve.
- Describe how fetal haemoglobin differs from adult haemoglobin, and the double Bohr shift.
- Explain the terms hypoventilation and hyperventilation.
- State the normal blood pH range.
- Define what is meant by a buffer and give four examples of buffers in the blood and their relative importance.
- Explain what is meant by an acid–base disturbance, and account for the four deviations.
- List the causes for respiratory acidosis and alkalosis.
- List the causes for metabolic acidosis and alkalosis.
- Define hypoxia and know the four different types of hypoxia and their clinical importance.

OVERVIEW

The pulmonary circulation is a highly specialized system which is adapted to accommodate the entire cardiac output both at rest and during exercise. It is able to do this because it is:

- A low-pressure, low-resistance system.
- Able to recruit more vessels with only a slight increase in arterial pulmonary pressure.

However, good perfusion is not enough to ensure that the blood is adequately oxygenated. The most important determinant in arterial blood gas composition is the way in which ventilation and perfusion are matched to each alveolus. Mismatching of ventilation : perfusion is a central fault in many common lung diseases.

The ability of the lungs to change minute ventilation, and therefore alter the rate of excretion of CO_2, gives the respiratory system a key role in maintaining the body's acid–base status. This chapter therefore also reviews the fundamentals of acid–base balance and discusses the common acid–base disturbances.

PULMONARY BLOOD FLOW

Outline of pulmonary circulation

An outline of the pulmonary blood flow was given in Figure 3.14. Venous blood returning from the body enters the right atrium and passively fills the right ventricle during diastole. During systole, the right ventricle contracts, ejecting its contents into the pulmonary artery (note the pulmonary artery contains deoxygenated blood).

Blood flows along the pulmonary arteries and arterioles, which closely follow the course of the airways. Blood enters the pulmonary capillaries (situated within the walls of the alveoli) and gaseous exchange takes place. Blood then returns to enter the left atrium through postcapillary venules and pulmonary veins (which contain oxygenated blood).

Mechanics of the circulation

The flow of blood through the pulmonary vasculature is slightly less than the systemic output of the left ventricle. This is because a proportion of the coronary circulation from the aorta drains directly into the left ventricle. In addition, the bronchial circulation from the aorta drains into pulmonary veins, thus bypassing the lungs. However, we can consider the flow through the pulmonary artery to be equal to cardiac output.

Pressures within the pulmonary circulation are much lower than in equivalent regions within the systemic circulation (Fig. 5.1). Because the volume of blood flowing through both circulations is approximately the same, the pulmonary circulation must offer lower resistance.

Pulmonary capillaries and arterioles cause the main resistance to flow in the pulmonary circulation. This low resistance is achieved in two ways:

- A large number of resistance vessels exist, which are usually dilated; thus, the total area for flow is very large.
- Small muscular arteries contain much less smooth muscle than equivalent arteries in the systemic circulation; they are more easily distended.

Many other factors affect pulmonary blood flow and pulmonary vascular resistance. These are discussed below.

Hydrostatic pressure

Hydrostatic pressure has three effects.

- It distends blood vessels: as hydrostatic pressure rises, distension of the vessel increases.

Pulmonary ΔP is small compared with the systemic circulation, so R must be small to achieve the same flow rate.

Flow = Driving force/resistance = $\Delta P/R$

Poiseuille's law tells us that the calibre of a vessel significantly affects resistance to flow and hence the flow rate through a vessel when a particular pressure difference is applied. The pulmonary circulation is therefore a low-pressure, low-resistance system.

Fig. 5.1 The pulmonary arterial and left atrial pressures are measured during cardiac catheterization, the former directly, the latter by wedging the arterial catheter into a branch of the pulmonary artery. The capillary pressure is computed by a standard equation. (After Berne & Levy 1993, with permission of Mosby.)

Fig. 5.1 Pressures within the pulmonary circulation

Site	Pressure (mmHg)	Pressure (cmH$_2$O)
Pulmonary artery		
Systolic/diastolic pressure	24/9	33/11
Mean pressure	14	19
Arteriole (mean pressure)	12	16
Capillary (mean pressure)	10.5	14
Venule (mean pressure)	9.0	12
Left atrium (mean pressure)	8.0	11

- It is capable of opening previously closed capillaries (recruitment).
- It causes flow to occur; in other words, a pressure difference (ΔP) between the arterial and venous ends of a vessel provides the driving force for flow (see Fig. 5.2).

In situations where increased pulmonary flow is required (e.g. during exercise), the cardiac output is increased, which raises pulmonary vascular pressure. This causes recruitment of previously closed capillaries and distension of already open capillaries (Fig. 5.3). In turn, this reduces the pulmonary vascular resistance to flow; it is for this reason that resistance to flow through the pulmonary vasculature decreases with increasing pulmonary vascular pressure.

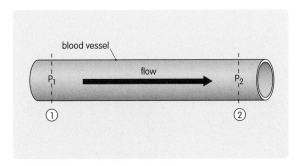

Fig. 5.2 Hydrostatic pressure in terms of driving force. $P_2 - P_1$ i.e. ΔP provides the driving force of the flow.

Remember, any resistance to flow causes a drop in pressure; therefore, the hydrostatic pressure in postcapillary venules will be less than that within the capillaries.

Pressure outside pulmonary blood vessels

Pressure outside a vessel can tend either to compress or collapse the vessel if the pressure is positive, or to aid the distension of the vessel if the pressure is negative.

The tendency for a vessel to distend or collapse is also dependent on the pressure inside the lumen. Thus, it is the pressure difference across the wall (or the transmural pressure) which determines whether a vessel compresses or distends (Fig. 5.4).

Pulmonary vessels can be considered in two groups (Fig. 5.5): alveolar and extra-alveolar vessels.

Alveolar vessels

Recall that there is a dense network of capillaries in the alveolar wall; these are the alveolar vessels. External pressure is alveolar pressure (normally atmospheric pressure). As the lungs expand, these vessels are compressed. The diameter of these vessels (capillaries) is dependent on the transmural pressure (i.e. the difference between hydrostatic pressure within the capillary lumen and pressure within the alveolus). If the alveolar pressure is greater than capillary hydrostatic pressure, the capillary will tend to collapse.

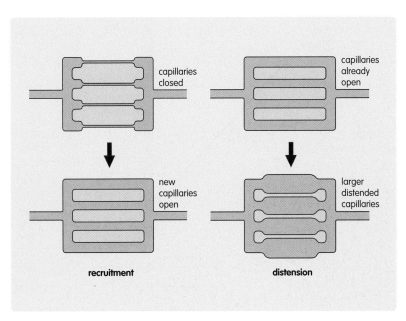

Fig. 5.3 In order to minimize pulmonary vascular resistance when pulmonary arterial pressure increases, new vessels are recruited and vessels that are already open are distended.

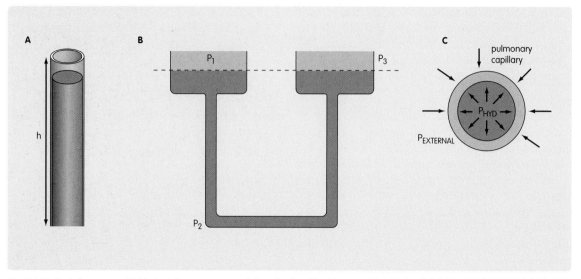

Fig. 5.4 Hydrostatic pressure. (A) Hydrostatic pressure = $\rho \bullet g \bullet h$ (ρ = density of liquid; g = gravity; h = height). (B) $P_2 > P_1$ because of the height of the column of liquid. $P_3 = P_1$ because they are at the same height. (C) Hydrostatic pressure tends to distend pulmonary vessels, whereas the external pressure tends to collapse them.

Fig. 5.5 Diagram of (A) alveolar vessels, which are subject to external pressures of alveolar gas, and (B) extra-alveolar vessels contained within lung tissue, subject to intrapleural pressure.

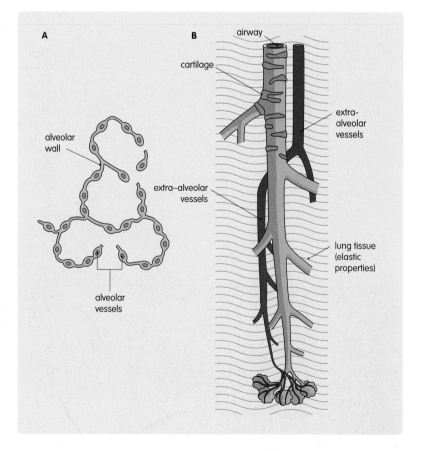

Vessels in the top of the lung may collapse as the alveoli expand. This is much more likely during diastole when the venous (capillary) pressure falls below alveolar pressure (Fig. 5.4).

Extra-alveolar vessels

Extra-alveolar vessels are arteries and veins contained within the lung tissue. As the lungs expand, these vessels are distended by radial traction. The external pressure is similar to intrapleural pressure (subatmospheric – negative).

Because extra-alveolar vessels have an external pressure that is almost always negative, transmural pressure tends to distend these vessels. During inspiration, intrapleural pressure and thus the pressure outside the extra-alveolar vessels become even more negative, causing these vessels to distend even further, reducing vascular resistance and increasing pulmonary blood flow. At large lung volumes, the effect of radial traction is greater and the extra-alveolar vessels are distended more.

Lung volume

Extra-alveolar vessels are distended by increased radial traction associated with increased lung volumes. The capillary, however, is affected in several ways.

Hydrostatic pressure within the capillaries during deep inspiration is lowered. This is caused by a negative intrapleural pressure around the heart. This changes the transmural pressure and the capillaries tend to be compressed, increasing pulmonary vascular resistance (Fig. 5.6).

At large lung volumes, the alveolar wall is stretched and becomes thinner, compressing the capillaries and increasing vascular resistance.

The factors affecting the capillary blood flow are:
- Hydrostatic pressure.
- Alveolar air pressure.
- Lung volume.
  The factors affecting extra-alveolar vessels are:
- Hydrostatic pressure.
- Intrapleural pressure.
- Lung volume.
- Smooth muscle tone.

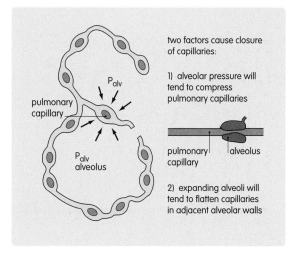

Fig. 5.6 Alveolar pressure and capillary compression. The transmural pressure is the difference between hydrostatic pressure inside the capillary and alveolar pressure outside the capillary. P_{alv} = pressure in the alveolus.

Smooth muscle within the vascular wall

Smooth muscle in the walls of extra-alveolar vessels tends to reduce their diameter. Thus, the forces caused by radial traction and hydrostatic pressure within the lumen are trying to distend these vessels, whereas the tone of the vascular smooth muscle opposes this action. Drugs that lead to contraction of smooth muscle therefore increase pulmonary vascular resistance.

Measurement of pulmonary blood flow

Pulmonary blood flow can be measured by three methods:

- Fick principle (Fig. 5.7).
- Indicator dilution method: a known amount of dye is injected into venous blood and its arterial concentration is measured.
- Uptake of inhaled soluble gas (e.g. N_2O): the gas is inhaled and arterial blood values measured.

Both the first and second methods give average blood flow, whereas the third method measures instantaneous flow. The third method relies upon N_2O transfer across the gas-exchange surface being perfusion limited.

Fick theorized that because of the laws of conservation of mass, the difference in oxygen concentration

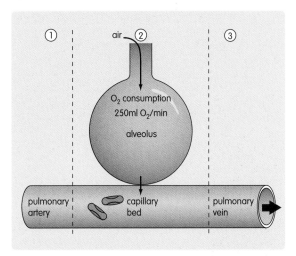

Fig. 5.7 Fick principle for measuring pulmonary blood flow. Fick theorized that the difference in oxygen content between pulmonary venous blood and pulmonary arterial blood must be due to uptake of oxygen in the pulmonary capillaries, therefore the pulmonary blood flow can be calculated.

between mixed-venous blood returning to the pulmonary capillary bed $[O_2]_{pv}$ and arterial blood leaving the heart $[O_2]_{pa}$ must be caused by uptake of oxygen within the lungs. This uptake must be equal to the body's consumption of oxygen (see Fig. 5.7).

Distribution of blood within the lung

Blood flow within the normal, healthy upright lung is not uniform. Blood flow at the base of the lung is greater than at the apex. This is because the lungs are vertical in an upright human, so they are under the influence of gravity and the pulmonary vessels at the lung base will therefore have a greater hydrostatic pressure than vessels at the apex.

The hydrostatic pressure exerted by a vertical column of fluid is given by the relationship:

$P = \rho \bullet g \bullet h$

where ρ = density of the fluid, h = height of the column and g = acceleration due to gravity.

From the equation above, it can be seen that:

- Vessels at the lung base are subjected to a higher hydrostatic pressure.
- The increase in hydrostatic pressure will distend these vessels, lowering the resistance to blood flow. Thus, pulmonary blood flow in the bases will be greater than in the apices.

Ventilation also increases from apex to base, but is less affected than blood flow because the density of air is much less than that of blood. In diastole, the hydrostatic pressure in the pulmonary artery is 11 cmH$_2$O. The apex of each lung is approximately 15 cm above the right ventricle, and the hydrostatic pressure within these vessels is lowered or even zero. Vessels at the apex of the lung are therefore narrower or even collapse because of the lower hydrostatic pressure within them.

Pattern of blood flow

The distribution of blood flow within the lung can be described in three zones (Fig. 5.8).

Zone 1 (at the apex of the lung)

In zone 1, arterial pressure is less than alveolar pressure: capillaries collapse and no flow occurs. Note that under normal conditions, there is no zone 1 because there is sufficient pressure to perfuse the apices.

Zone 2

In zone 2, arterial pressure is greater than alveolar pressure, which is greater than venous pressure. Postcapillary venules open and close depending on hydrostatic pressure (i.e. hydrostatic pressure difference in systole and diastole). Flow is determined by the arterial–alveolar pressure difference (transmural pressure).

Zone 3 (at the base of the lung)

In zone 3, arterial pressure is greater than venous pressure, which is greater than alveolar pressure. Blood flow is determined by arteriovenous pressure difference as in the systemic circulation.

Control of pulmonary blood flow

We have explored how the pulmonary circulation adapts to changes of hydrostatic pressure and how it can recruit capillaries during exercise. These effects are passive and caused by changes in hydrostatic pressure. The pulmonary blood flow can also be controlled by other local mechanisms to improve efficiency of gaseous exchange. As in the systemic circulation, other mediators such as thromboxane, histamine and prostacylin also alter pulmonary vascular tone.

Contraction and relaxation of smooth muscle contained within the walls of arteries, arterioles and veins is the mechanism for active control of pulmonary blood flow.

Fig. 5.8 Zones of pulmonary blood flow.

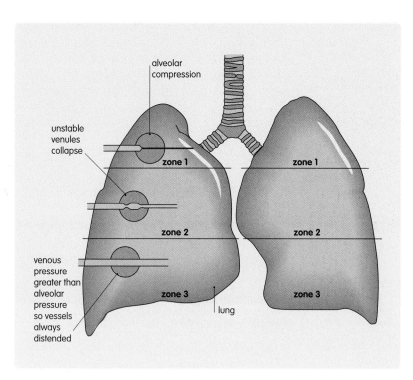

An important mechanism of control, particularly in disease, is hypoxic vasoconstriction.

Hypoxic vasoconstriction

The aim of breathing is to oxygenate the blood sufficiently. This is achieved by efficient gaseous exchange between alveolar gas and the bloodstream. If an area of lung is poorly ventilated and the alveolar partial pressure of oxygen (alveolar oxygen tension) is low, perfusion of this area with blood will lead to inefficient gaseous exchange. It would be more beneficial to perfuse an area that is well ventilated. This is the basis behind hypoxic vasoconstriction. Small pulmonary arteries and arterioles are in close proximity to the gas-exchange surface, and vessels in and around the alveolar wall are surrounded by alveolar gas. Oxygen passes through the alveolar walls into the smooth muscle of the blood vessel by diffusion. The extremely high oxygen tension to which these smooth muscles are normally exposed acts to dilate the pulmonary vessels. In contrast, if the alveolar oxygen tension is low, pulmonary blood vessels are constricted, which leads to reduced blood flow in the area of lung which is poorly ventilated and diversion to other regions where alveolar oxygen tension is high.

It should be noted that it is the partial pressure of oxygen in the alveolus (P_AO_2) and not in the pulmonary artery (P_aO_2) that causes this response.

The actual mechanism and the chemical mediators involved in hypoxic vasoconstriction are not known. Many mediators have been investigated and nitric oxide has been shown to reverse the vasoconstriction. Factors that regulate pulmonary vascular tone are shown in Figure 5.9.

In summary:

- The aim of ventilation is to oxygenate blood sufficiently and blow off carbon dioxide.
- High levels of alveolar oxygen dilate pulmonary vessels.
- Low levels of alveolar oxygen constrict pulmonary blood vessels.
- This aims to produce efficient gaseous exchange.

Higher than normal alveolar carbon dioxide partial pressures also cause pulmonary blood vessels to constrict, thus reducing blood flow to an area that is not well ventilated.

Pulmonary water balance

Figure 5.10 shows the structure of the alveolar–capillary membrane. Note that on one side there is

Fig. 5.9 Factors that regulate vascular tone

Vasodilatation	Vasoconstriction
Nitric oxide	Histamine
Prostacyclin	Serotonin
Prostaglandin	Thromboxane
Bradykinin	Leukotrienes
Acetylcholine	Platelet activating factor
	Angiotensin II

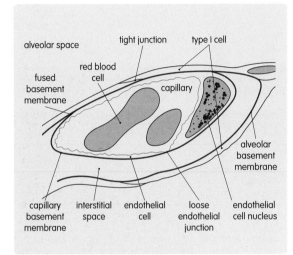

Fig. 5.10 The alveolar–capillary membrane. *Note that the basement membranes of the alveolus and capillary are fused on one side; on the other is the interstitial space.* (After Seaton, Leitch & Seaton 2000, with permission of Blackwell Science.)

the interstitial space whilst on the other the epithelial and endothelial membranes are fused and there is only a tiny membrane between pulmonary capillary blood and the alveolus. It is essential for gas exchange that this surface is kept dry; the mechanisms by which liquid is prevented from entering are discussed below.

Fluids in the pulmonary capillary and interstitial spaces obey Starling's forces (Fig. 5.11). In addition, surfactant lowers the surface tension of the alveolar lining fluid, thus reducing the transudation of liquid into the alveolus by increasing the interstitial pressure from –23 mmHg to –4 mmHg. Hydrostatic pressure within the capillary tends to force fluid out into the interstitial space. The colloid osmotic pressure difference between interstitial space and capillary tends to force fluid into the capillary.

The resultant fluid flow from capillary to interstitial space is small, and normally fluid drains to lymphatics and the perivascular space. Under pathological conditions, fluid can reside either in the interstitial space (interstitial oedema) or in the alveoli (alveolar oedema). This may be due to an increase in:

- Hydrostatic pressure in the pulmonary capillaries.
- Permeability of the capillaries.

Adult respiratory distress syndrome (ARDS) is non-cardiogenic pulmonary oedema caused by capillaries which have become acutely inflamed and 'leaky'.

THE VENTILATION:PERFUSION RELATIONSHIP

Basic concepts

To achieve efficient gaseous exchange, it is essential that the flow of gas (ventilation: $\dot{V}$) and the flow of blood (perfusion: $\dot{Q}$) are closely matched.

The ideal situation would be where:

- All alveoli are ventilated equally with gas of identical composition and pressure.
- All pulmonary capillaries in the alveolar wall are perfused with equal amounts of mixed-venous blood.

Unfortunately, this is not the case. Ventilation is not uniform throughout the lung; neither is perfusion.

The partial pressure of oxygen in the alveoli determines the amount of oxygen transferred to the blood. Two factors affect the partial pressure of oxygen in the alveoli: the amount of ventilation (i.e. the addition of oxygen to the alveolar compartment) and the perfusion of blood through pulmonary capillaries (i.e. the removal of oxygen from the alveolar compartment).

It is the ratio of ventilation to perfusion that determines the concentration of oxygen in the alveolar compartment.

Ventilation:perfusion ratio

By looking at the ventilation:perfusion ratio, we can see how well ventilation and perfusion are matched. By definition:

$$\text{Ventilation:perfusion ratio} = \dot{V}_A/\dot{Q}$$

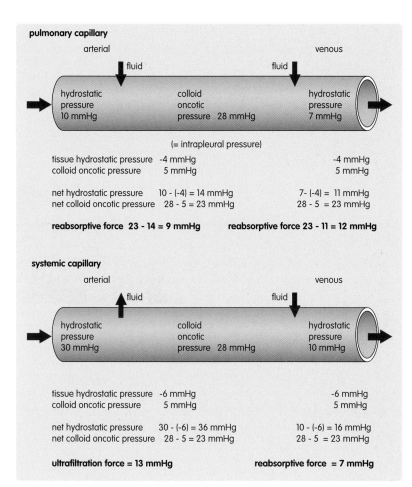

Fig. 5.11 Comparison of Starling's forces between pulmonary and systemic capillary beds. The resorptive force is positive and hence fluid is reabsorbed into the pulmonary capillary. Without surfactant in the alveoli, the tissue hydrostatic pressure could be −23 mmHg and the resorptive force would be −10 mmHg causing transudation of fluid into the alveolus.

where $\dot{V}_A$ = alveolar minute ventilation (usually about 4.2 L/min); $\dot{Q}$ = pulmonary blood flow (usually about 5.0 L/min).

Thus, normal $\dot{V}_A/\dot{Q}$ = 0.84 (i.e. approximately 1).

This is an average value across the lung. Different ventilation : perfusion ratios are present throughout the lung from apex to base (Fig. 5.12).

Extremes of ventilation : perfusion ratio

Looking at the ventilation : perfusion ratio, it can be seen that there are two extremes to this relationship. These extremes were introduced in Chapter 1. Either there is:

- No ventilation (a shunt): $\dot{V}_A/\dot{Q}$ = 0.
- No perfusion (dead space): $\dot{V}_A/\dot{Q}$ = •.

Right-to-left shunt

A right-to-left shunt is described when the pulmonary circulation bypasses the ventilation process (Fig. 5.13), by either:

- Bypassing the lungs completely (e.g. transposition of great vessels, see Ch. 3).
- Perfusion of an area of lung that is not ventilated.

The shunted blood will not have been oxygenated or been able to given up its carbon dioxide. Therefore, its levels of PO_2 and PCO_2 are those of venous blood. When added to the systemic circulation, this blood will proportionately decrease arterial PO_2; it is called the venous admixture.

A right-to-left shunt may cause a low arterial PO_2 but a normal PCO_2 – how can this be explained?

Some degree of venous admixture naturally occurs, for example when the blood from the bronchial circulation drains into the pulmonary veins.

Fig. 5.12 Distribution of ventilation (V_A) and perfusion (Q). Blood flow and ventilation are both higher at the lung base but the difference in blood flow is more striking. (After Widdicombe & Davies 1991, with permission of Edward Arnold.)

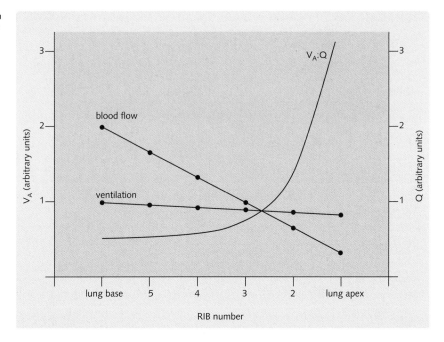

Fig. 5.13 Shunted blood. The shunted blood has a low oxygen concentration (i.e. of venous blood) and is known as the venous admixture.

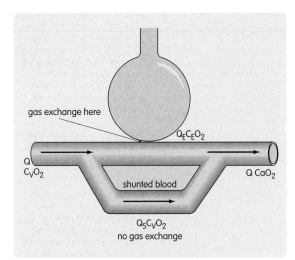

the shape of the oxyhaemoglobin dissociation curve (i.e. haemoglobin is already saturated in the well-ventilated areas). Only a small increase in oxygen content is seen because of increased dissolved oxygen from the overventilated areas. This small increase in PO_2 from overventilated areas is unable to increase the arterial PO_2 to its normal value. Thus, the mixed blood has a lower PO_2 and normal PCO_2.

In normal subjects, there is only a very small amount of shunting (about 1%). However, right-to-left shunting makes a significant contribution to abnormal gas exchange in some disease states, notably:

- Cyanotic congenital heart disease.
- Pulmonary oedema.
- Severe pneumonia.

The venous admixture has a low arterial PO_2 and high PCO_2. This initially causes the arterial PO_2 to be lowered and the arterial PCO_2 to be increased. This high PCO_2 causes an increase in ventilation, which reduces PCO_2 in those areas of lung that are well ventilated, giving them a lower than normal PCO_2. This reduction in PCO_2 lowers the arterial PCO_2 to its normal value. This additional ventilation in well-ventilated areas, however, has very little effect on the arterial oxygen content because of

Giving oxygen to patients with shunt does not increase arterial oxygen tension. This makes sense because:
- Shunted blood is not actually exposed to the oxygen.
- Haemoglobin is already saturated in well-ventilated areas.

Effect of $\dot{V}/\dot{Q}$ mismatch on blood gases

The easiest way to imagine how the ventilation: perfusion ratio affects the arterial oxygen concentration is to look at the extremes of ventilation: perfusion.

Ventilation but no perfusion

If a unit of lung is ventilated but not perfused, that unit will have a PO_2 and PCO_2 of inspired gas, because no gas exchange with the blood has taken place (Fig. 5.14C). If the perfusion of the unit increases (lowering the $\dot{V}:\dot{Q}$ ratio), PCO_2 will rise and the PO_2 will fall (an example of lung normally perfused is shown in Fig. 5.14A).

Perfusion but no ventilation

If the perfusion is increased further and the ventilation reduced until the unit of lung is perfused but not ventilated, the gas within that unit will be in equilibrium with the blood perfusing the alveolar capillaries (venous blood), because no gas exchange has taken place (Fig. 5.14B). This relationship is also described in Figure 5.15; read the caption to work through the figure.

It should be noted that:

- PO_2 varies to a much greater extent than PCO_2 with small changes in the ventilation: perfusion ratio.

- Overall, variation in PO_2 is much greater than that of PCO_2.
- PCO_2 cannot rise above that of mixed-venous blood, assuming the ventilation: perfusion ratio applies to a small area of lung.

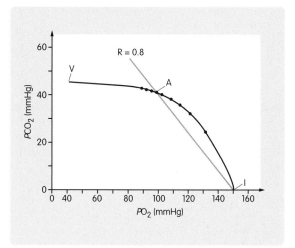

Fig. 5.15 The effect of altering the ventilation:perfusion ratio on both PO_2 and PCO_2. Point A represents normal arterial values of PO_2 and PCO_2 at a value of ventilation:perfusion ratio of 0.84. Increasing ventilation:perfusion ratios reduces PCO_2 but causes a corresponding rise in PO_2. Eventually point I is reached, where PCO_2 is zero and PO_2 is equal to that of inspired gas; this relates to a point of infinite ventilation:perfusion (i.e. there is no perfusion). Point V represents the opposite end of the ventilation:perfusion spectrum where the lung is not ventilated at all. The alveolar end capillary blood partial pressures of oxygen and carbon dioxide are of venous values. Thus values of ventilation:perfusion ratio greater than normal are to the right of point A and those that are less are to the left. (After Berne & Levy 1993, with permission of Mosby.)

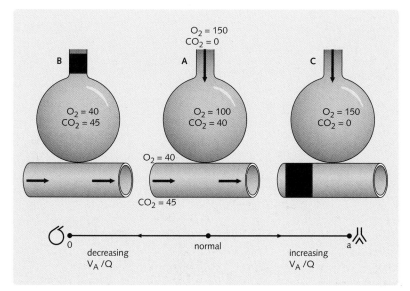

Fig. 5.14 The effect of altering the ventilation:perfusion ratio on the P_AO_2 and P_ACO_2 in a lung unit: (A) normal lung; (B) lung unit is not ventilated – O_2 falls and CO_2 rises within lung unit; (C) lung unit is not perfused – O_2 is not taken up and CO_2 does not diffuse into the alveolus.

Regional variation of ventilation and perfusion

Both ventilation and perfusion increase towards the lung base because of the effects of gravity.

Because the blood has a greater density than air, the gravitational effects on perfusion are much greater than on ventilation. This leads to a regional variation (see Fig. 5.12) in the ventilation:perfusion ratio from lung apex (high $\dot{V}/\dot{Q}$) to lung base (low $\dot{V}/\dot{Q}$).

These regional variations in the ventilation:perfusion ratio are caused by the lung being upright; thus, changes in posture will alter the ventilation:perfusion ratio throughout the lung. For example, when lying down, the posterior area of the lung has a low ventilation:perfusion ratio and the anterior area has a high ventilation:perfusion ratio.

The effect of high and low ventilation:perfusion ratios on carbon dioxide and oxygen in the alveolus and blood is highlighted in Figure 5.16 and described below.

At low ventilation:perfusion ratios (e.g. at the lung base)

Effect on carbon dioxide concentrations

Carbon dioxide diffuses from the blood to alveoli; however, because ventilation is low, carbon dioxide is not taken away as rapidly. Thus, carbon dioxide tends to accumulate in the alveolus until a new, higher steady-state P_ACO_2 is reached.

Diffusion occurs only until equilibrium is achieved, when P_aCO_2 is equal to P_ACO_2. If there

were no ventilation, the P_ACO_2 of this lung unit would rise quickly to meet mixed-venous P_vCO_2, and no diffusion could take place.

Assuming that the overall lung function is normal, this regional variation in P_ACO_2 will not affect overall P_vCO_2. Thus, reducing the ventilation:perfusion ratio will not increase P_aCO_2 above the mixed-venous value.

Effect on oxygen concentrations

Oxygen diffuses from the alveolus into the blood; however, because ventilation is low, oxygen taken up by the blood and metabolized is not replenished fully by new air entering the lungs. Oxygen in the alveolus is depleted until a new, lower steady-state P_AO_2 is reached. Because diffusion continues until equilibrium is achieved, the P_aO_2 of this unit will also be low (Fig. 5.16A).

At high ventilation:perfusion ratios (e.g. at the lung apex)

Effect on carbon dioxide concentrations

The carbon dioxide diffusing from the blood is nearly all removed; carbon dioxide in the alveolus is depleted until a new, lower steady-state P_ACO_2 is reached. Diffusion continues until equilibrium is achieved: P_aCO_2 will also be low.

If we take this to the extreme, then as ventilation:perfusion ratios tend to infinity, P_ACO_2 tends to zero.

Effect on oxygen concentrations

Oxygen diffusing from the alveolar gas is not taken away by the blood in such large amounts because

Fig. 5.16 Ventilation and perfusion at lung base (A) and apex (B). At the lung base perfusion is high and the $\dot{V}/\dot{Q}$ ratio is low. This reduces alveolar O_2 and raises CO_2. At the apex the $\dot{V}/\dot{Q}$ ratio is higher, leading to a high alveolar O_2 and more CO_2 blown off.

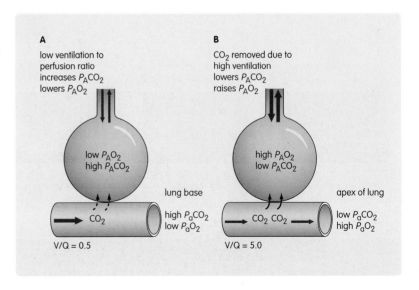

A
low ventilation to perfusion ratio increases P_ACO_2 lowers P_AO_2

low P_AO_2
high P_ACO_2

CO_2

lung base

high P_aCO_2
low P_aO_2

V/Q = 0.5

B
CO_2 removed due to high ventilation lowers P_ACO_2 raises P_AO_2

high P_AO_2
low P_ACO_2

apex of lung

CO_2 CO_2

low P_aCO_2
high P_aO_2

V/Q = 5.0

the relative blood flow is reduced; in addition, oxygen is replenished with each breath. Thus, oxygen tends to accumulate in the alveolus until a new steady-state concentration is reached (Fig. 5.16B).

Diffusion occurs until a new higher equilibrium is achieved; thus, P_aO_2 is also higher.

How do regional variations in $\dot{V}/\dot{Q}$ affect overall gas exchange?

As mentioned previously, a normal healthy lung is not ventilated or perfused uniformly and ventilation:perfusion ratios vary (Fig. 5.17). The actual difference between gaseous exchange in a healthy lung and in an ideal lung is perhaps smaller than one might expect. The ideal lung is capable of only 2–3% more gaseous exchange.

However, if the ventilation:perfusion inequality from lung apex to base becomes more severe, the transfer of oxygen and carbon dioxide will be significantly affected. The majority of the blood will come from poorly ventilated areas at the lung base, where P_AO_2 is low; thus P_aO_2 will be low. P_aCO_2 will similarly be raised at the base of the lung.

The non-linear shape of the oxyhaemoglobin dissociation curve does not allow areas with high ventilation:perfusion ratios to compensate for areas of low ratio.

Ventilation:perfusion distributions

If we look at the variation in ventilation and blood flow in relation to $\dot{V}/\dot{Q}$ in the normal lung (Fig. 5.18), it should be noted that:

- Where the ventilation:perfusion ratio is high, absolute values of ventilation are low.
- Where the ventilation:perfusion ratio is low, absolute values of blood flow are also low.

Thus, the majority of blood flow and ventilation go to areas of lung that have a ventilation:perfusion ratio that is close to the average value. In the diseased lung this might not be the case and blood may flow to areas where ventilation:perfusion ratios are extremely low; this is effectively a shunt.

Areas with extremely high ventilation:perfusion ratios may be ventilated to high absolute values and receive very poor blood flow. This is effectively wasted ventilation (Fig. 5.19).

Measurement of ventilation and perfusion

Ventilation:perfusion scans

In clinical practice, ventilation:perfusion ratios are assessed primarily by means of radioisotope scans.

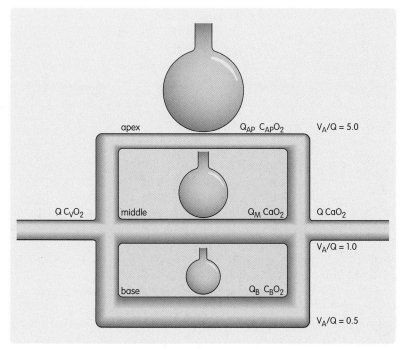

Fig. 5.17 Ventilation and perfusion at the lung apex, middle and base.

Fig. 5.18 Normal human ventilation : perfusion curves. *Note that ventilation and perfusion are matched in health. At the average V̇/Q̇ ratio of 0.8, blood flows to the areas that are well ventilated.* (After West 1995, with permission of Lippincott, Williams & Wilkins.)

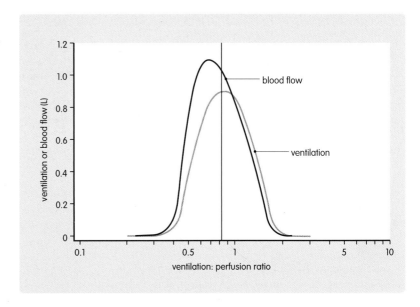

Fig. 5.19 Ventilation : perfusion curves for patient with chronic bronchitis. (From West 1995, with permission of Lippincott, Williams & Wilkins.)

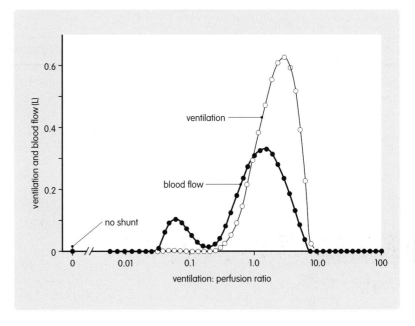

Ventilation is detected by inhalation of a gas or aerosol labelled with the radioisotope, ^{133}Xe. The distribution of pulmonary blood flow is tested with an intravenous injection of ^{99m}Tc-labelled macro-aggregated albumin (MAA). These radioactive particles are larger than the diameter of the pulmonary capillaries and they remain lodged for several hours. A gamma camera is then used to detect the position of the MAA.

The two scans are then assessed together for 'filling defects' or areas where ventilation and perfusion are not matched. The technique is primarily used to detect pulmonary emboli. Spiral CT scans are now superseding this technique. Figure 5.20 shows a lung scan following pulmonary embolism.

Multiple inert gas procedure

As noted above, radioisotope scans can allow only a broad comparison to be made between areas of ventilation and perfusion in the lungs. The multiple inert gas procedure measures the actual ratio of

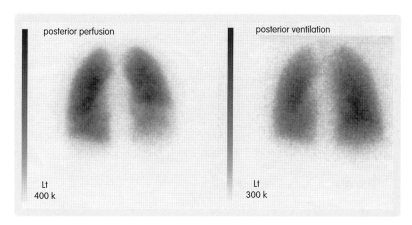

Fig. 5.20 Ventilation : perfusion scan following pulmonary embolus. (Courtesy of Ivor Jones and the Nuclear Medicine staff, Derriford Hospital, Plymouth.)

posterior perfusion

Lt
400 k

posterior ventilation

Lt
300 k

ventilation : perfusion, but is a much more complicated technique. In the multiple inert gas procedure, six inert gases are infused into the venous bloodstream. Each gas has a different partition coefficient in gas and blood (i.e. different solubility in gas and blood).

Steady state is reached by a constant rate of infusion and expiration. From component balances for each gas of amount infused and amount expired the ventilation : perfusion distribution is calculated.

Amount infused = $P_{in} \times S \times Q$
Amount expired = $P_{ex} \times V$

where S = solubility of the gas.

Thus, ventilation and perfusion can be calculated giving a ventilation : perfusion distribution.

GAS TRANSPORT IN THE BLOOD

Oxygen transport

Oxygen is carried in the blood in two forms:

- Dissolved in plasma.
- Bound to haemoglobin.

Dissolved oxygen

To meet the metabolic demands of the body, large amounts of oxygen must be carried in the blood. We have seen that the amount of gas dissolved in solution is proportional to the partial pressure of the gas (Henry's law). The solubility of oxygen in the blood is low: 0.000225 mL of oxygen per kilopascal per millilitre of blood. With normal arterial P_aO_2

(100 mmHg; 13.3 kPa), for each 100 mL of blood there is only 0.003 mL of dissolved oxygen.

Normal cardiac output is 5.0 L/min; it is therefore capable of supplying:

$5 \times 1000 \times 0.003 = 15$ mL of oxygen per minute

At rest, the body requires approximately 250 mL of oxygen per minute. Thus, if all the oxygen in the blood were carried in the dissolved form, cardiac output would meet only 6% of the demand.

In fact, in contrast to the tiny amounts calculated above, the oxygen content of blood is approximately 200 mL of oxygen per litre of arterial blood. Therefore, most of the oxygen must be carried in chemical combination, not in simple solution. Oxygen is combined with haemoglobin.

Haemoglobin

Haemoglobin (Hb) is found in red blood cells and is a conjugate protein molecule, containing iron within its structure. The molecule consists of four polypeptide subunits, two α and two β. Associated with each polypeptide chain is a haem group that acts as a binding site for oxygen (Fig. 5.21).

The haem group consists of a porphyrin ring containing iron and is responsible for binding of oxygen:

- Haemoglobin contains iron in a ferrous (Fe^{2+}) or ferric (Fe^{3+}) state.
- Only haemoglobin in the ferrous form can bind oxygen.
- Methaemoglobin (containing iron in a ferric state) cannot bind oxygen.

The quaternary structure of haemoglobin determines its ability to bind oxygen.

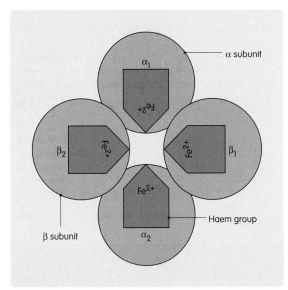

Fig. 5.21 Schematic diagram of haemoglobin: α subunit consists of a polypeptide chain of 141 amino acids and one haem group; β subunit consists of a polypeptide chain of 146 amino acids and one haem group.

In its deoxygenated state, haemoglobin (known as reduced haemoglobin) has a low affinity for oxygen. The binding of one oxygen molecule to haemoglobin causes a conformational change in its protein structure; this positive cooperativity allows easier access to the other oxygen-binding sites, thus increasing haemoglobin's affinity for further binding of oxygen. Haemoglobin is capable of binding up to four molecules of oxygen.

$$Hb + 4O_2 = Hb(O_2)_4$$

It should be noted that during this reaction the iron atom of the haem group remains in the ferrous Fe^{2+} form. It is not oxidized to the ferric Fe^{3+} form. The interaction of oxygen with haemoglobin is oxygenation not oxidation.

The main function of haemoglobin is to take up oxygen at the alveolar capillary membrane and to transport the oxygen within the blood and release it into the tissues. However, haemoglobin also has other functions:

- Buffering of H^+ ions.
- Transport of CO_2 as carbamino compounds.

Haemoglobin binding

Haemoglobin has four binding sites; the amount of oxygen carried by haemoglobin in the blood depends on how many of these binding sites are occupied. Therefore, the haemoglobin molecule can be said to be saturated or partially saturated:

- Saturated – all four binding sites are occupied by O_2.
- Partially saturated – some oxygen has bound to haemoglobin, but not all four sites are occupied.

If completely saturated, each gram of haemoglobin can carry 1.34 mL of oxygen. There are 150 g of haemoglobin per litre of the blood; therefore, the maximum binding of oxygen to haemoglobin we could expect is:

150 × 1.34 = 201 mL of oxygen per litre of blood

In addition, there is approximately 10 mL of O_2 in solution. The total (21 mL) is called the oxygen capacity; the haemoglobin is said to be 100% saturated (SO_2 = 100%). The actual amount of oxygen bonded to haemoglobin and dissolved in the blood at any one time is called the oxygen content.

The oxygen saturation (SO_2) of the blood is defined as the amount of oxygen carried in the blood, expressed as a percentage of oxygen capacity:

$$SO_2 = O_2 \text{ content}/O_2 \text{ capacity} \times 100$$

Cyanosis

Haemoglobin absorbs light of different wavelengths depending on whether it is in the reduced or oxygenated form. Oxyhaemoglobin appears bright red, whereas reduced haemoglobin appears purplish, giving a bluish pallor to skin. This is called cyanosis, which can be described as either central or peripheral. Cyanosis depends on the absolute amount of deoxygenated haemoglobin in the vessels, not the proportion of deoxygenated : oxygenated haemoglobin. In central cyanosis, there is more than 5 g/dL deoxygenated haemoglobin in the blood and this can be seen in the peripheral tissues (e.g. lips, tongue). Peripheral cyanosis is due to a local cause (e.g. vascular obstruction of a limb).

It follows that an anaemic patient with low haemoglobin may become dangerously desaturated without appearing cyanosed!

Oxygen dissociation curve

How much oxygen binds to haemoglobin is dependent upon the partial pressure of oxygen in the blood. This relationship is represented by the oxygen dissociation curve (Fig. 5.22A); this is an equilibrium curve at specific conditions:

- 150 g of haemoglobin per litre of blood.
- pH 7.4.
- Temperature 37°C.

Factors affecting the oxygen dissociation curve

The shape of the curve, and therefore oxygen delivery to the tissues, is affected by a number of factors including:

- pH.
- CO_2.
- Temperature.
- Other forms of haemoglobin.

These factors shift the oxygen dissociation curve to the right or to the left:

- A shift to the right allows easier dissociation of oxygen (i.e. lower oxygen saturation at any particular PO_2) and increases the oxygen release from oxyhaemoglobin.
- A shift to the left makes oxygen binding easier (i.e. higher oxygen saturation at any particular PO_2) and increases the oxygen uptake by haemoglobin.

The following factors shift the curve to the right (Fig. 5.22B):

- Increased PCO_2 and decreased pH (increased hydrogen ion concentration), known as the Bohr shift.
- Increased temperature.

If you cannot remember how the above factors affect the oxygen dissociation curve, it is helpful to think of exercising muscle. It would be useful if its blood supply gave up oxygen more easily (right shift of the curve).

An exercising muscle produces carbon dioxide (increased carbon dioxide), which forms carbonic acid in the blood, which in turn dissociates to form hydrogen ions (lowers the pH). Exercising muscle is hot (increased temperature) and uses up oxygen, forming more reduced haemoglobin in red blood cells (increased 2,3-DPG concentration).

- Increase in 2,3-diphosphoglycerate (2,3-DPG), which binds to the β chains.

2,3-DPG is a product of anaerobic metabolism. Red blood cells possess no mitochondria and therefore carry out anaerobic metabolism to produce energy. 2,3-DPG binds more strongly to reduced haemoglobin than to oxyhaemoglobin. Concentrations of 2,3-DPG increase in chronic hypoxia, e.g. in patients with chronic lung disease, or at high altitude.

Other forms of haemoglobin

Myoglobin

Myoglobin is an iron-containing molecule found within skeletal muscle and cardiac muscle. It consists of a single polypeptide chain with a haem group:

- Myoglobin is capable of binding oxygen.
- It acts as a temporary store of oxygen within skeletal muscle.
- Myoglobin has a higher affinity for oxygen than does normal adult haemoglobin (HbA), seen as a shift to the left of the dissociation curve (Fig. 5.23).
- Myoglobin is unsuitable for oxygen transport, because it binds oxygen at partial pressures below those of mixed-venous blood (< 40 mmHg) and so could not readily release O_2 to the tissues.

Fetal haemoglobin (HbF)

Fetal haemoglobin differs from adult haemoglobin by having two γ chains instead of two β chains (Fig. 5.23).

Fetal haemoglobin has a higher affinity for oxygen because its γ chains bind 2,3-DPG less avidly than the β chains of adult haemoglobin and are therefore able to bind oxygen at lower partial pressures (maternal venous P_vO_2 is low: < 40 mmHg).

Release of carbon dioxide from fetal haemoglobin causes a shift to the left of the fetal oxyhaemoglobin dissociation curve, thus increasing its affinity for oxygen. This released carbon dioxide binds to maternal haemoglobin, causing a shift to the right of maternal haemoglobin, thus reducing the affinity of the latter for oxygen. Oxygen is therefore released by maternal haemoglobin and bound by fetal haemoglobin. This is known as the double Bohr shift.

Haemoglobin S

Haemoglobin S (HbS) is a form of haemoglobin found in sickle cell anaemia. Sickle cell anaemia is

Fig. 5.22 (A) Oxyhaemoglobin dissociation curve. (B) The effect of temperature, PCO_2, pH and 2,3-DPG on the oxyhaemoglobin dissociation curve.

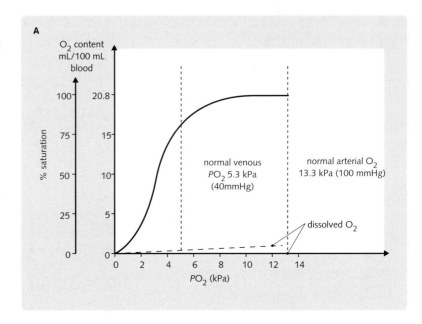

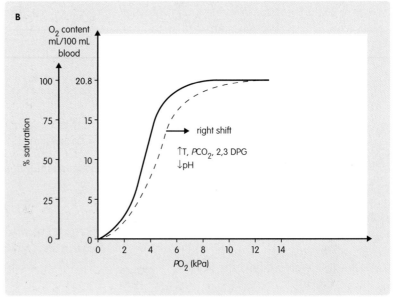

an autosomal recessive disorder in which there is a defect in the β-globulin chain of the haemoglobin molecule.

There is a substitution of the amino acid valine for glutamine at position 6 of the β chain, forming HbS. The heterozygote has sickle cell trait and the homozygote sickle cell anaemia. The abnormal HbS molecules polymerize when deoxygenated and cause the red blood cells containing the abnormal haemoglobin to sickle. The fragile sickle cells haem-

olyse and may block vessels, leading to ischaemia and infarction.

The heterozygous patient may have painful crises with bone and abdominal pain; there may also be intrapulmonary shunting.

Thalassaemia

The thalassaemias are autosomal recessive disorders due to decreased production of either the α or the β chain of haemoglobin.

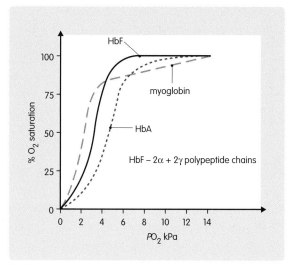

Fig. 5.23 Comparison of oxygen dissociation curves for myoglobin, fetal haemoglobin (HbF) and adult haemoglobin (HbA). (After Berne & Levy 1993, with permission of Mosby.)

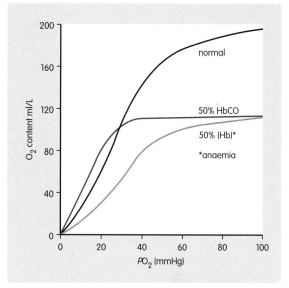

Fig. 5.24 Oxyhaemoglobin curve showing effects of anaemia and carbon monoxide poisoning (50% HbCO and anaemia compared with normal haemoglobin). (After Berne & Levy 1993, with permission of Mosby.)

There are two genes for the β chain and, depending on the number of normal genes, the thalassaemia is quoted as major or minor. There are four genes which code for the α chain, leading to various clinical disorders depending on the genetic defect.

HbA$_2$ is present in a small amount in the normal population and consists of two α and two β chains. It is markedly raised in β thalassaemia minor.

Carboxyhaemoglobin (carbon monoxide poisoning)

Carbon monoxide (CO) displaces oxygen from oxyhaemoglobin because the affinity of haemoglobin for carbon monoxide is more than 200 times that for oxygen. This changes the shape of the oxyhaemoglobin dissociation curve. Note that in Figure 5.24, showing the effects of carbon monoxide poisoning:

- In this instance, oxygen capacity is 50% of normal (i.e. 50% HbO$_2$ and 50% HbCO). The actual value will depend on the partial pressure of CO (e.g. with a PCO of 16 mmHg, 75% of Hb will be in the form of HbCO).
- Saturation is achieved at a PO_2 of <40 mmHg (below venous PO_2).
- HbCO causes a shift to the left for the oxygen dissociation curve (i.e. HbCO has a higher affinity for oxygen than normal HbO$_2$).
- Carbon monoxide binds to two of the four available haem groups.

- Carbon monoxide takes a long time to be cleared, but this can be speeded up by ventilation with 100% oxygen.
- The patient is not cyanosed, because HbCO is cherry-red.

Carbon dioxide transport

There are three ways in which carbon dioxide can be transported in the blood:

- Dissolved in plasma.
- As bicarbonate ions.
- As carbamino compounds.

Dissolved carbon dioxide

The solubility of carbon dioxide in the blood is much greater than that of oxygen (20 times greater); so, unlike oxygen, a significant amount (approximately 10%) of carbon dioxide is carried in solution.

Solubility of carbon dioxide = 5.2 mL of carbon dioxide per kilopascal per litre of blood.
Normal P_aCO_2 = 5.3 kPa.
So, normal dissolved carbon dioxide = 27.4 mL of carbon dioxide per litre of blood.

Bicarbonate ions

Approximately 60% of carbon dioxide is transported as bicarbonate ions. Dissolved carbon dioxide interacts with water to form carbonic acid as follows:

$$CO_2 + H_2O \rightleftharpoons H_2CO_3$$
(1)

Carbonic acid rapidly dissociates into ions:

$$H_2CO_3 \rightleftharpoons H^+ + HCO_3^-$$
(2)

The total reaction being:

$$CO_2 + H_2O \rightleftharpoons H_2CO_3 \rightleftharpoons H^+ + HCO_3^-$$

The first reaction is very slow in plasma, but within the red blood cell is dramatically speeded up by the enzyme, carbonic anhydrase. Reaction (2) is very fast, but if allowed to proceed alone, a large amount of H^+ would be formed, slowing down or halting the reaction. Haemoglobin has the property that it can bind H^+ ions and act as a buffer, thus allowing the reaction to go on rapidly.

$$H^+ + HbO_2^- \rightleftharpoons HHb + O_2$$
$$H^+ + Hb^- \rightleftharpoons HHb$$

Reduced Hb can bind H^+ more actively; this is because reduced Hb is less acidic. The buffering capacities of haemoglobin and oxyhaemoglobin are conferred by the imidazole groups of the 36 histidine residues in the haemoglobin molecule. The imidazole groups dissociate less readily in the deoxygenated form of haemoglobin, which is therefore a weaker acid and so a better buffer. This action reduces H^+ ions in the plasma and also pulls the second reaction to the right.

The bicarbonate produced in the red blood cells diffuses down its concentration gradient into the plasma in exchange for chloride ions (Cl^-). This process is known as the chloride shift (see Fig. 5.25).

Carbamino compounds

Carbon dioxide is capable of combining with proteins, interacting with their terminal amine groups to form carbamino compounds (Fig. 5.25). The most important protein involved is haemoglobin, as it is the most abundant in the blood. It is also important to note that:

• The interaction of carbon dioxide and haemoglobin is rapid.
• No enzyme is involved.
• Haemoglobin binds carbon dioxide in its deoxygenated state (reduced haemoglobin).
• Approximately 30% of carbon dioxide is carried as carbamino compounds.

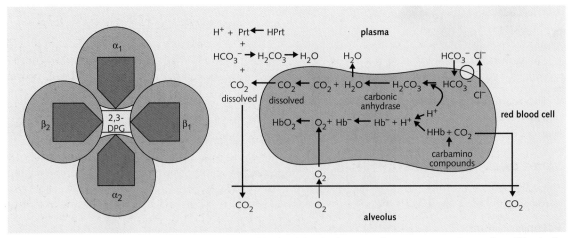

Fig. 5.25 The exchange of CO_2 and O_2 that occurs between the blood and the alveolar air. Bicarbonate ions (HCO_3^-) enter the red blood cell in exchange for chloride ions (which are transported out). Carbonic acid is formed once the O_2 is bound to Hb. Carbonic acid is converted to CO_2 and H_2O. The CO_2 is then excreted from the cell. CO_2 stored in carbamino compound form can be excreted from the cell passively without the involvement of an enzyme. (After Berne & Levy 1993, with permission of Mosby.)

Haldane effect

Carriage of carbon dioxide is increased in deoxygenated blood because of two factors:

- Reduced haemoglobin has a greater affinity for carbon dioxide than does oxyhaemoglobin.
- Reduced haemoglobin is less acidic (i.e. a better proton acceptor: H^+ buffer) than oxyhaemoglobin.

The Haldane effect minimizes changes in pH of the blood when gaseous exchange occurs. The decrease in pH due to the oxygenation of Hb is offset by the increase that results from the loss of CO_2 to the alveolar air. The reverse occurs in the tissues. This is an important effect because:

- In peripheral capillaries, the unloading of oxygen from haemoglobin aids the binding of carbon dioxide to haemoglobin.
- In pulmonary capillaries, the loading of oxygen on haemoglobin reduces the binding of carbon dioxide to haemoglobin.

This allows efficient gaseous exchange of carbon dioxide in the tissues and the lungs.

Carbon dioxide dissociation curve

The carriage of carbon dioxide is dependent upon the partial pressure of carbon dioxide in the blood. This relationship is described by the carbon dioxide dissociation curve (Fig. 5.26). Compared with the oxygen dissociation curve:

- The carbon dioxide curve is more linear.
- The carbon dioxide curve is much steeper than the oxygen curve (between venous and arterial partial pressure of respiratory gases).
- The carbon dioxide curve varies according to oxygen saturation of haemoglobin.

Two main carbon dioxide dissociation curves, for mixed-venous and arterial blood, can be drawn (Fig. 5.26).

Stores of oxygen and carbon dioxide

There are only small stores (approximately 1550 mL) of oxygen in body tissues as follows:

- Lungs – 450 mL.
- Blood – 850 mL.
- Myoglobin – 200 mL.
- Tissue fluids – 50 mL.

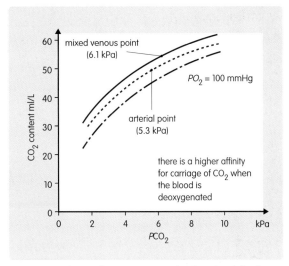

Fig. 5.26 Ventilation effects on oxygen and carbon dioxide levels in the blood.

On the other hand, carbon dioxide has vast stores (approximately 120 L):

- Blood carbonates.
- Bone carbonates.
- Tissue carbonates (including fat tissue).

A change in ventilation will affect both P_aO_2 and P_aCO_2. Because oxygen stores are small in comparison with those of carbon dioxide, a short-term variation in ventilation will affect P_aO_2. A persistent change in ventilation will be shown by a change in P_aCO_2. Clinically, ventilation is assessed by measurement of P_aCO_2.

Hypoventilation and hyperventilation

If P_aCO_2 is a measure of ventilation, it is appropriate in a review of carbon dioxide transport to consider two key concepts in respiratory medicine: hypoventilation and hyperventilation.

For the body to function normally, ventilation must meet the metabolic demand of the tissues (Fig. 5.27).

Thus, metabolic tissue consumption of oxygen must be equal to the oxygen taken up in the blood from alveolar gas. Or, metabolic tissue production of carbon dioxide must be equal to the amount of carbon dioxide blown off at the alveoli.

Hypoventilation

The term hypoventilation refers to a situation when ventilation is insufficient to meet metabolic demand.

Fig. 5.27 Comparison of hyperventilation and hypoventilation

Hyperventilation	Hypoventilation
Causes	**Causes**

anxiety
brainstem lesion
drugs
	obstruction:
	  asthma
	  chronic obstructive airways disease
	  foreign body (e.g. peanut)
	brainstem lesion
	pneumothorax or lung collapse
	trauma (e.g. fractured rib)
	drugs, notably opioids

Consequences	**Consequences**
ventilation too great for metabolic demand too much CO_2 blown off from lungs P_aCO_2 <40 mmHg	ventilation is too low for metabolic demand not enough CO_2 is blown off at the lungs P_aCO_2 >45 mmHg

Fig. 5.28 The alveolar ventilation equation

The alveolar ventilation equation: states that the alveolar P_ACO_2 is inversely proportional to the alveolar ventilation (as long as CO_2 production is constant)

$$P_ACO_2 = K \cdot \dot{V}CO_2/\dot{V}_A$$

$\dot{V}CO_2$=the volume of CO_2 exhaled
$\dot{V}_A$ is alveolar ventilation
K is a constant.

CO_2 exhaled ($\dot{V}CO_2$)=minute ventilation ($\dot{V}E$) x the fractional concentration of CO_2 in the expired air (F_ECO_2).
CO_2 produced in the tissues=exhaled CO_2

$$\dot{V}CO_2 = \dot{V}_E \, F_ECO_2$$

CO_2 expired=the amount of CO_2 released at the alveoli, so:
$$\dot{V}CO_2 = \dot{V}A \cdot F_ACO_2$$

Where $\dot{V}_A$=alveolar ventilation; F_ACO_2=fractional concentration of CO_2 at the alveoli.

$$F_ACO_2 = \dot{V}CO_2/V_A$$

Using Dalton's law, relating the partial pressure to fractional concentration:

$$P_ACO_2 \propto \dot{V}CO_2/\dot{V}_A$$

Or:

$$P_ACO_2 = K \cdot \dot{V}CO_2/\dot{V}_A$$

Hyperventilation

The term hyperventilation refers to a situation where ventilation is excessive to metabolic demand.

The alveolar ventilation equation (see Fig. 5.28 for derivation) states that if carbon dioxide produced in the tissues equals carbon dioxide exhaled (as is usual at rest) then alveolar PCO_2 (i.e. P_ACO_2) is inversely proportional to the alveolar ventilation:

$$P_ACO_2 = K \times \dot{V}CO_2/\dot{V}_A$$

where $\dot{V}CO_2$ is the volume of CO_2 exhaled, $\dot{V}_A$ is the alveolar ventilation and K is a constant.

We can see that this makes sense: increasing alveolar ventilation increases the concentration of CO_2 blown off from the lungs.

Because alveolar gas is in equilibrium with the blood, P_ACO_2 can be estimated as P_aCO_2. Thus, it can be seen how ventilation will affect partial pressures of carbon dioxide and that hypoventilation and hyperventilation can be shown clinically by the partial pressure of carbon dioxide in the blood.

In order to relate P_ACO_2 to P_AO_2, so that we can see how hyperventilation and hypoventilation affect alveolar oxygen, we use the alveolar gas equation:

$$P_AO_2 = P_IO_2 - (P_ACO_2/R) + K$$

where P_IO_2 = partial pressure of oxygen in inspired air and R = respiratory exchange ratio (or the ratio of CO_2 production to O_2 consumption: normally about 0.8).

Hypercapnia and hypocapnia

Hypercapnia

A high partial pressure (concentration) of carbon dioxide in the blood ($P_aCO_2 > 45$ mmHg) is termed hypercapnia (Fig. 5.29).

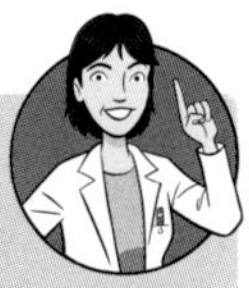

> Hyperventilation is an increase in breathing rate above the level needed to keep P_aCO_2 constant. It should not be confused with hyperpnoea which occurs in exercise when the CO_2 production is increased from respiring muscle and the increase in ventilation is in order to stop the P_aCO_2 from rising.

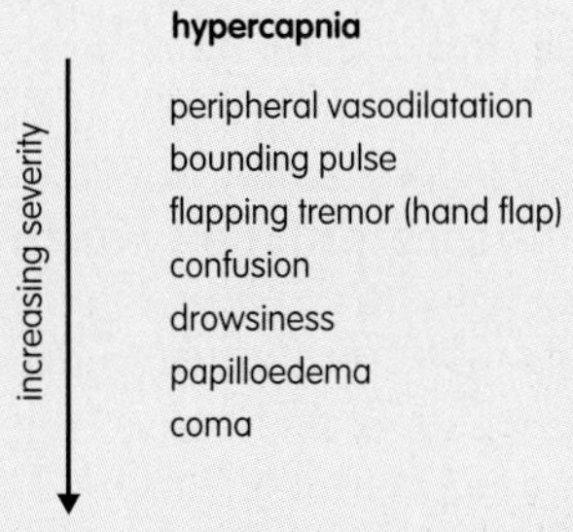

increasing severity

hypercapnia

peripheral vasodilatation
bounding pulse
flapping tremor (hand flap)
confusion
drowsiness
papilloedema
coma

Fig. 5.29 Clinical signs of hypercapnia.

Hypocapnia

A low partial pressure of carbon dioxide in the blood ($P_aCO_2 < 40$ mmHg) is termed hypocapnia.

Respiratory failure

Hypercapnia and hypocapnia are important concepts in the assessment of respiratory failure (see Ch. 8). Respiratory failure is defined as a $P_aO_2 < 8$ kPa (60 mmHg) and is divided into type I and type II depending on the P_aCO_2.

In type I respiratory failure, $P_aCO_2 < 6.5$ kPa. P_aO_2 is low (hypoxaemic), but P_aCO_2 may be normal or low; this represents a ventilation : perfusion mismatch.

In type II respiratory failure, $P_aCO_2 > 6.5$ kPa. Both P_aO_2 and P_aCO_2 indicate that the lungs are not well ventilated.

The significance of this classification is that in type II respiratory failure the patient may have developed tolerance to increased levels of P_aCO_2; in other words, the drive for respiration no longer relies on hypercapnic drive (high P_aCO_2) but on hypoxic drive (low P_aO_2). Thus, if the patient is given high-concentration oxygen therapy the hypoxic drive for ventilation may decrease and the patient may stop breathing and die.

Hypoxia

This is a condition in which the metabolic demand for oxygen cannot be met by the circulating blood.

Causes of hypoxia

Many cells can respire anaerobically; however, the neurons in the brain cannot and therefore need a constant supply of oxygen to maintain normal function. A severe shortage of oxygen to the brain can lead to unconsciousness and even death. Therefore, treatment of hypoxic patients is critically important.

There are four principal types of hypoxia:

- Hypoxic hypoxia.
- Anaemic hypoxia.
- Stagnant hypoxia (or static hypoxia).
- Cytotoxic hypoxia (or histotoxic hypoxia).

Hypoxic hypoxia

This occurs when the arterial P_aO_2 is significantly reduced, so that haemoglobin in the blood exiting the lungs is not fully saturated with oxygen. Hypoxic hypoxia can be produced in many ways but the end result is the same with the lowering of oxygen content in the systemic blood. Figure 5.30 highlights the main causes of hypoxic hypoxia.

Note that even if the P_AO_2 is normal, the P_aO_2 can still be reduced. This is highlighted in cases where there is a reduced diffusing capacity. A reduced diffusion rate can occur if the distance for gaseous exchange is increased. This can happen in pulmonary oedema when there is increased accumulation of interstitial fluid between the epithelial cells of the alveoli and the endothelial cells of the capillary. Once the pressure in the capillaries is above 20 mmHg, this causes fluid leakage into the interstitial space; however, in more severe situations the accumulation of fluid can rupture the membranes and lead to fluid in the alveoli.

The haemoglobin saturation is reduced in patients with hypoxic hypoxia. Most forms of hypoxic hypoxia can be corrected if patients are given hyperbaric oxygen to breathe. The high concentration of oxygen will increase the P_AO_2 and thus the P_aO_2, improving the oxygen saturation status of haemoglobin. In patients with right-to-left shunt, hyperbaric oxygen may not have any benefit, because the P_AO_2 will be normal, but since the blood is being shunted away from the alveoli the P_aO_2 will remain low.

Anaemic hypoxia

This occurs when there is a significant reduction in the concentration of haemoglobin, so the oxygen content of the arterial blood will be abnormally reduced. There are numerous causes of anaemia. It can be due to:

- Blood loss (e.g. large haemorrhage).
- Reduced synthesis of haemoglobin (e.g. vitamin B_{12} deficiency, folate deficiency).
- Abnormal haemoglobin synthesis due to a genetic defect (e.g. sickle cell anaemia).

As mentioned previously, anaemic hypoxia can also be caused by carbon monoxide poisoning.

The P_AO_2 in anaemic patients is usually normal and the haemoglobin saturation is also normal. Patients become hypoxic because there is a reduction in the oxygen content in the blood as there is less haemoglobin than normal. Treating anaemic patients with hyperbaric oxygen will be of limited benefit because the blood leaving the lung will already be fully saturated. Anaemic patients will not appear to be cyanosed because the amount of de-oxygenated blood leaving the respiring tissue will not be higher than normal.

Stagnant hypoxia

This is the result of a low blood flow, and hence a reduction in oxygen supply, to the tissues. This may occur with a reduced blood flow along an artery to a specific organ, with only that organ being affected; alternatively reduced blood flow to all organs can occur if the cardiac output is significantly reduced (e.g. due to heart failure). There is usually nothing wrong with the lungs in terms of ventilation and perfusion in stagnant hypoxia, so the P_AO_2 and the P_aO_2 will be normal. Since the blood flow to the respiring tissues is slow, the tissues will try to extract as much available oxygen as possible from the arterial supply and so the venous PO_2 will be lowered and hence give rise to peripheral cyanosis.

Treatment with hyperbaric oxygen will not be beneficial to these patients as the blood leaving the lung will already be fully saturated. Only a slight rise in the level of oxygen dissolved within the blood plasma will occur.

Cytotoxic hypoxia

This occurs when the respiring cells within the tissues are unable to use oxygen, mainly due to poisoning of the oxidative enzymes of the cells. For example in cyanide poisoning, cyanide combines with the cytochrome chain and prevents oxygen being used in oxidative phosphorylation.

In cytotoxic hypoxia both the P_AO_2 and the P_aO_2 are normal and so again treating these patients with oxygen will be of limited value. Since the oxygen is unable to be utilized by the tissues, the venous PO_2

Fig. 5.30 Causes of hypoxic hypoxia

Physiological
- at high altitude where there is a low oxygen tension in inspired air, the P_AO_2 and accordingly the P_aO_2 will fall

Pathological
- hypoventilation:
  - respiratory muscle weakness, e.g. COPD, myasthenia gravis and poliomyelitis patients
  - iatrogenic causes, e.g. general anaesthetics and analgesics (opiates) which act upon the respiratory centres in the medulla to decrease respiratory muscle activity
- abnormal $\dot{V}/\dot{Q}$ matching, e.g. airway obstruction, pulmonary embolism
- impaired diffusing capacity, e.g. pulmonary oedema as seen in left ventricular failure
- right-left shunting, e.g. cyanotic congenital heart diseases, severe pneumonia

Carbon monoxide poisoning causes anaemic hypoxia and not cytotoxic hypoxia (commonly confused by medical students). The carbon monoxide prevents the binding of oxygen to haemoglobin rather than interfering with the use of oxygen by the respiring cells.

will be abnormally high and cyanosis will not occur in these patients.

ACID–BASE BALANCE

Normal pH

The pH of the intracellular and extracellular compartments must be tightly controlled for the body to function efficiently, or at all. The normal arterial pH lies within a relatively narrow range: 7.35–7.45 ($[H^+]$ range, 45–35 mmol/L). An acid–base disturbance arises when arterial pH lies outside this range. If the blood pH is less than 7.35, an acidosis is present; if pH is greater than 7.45, the term alkalosis is used. Although a larger variation in pH can be tolerated (pH 6.8–7.8) for a short time, recovery is often impossible if blood remains at pH 6.8 for long.

Such a tight control on blood pH is achieved by a combination of blood buffers and the respiratory and renal systems which make adjustments to return pH towards its normal levels.

Key concepts in acid–base balance

Metabolic production of acids

Products of metabolism (carbon dioxide, lactic acid, phosphate, sulphate, etc.) form acidic solutions, thus increasing the hydrogen ion concentration and reducing pH. We also have an intake of acids in our diet (approximately 50–100 mmol H^+ per day).

We rely on three methods to control our internal hydrogen ion concentration:

- Dilution of body fluids.
- The physiological buffer system.
- Excretion of volatile and non-volatile acids.

Buffers

A buffer is a substance that can either bind or release hydrogen ions, therefore keeping the pH relatively constant even when considerable quantities of acid or base are added. There are four buffers of the blood:

- Haemoglobin.
- Plasma proteins.
- Phosphate.
- Bicarbonate.

It is the bicarbonate system that acts as the principal buffer and which is of most interest in respiratory medicine.

We have already seen that CO_2 dissolves in water and reacts to form carbonic acid and that this dissociates to form bicarbonate and protons:

$$CO_2 + H_2O \rightleftharpoons H_2CO_3 \rightleftharpoons H^+ + HCO_3^-$$

This equilibrium tells us that changes in either CO_2 or HCO_3^- will have an effect on pH. For example, increasing CO_2 will drive the reaction to the right, increasing hydrogen ion concentration.

As changes in CO_2 and bicarbonate can alter pH, controlling these elements allows the system to control acid–base equilibrium. This is why the bicarbonate buffer system is so useful; the body has control over both elements:

- Carbon dioxide is regulated through changes in ventilation.
- Bicarbonate concentrations are determined by the kidneys.

The Henderson–Hasselbalch equation

We can calculate the pH resulting from the dissociation of carbonic acid by using the Henderson–Hasselbalch equation. In its simplest form this states:

$$[H^+] \propto PCO_2/[HCO_3^-]$$

The effect on pH of changing carbon dioxide or bicarbonate is now even clearer: if carbon dioxide rises, and there is no change in bicarbonate, then the hydrogen ion concentration will rise.

Acid–base disturbances

As noted above, blood pH can either be higher than normal (alkalosis) or lower (acidosis). From the Henderson–Hasselbalch equation we can see that an acidosis could be caused by either:

- A rise in PCO_2.
- A fall in HCO_3^-.

Similarly alkalosis could occur through:

- A fall in PCO_2.
- A rise in HCO_3^-.

Where the primary change is in CO_2 we term the disturbance respiratory, whereas a disturbance in bicarbonate is termed metabolic. This allows us to classify four types of disturbance:

- Respiratory alkalosis.
- Respiratory acidosis.
- Metabolic alkalosis.
- Metabolic acidosis.

The disturbance was described as *primary* because the kidneys and lungs may try to return the acid–base disturbance towards normal values. This is called compensation and means that even in respiratory disturbances it may not be just CO_2 that is abnormal; bicarbonate may have altered too. Similarly, CO_2 may be abnormal in a metabolic disturbance. The ways in which the two systems compensate are:

- The respiratory system alters ventilation; this happens quickly.

- The kidney alters excretion of bicarbonate; this takes 2–3 days.

It is now clear that lung disease that affects gas exchange and therefore PCO_2 will have major effects on the body's acid–base status. It is also clear that whilst the respiratory system can act quickly to compensate for metabolic disturbances, it will take time for compensation to take place in respiratory disease; the renal system cannot act as quickly. We see this in clinical practice: a change in bicarbonate is characteristic of chronic lung disease, rather than acute lung disease.

Assessing acid–base disturbances

Assessing acid–base disorders is relatively simple if you approach the problem in stages (Fig. 5.31).

1. Start with the pH, is it outside the normal range?
2. If there is an acidosis or alkalosis, can it be explained by a change in CO_2?
3. If so, then it is a primary disturbance due to a respiratory cause.
4. Now look at bicarbonate – has this changed to return the ratio to normal?
5. If so, it is a respiratory disorder with metabolic compensation.

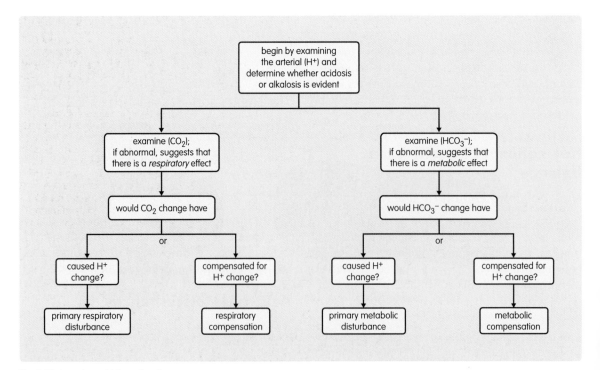

Fig. 5.31 Assessing acid–base disorders.

Davenport diagram

The Davenport diagram (Fig. 5.32) demonstrates the relationship between plasma [HCO_3^-], pH and PCO_2 in a graphical form.

Respiratory acidosis

Respiratory acidosis results from an increase in PCO_2 caused by:

- Hypoventilation (less CO_2 is blown off).
- Ventilation : perfusion mismatch.

From the Henderson–Hasselbalch equation, we see that an increase in PCO_2 causes an increase in hydrogen ion concentration (i.e. a reduction in pH). Thus, plasma bicarbonate concentration increases to compensate for the increased hydrogen ion concentration (Fig. 5.33).

Renal compensation

The increase in hydrogen ion concentration in the blood results in increased filtration of hydrogen ions at the glomeruli, thus:

Throughout the following text, it is easiest to follow the principles of acid–base balance by using the Davenport diagram.

- Increasing HCO_3^- reabsorption.
- Increasing HCO_3^- production.

Thus, plasma HCO_3^- rises compensating for the increased [H^+], i.e. renal compensation raises pH towards normal.

Causes of respiratory acidosis

Mechanisms reducing ventilation or causing $\dot{V}/\dot{Q}$ mismatch include:

- COPD.
- Asthma.
- Blocked airway (by tumour or foreign body).
- Spontaneous lung collapse, brainstem lesion.
- Injury to the chest wall.

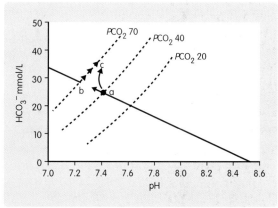

Fig. 5.33 Respiratory acidosis causes increases in PCO_2 and HCO_3^-, and reduction in pH, shown as a move from a to b. The kidneys compensate by increasing HCO_3^- reabsorption and production, shown from point b to point c. Arrow a–c show the real-life situation.

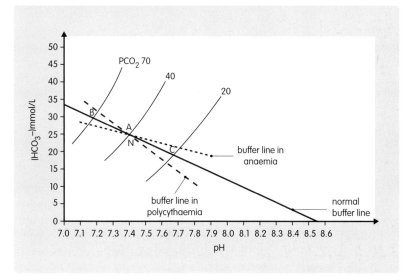

Fig. 5.32 The relationship between plasma [HCO_3^-], pH and PCO_2. A buffer line runs from points A to B. Any change in PCO_2 will have an equivalent rise or fall in [HCO_3^-] because of bicarbonate buffering of hydrogen ions; this can be shown by moving up and down the buffer line. Point N shows the normal plasma pH and [HCO_3^-]. Lines running perpendicular to the buffer line are of constant PCO_2.

Drugs that reduce respiratory drive (ventilation) include morphine, barbiturates and general anaesthetics.

Respiratory alkalosis

Respiratory alkalosis results from a decrease in PCO_2 generally caused by alveolar hyperventilation (more carbon dioxide is blown off). This causes a decrease in hydrogen ion concentration and thus an increase in pH (Fig. 5.34).

Renal compensation

The reduction in hydrogen ion concentration in the blood results in decreased hydrogen ion filtration at the glomeruli, thus:

- Reducing HCO_3^- reabsorption.
- Reducing HCO_3^- production.

Thus, plasma HCO_3^- falls, compensating for the reduced $[H^+]$; i.e. renal compensation reduces pH towards normal.

Causes of respiratory alkalosis

The causes of respiratory alkalosis include:

- Increased ventilation – caused by hypoxic drive in pneumonia, diffuse interstitial lung diseases, high altitude, mechanical ventilation, etc.
- Hyperventilation – brainstem damage, infection causing fever, drugs (e.g. aspirin), hysterical overbreathing.

Metabolic acidosis

Metabolic acidosis results from an excess of hydrogen ions in the body, which reduces bicarbonate concentration (shifting the equation below to the left). Respiration is unaffected; therefore, PCO_2 is initially normal (Fig. 5.35).

Respiratory compensation

$$CO_2 + H_2O \rightleftharpoons H_2CO_3 \rightleftharpoons H^+ + HCO_3^-$$

The reduction in pH is detected by the peripheral chemoreceptors. This causes an increase in ventilation, which lowers PCO_2. Also:

Mr Wood, who was recently diagnosed with COPD and is a heavy smoker, came into hospital appearing cyanosed. His blood gases showed a pH = 7.35; PCO_2 = 11 kPa; PO_2 = 5 kPa and HCO_3^- = 35 mmol/L.

Mr Wood's blood gases showed a respiratory acidosis with renal compensation. The underlying cause was a chest infection demonstrated by chest X-ray and sputum culture (positive for *Haemophilus influenzae*) which decreased the ventilation rate and impaired gaseous exchange. Careful oxygen therapy, rehydration and antibiotic therapy helped resolve the infection.

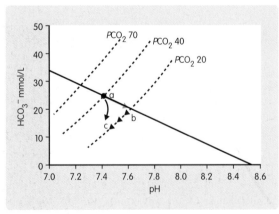

Fig. 5.34 Respiratory alkalosis causes reduced PCO_2 and HCO_3^-, and increases the pH, shown as a move from point a to point b. The kidneys compensate by reducing the rate of renal excretion of H^+ so that less HCO_3^- is reabsorbed or produced by the kidney. This is shown as a move from point b to point c. The real-life situation is shown from point a to c.

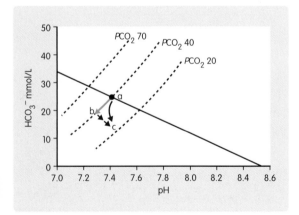

Fig. 5.35 Metabolic acidosis causes a rise in H^+, reduced HCO_3^- and reduced pH, shown as a move from point a to point b. The lungs compensate by blowing off CO_2 and therefore increasing the pH, shown as a move from point b to point c. The arrow a–c shows the real-life situation.

- The above equation is driven further to the left, reducing hydrogen ion concentration and bicarbonate.
- The decrease in hydrogen ion concentration raises pH towards normal.

Respiratory compensation cannot fully correct the values of PCO_2, $[HCO_3^-]$ and $[H^+]$, as there is a limit to how far PCO_2 can fall with hyperventilation. Correction can be carried out only by removing the excess hydrogen ions from the body or restoring the lost bicarbonate (i.e. correcting the metabolic fault).

Causes of metabolic acidosis

Causes of metabolic acidosis are:

- Exogenous acid loading (e.g. aspirin overdose).
- Endogenous acid production (e.g. ketogenesis in diabetes).
- Loss of HCO_3^- from the kidneys or gut (e.g. diarrhoea).
- Metabolic production of hydrogen ions. The kidneys may not be able to excrete the excess hydrogen ions immediately, or at all (as in renal failure).

Metabolic alkalosis

Metabolic alkalosis results from an increase in bicarbonate concentration or a fall in hydrogen ion concentration. Removing hydrogen ions from the right of the equation (below) drives the reaction to the right, increasing bicarbonate concentration. Decrease in hydrogen ion concentration raises pH; initially, PCO_2 is normal (Fig. 5.36).

Respiratory compensation

$$CO_2 + H_2O \rightleftharpoons H_2CO_3 \rightleftharpoons H^+ + HCO_3^-$$

The increase in pH is detected by the peripheral chemoreceptors. This causes a decrease in ventilation which raises PCO_2. Also:

- The above equation is driven further to the right, increasing hydrogen ion and bicarbonate concentrations.
- The decrease in hydrogen ion concentration raises pH towards normal.

Respiratory compensation is through alveolar hypoventilation but ventilation cannot reduce enough to correct the disturbance. This can only be carried out by removing the problem either of

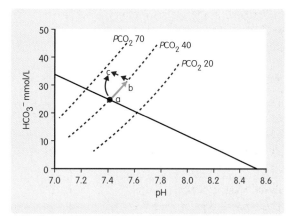

Fig. 5.36 Metabolic alkalosis due to loss of H^+ ions and increase in HCO_3^- with increase in pH, shown as a move from point a to point b. The lungs compensate by reducing ventilation and increase PCO_2, shown as a move from point b to point c. The arrow from point a to point c shows the real situation.

reduced hydrogen ion concentration or increased bicarbonate concentration. This is done by reducing renal hydrogen ion secretion.

More bicarbonate is excreted because more is filtered at the glomerulus and less is reabsorbed in combination with hydrogen ions.

Causes of metabolic alkalosis

The causes of metabolic alkalosis include:

- Vomiting (hydrochloric acid loss from the stomach).
- Ingestion of alkaline substances.
- Potassium depletion (e.g. diuretic, excess aldosterone).

John, an 18-year-old man, was found by the roadside having been vomiting. On his way to hospital he becomes severely short of breath. On examination, he had pinpoint pupils. Blood gases results showed: pH = 7.35; PCO_2 = 9 kPa; PO_2 = 6 kPa and HCO_3^- = 38 mmol/L.

John had taken an opiate overdose. His pH was in the normal range because at first he was vomiting (i.e. losing acid), therefore causing a metabolic alkalosis. But suddenly he went into respiratory depression, which can be caused by opiate use, and will cause a respiratory acidosis. Thus the alkalosis and the subsequent acidosis balanced the pH. John was treated with oxygen, naloxone (opiate antagonist) and fluid rehydration therapy.

Control of respiratory function

6

Objectives

By the end of this chapter you should be able to:

- Describe what is meant by feedback and feed-forward control.
- Discuss the central control of breathing with reference to the pontine respiratory group, and the dorsal and ventral respiratory groups of the medulla.
- List the different types of receptors involved in control.
- Describe the factors that stimulate central and peripheral chemoreceptors.
- Outline the responses of the respiratory system to changes in carbon dioxide concentration, oxygen concentration and pH.
- Discuss the mechanisms thought to influence the control of ventilation in exercise.
- Discuss the changes that occur in response to high altitude.

CONTROL OF VENTILATION

Basics of control

Every control system needs certain key elements for it to function correctly. These are:

- A control variable – a variable to be kept within certain limits (e.g. P_aCO_2 or P_aO_2).
- A desired value for that control variable, often quoted as normal physiological range (e.g. P_aCO_2 of around 40 mmHg).
- A measured value for the control variable (e.g. actual P_aCO_2 = 46 mmHg, 35 mmHg, etc.).
- Sensors to detect the measured value or a difference from the desired value (e.g. muscle spindle stretch receptors or chemoreceptors).
- Effectors (e.g. respiratory muscles, which alter ventilation and thus change P_aCO_2).
- A controller that relates the measured value to the desired value and changes output to the effectors (respiratory muscles), altering ventilation.

There are two types of control system: feedback and feed-forward:

- Feedback control – the system detailed below (Fig. 6.1), in which the controller looks at the measured value of the control variable (e.g. P_aCO_2) and relates this to the desired value. Adjustments to the system are then made.

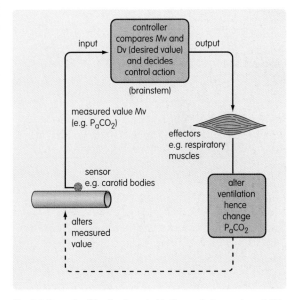

Fig. 6.1 Example of feedback control in the respiratory system. P_aCO_2 is used as the control variable.

- Feed-forward control – the system detailed below (Fig. 6.2), which anticipates the effects of external factors to the system and makes adjustments to the system in an attempt to control their effect. An example of this is behavioural control of breathing when we sing.

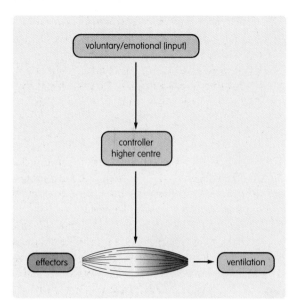

Fig. 6.2 Example of feed-forward control in the respiratory system. Higher centres predict the effect of external changes (e.g. emotion or singing) and alter the output to the effectors (respiratory muscles) to achieve the required ventilation.

Control within the respiratory system

When considering control of breathing, the main control variable is P_aCO_2 (we try to control this value near to 40 mmHg). This can be carried out by adjusting the respiratory rate, the tidal volume, or both.

By controlling P_aCO_2 we are effectively controlling alveolar ventilation (see Ch. 3) and thus P_ACO_2.

Although P_aCO_2 is the main control variable, P_aO_2 is also controlled, but normally to a much lesser extent than P_aCO_2. However, the P_aO_2 control system can take over and become the main controlling system when the P_aO_2 drops below 50 mmHg.

Control can seem to be brought about by:

- Metabolic demands of the body (metabolic control) – tissue oxygen demand and acid–base balance.

Note that we move between P_aO_2 and P_AO_2 here and throughout the chapter. Remember that these are different – if you are unclear, the abbreviations are explained on page 8.

- Behavioural demands of the body (behavioural control) – singing, coughing, laughing (i.e. control is voluntary).

These are essentially feedback and feed-forward control systems, respectively. The behavioural control of breathing overlays the metabolic control. Its control is derived from higher centres of the brain. The axons of neurons whose cell bodies are situated in the cerebral cortex bypass the respiratory centres in the brainstem and synapse directly with lower motor neurons that control respiratory muscles. This system will not be dealt with in this text; we shall deal only with the metabolic control of respiration.

Metabolic control of breathing

Metabolic control of breathing is a function of the brainstem (pons and medulla). The controller can be considered as specific groups of neurons (previously called respiratory centres).

Pontine neurons

Those located in the pons are the pontine respiratory group and consist of two groups of neurons:

- Expiratory neurons in the nucleus parabrachialis medialis.
- Inspiratory neurons in the lateral parabrachial nucleus and Kölliker's fuse nucleus.

The role of the pontine respiratory group (PRG) is to regulate (i.e. affect the activity of) the dorsal respiratory group (DRG) and possibly the ventral respiratory group (VRG, neuron groups in the medulla).

Medullary neurons

It is believed that the medulla is responsible for respiratory rhythm.

Three groups of neurons associated with respiratory control have been identified in the medulla:

- The dorsal respiratory group, situated in the nucleus tractus solitarius.
- The ventral respiratory group, situated in the nucleus ambiguus and the nucleus retroambigualis.
- The Bötzinger complex, situated rostral to the nucleus ambiguus.

These groups receive sensory information, which is compared with the desired value of control;

adjustments are made to respiratory muscles to rectify any deviation from ideal.

The dorsal respiratory group (Fig. 6.3) contains neuron bodies of inspiratory upper motor neurons. These inhibit the activity of expiratory neurons in the ventral respiratory group and have an excitatory effect on lower motor neurons to the respiratory muscles, increasing ventilation.

Ventral respiratory group neurons in the nucleus ambiguus (Fig. 6.4) are again inspiratory upper motor neurons.

Ventral respiratory group neurons in the rostral part of the nucleus retroambigualis (Fig. 6.5) contain inspiratory upper motor neurons which go on to supply through their lower motor neurons external intercostal muscles and accessory muscles.

Ventral respiratory group neurons in the caudal part of the nucleus retroambigualis (Fig. 6.6) are expiratory upper motor neurons.

The Bötzinger complex (Fig. 6.7) contains only expiratory neurons. Its sensory input is through the nucleus tractus solitarius. It has two functions:

- Inhibition of inspiratory neurons of the dorsal and ventral respiratory groups.
- Excitation of expiratory neurons in the ventral respiratory group.

Two main theories exist as to how the medulla influences respiratory rhythm:

- Dorsal respiratory group inspiratory pacemaker – neurons discharge in a phasic manner, inhibiting expiratory neurons.
- Neural networks – local re-excitation causes phasic firing in both inspiratory and expiratory neurons with reciprocal inhibition.

Effectors (muscles of respiration)

The muscles involved in respiration have been described in Chapter 4. The major muscle groups involved are the diaphragm, internal and external intercostals, and abdominal muscles.

Effectors carry out the control action for the central controller. Thus, the strength of contraction and coordination of these muscles is set by the central controller. If the muscles are not coordinated, this will result in abnormal breathing patterns.

Sensors (receptors)

Sensors report current values or discrepancies from ideal values for the various variables being controlled (e.g. P_aCO_2, P_aO_2 and pH) to the central controller.

There are many types of sensors and receptors involved with respiratory control:

- Chemoreceptors – central and peripheral.
- Lung receptors – slowly adapting stretch receptors, rapidly adapting stretch receptors and C-fibres.

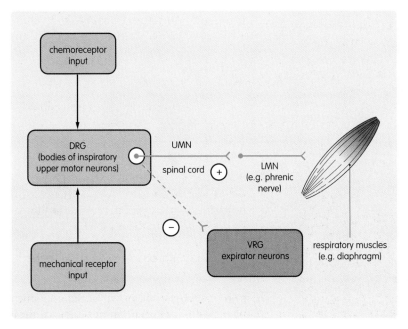

Fig. 6.3 Dorsal respiratory group. *Note the output to respiratory muscle and inhibition of expiratory neurons in the ventral respiratory group.* UMN = upper motor neuron; LMN = lower motor neuron; VRG = ventral respiratory group; DRG = dorsal respiratory group.

Fig. 6.4 Ventral respiratory group in the nucleus ambiguus. LMN = lower motor neuron; UMN = upper motor neuron; VRG = ventral respiratory group.

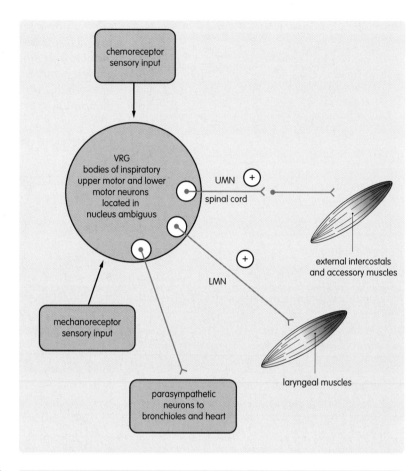

Fig. 6.5 Ventral respiratory group located in rostral nucleus retroambigualis. UMN = upper motor neuron; LMN = lower motor neuron; VRG = ventral respiratory group.

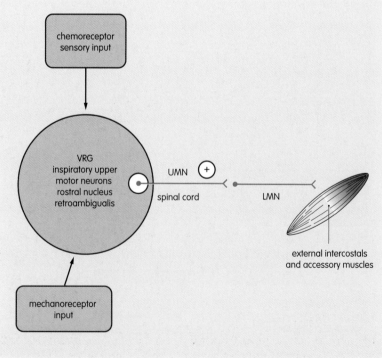

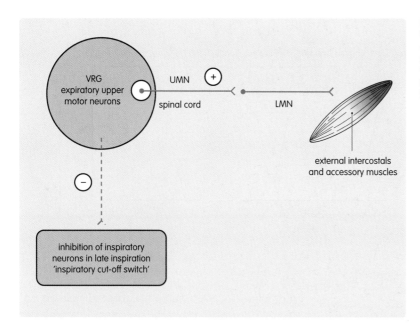

Fig. 6.6 Ventral respiratory group located in caudal nucleus retroambigualis (expiratory neurons). LMN = lower motor neuron; UMN = upper motor neuron; VRG = ventral respiratory group. (After Scott & Scott PP 1985, with permission of BC Decker.)

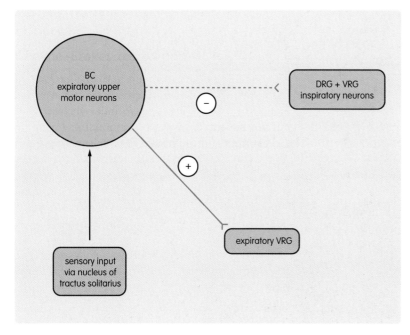

Fig. 6.7 Bötzinger complex (BC); located first rostral to nucleus ambiguus and consisting entirely of expiratory neurons. PRG = pontine respiratory group; DRG = dorsal respiratory group; VRG = ventral respiratory group. (After Greene, Johnson & Maricic 1993, with permission of Mosby.)

- Receptors in the chest wall – muscle spindles and Golgi tendon organs.
- Other receptors – nasal, tracheal and laryngeal receptors, arterial baroreceptors, pain receptors.

Chemoreceptors

Chemoreceptors monitor blood gas tensions, P_aCO_2, P_aO_2 and pH, and help keep minute volume appropriate to metabolic demands of the body. Therefore, chemoreceptors respond to:

- Hypercapnia.
- Hypoxia.
- Acidosis.

There are both central and peripheral chemoreceptors.

105

Central chemoreceptors

Central chemoreceptors are tonically active and vital for maintenance of respiration; 80% of the drive for ventilation is a result of stimulation of the central chemoreceptors. When they are inactivated, respiration ceases. These receptors are readily depressed by drugs (e.g. opiates and barbiturates).

The receptors are located in the brainstem on the ventrolateral surface of the medulla, close to the exit of cranial nerves IX and X. They are anatomically separate from the medullary respiratory control centre.

Central chemoreceptors respond to hydrogen ion concentration within the surrounding brain tissue and cerebrospinal fluid.

- Raised hydrogen ion concentration increases ventilation.
- Lowered hydrogen ion concentration decreases ventilation.

Diffusion of ions across the blood–brain barrier is poor. Blood levels of hydrogen ions and bicarbonate have little effect in the short term on the concentrations of hydrogen ions and bicarbonate in the cerebrospinal fluid and thus have little effect on the central chemoreceptors.

Carbon dioxide, however, can pass freely by diffusion across the blood–brain barrier. On entering the cerebrospinal fluid, the increase in carbon dioxide increases the free hydrogen ion concentration. This increase in hydrogen ion concentration stimulates the central chemoreceptors. Thus:

- Central chemoreceptors are sensitive to P_aCO_2 not arterial hydrogen ion concentration.
- Central chemoreceptors are not sensitive to P_aO_2.
- Because there is less protein in the cerebrospinal fluid ($<0.4\,g/L$) than in the plasma ($60–80\,g/L$), a rise in P_aCO_2 has a larger effect on pH in the cerebrospinal fluid than in the blood (CSF has lower buffering capacity).

Long-standing raised P_aCO_2 causes the pH of the cerebrospinal fluid to return towards normal. This is because prolonged hypercapnia alters production of bicarbonate by the glial cells and allows bicarbonate to cross the blood–brain barrier. It can therefore diffuse freely into the CSF and alter the CSF pH.

Peripheral chemoreceptors

Figure 6.8 shows the location of chemoreceptors around the carotid sinus and aortic arch. These are

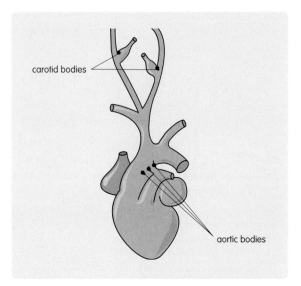

Fig. 6.8 Peripheral chemoreceptors. Carotid bodies are situated around the carotid sinus and are sensitive both to P_aCO_2 and P_aO_2. Aortic bodies are situated around the aortic arch and are sensitive only to P_aCO_2.

the carotid bodies and aortic bodies, respectively. Stimulation of peripheral chemoreceptors has both cardiovascular and respiratory effects. Of the two receptor groups, the carotid bodies have the greatest effect on respiration.

Carotid bodies

The carotid bodies contain two different types of cells: type I (glomus) cells and type II (sustentacular) cells. Type I cells are stimulated by hypoxia; they connect with afferent nerves to the brainstem. Type II cells are supportive (structural and metabolic), similar to glial cells of the central nervous system.

There is a rich blood supply to the carotid bodies (blood flow per mass of tissue far exceeds that to the brain); venous blood flow, therefore, remains saturated with oxygen.

The exact mechanism of action of the carotid bodies is not known. It is believed that type I (glomus) cells are activated by hypoxia and release transmitter substances that stimulate afferents to the brainstem.

Peripheral chemoreceptors are sensitive to:

- P_aO_2.
- P_aCO_2.
- pH.
- Blood flow.
- Temperature.

The carotid bodies are supplied by the autonomic nervous system, which appears to alter their sensitivity to hypoxia by regulating blood flow to the chemoreceptor:

- Sympathetic action vasoconstricts, increasing sensitivity to hypoxia.
- Parasympathetic action vasodilates, reducing sensitivity to hypoxia.

The relationship between P_aO_2 and the response from the carotid bodies is not a linear one. At a low P_aO_2 ($<50\,mmHg$), a further decrease in arterial oxygen tension significantly increases ventilation (Fig. 6.9). However, at levels of oxygen tension close to $100\,mmHg$, changes have little effect on ventilation. If P_aO_2 increases above $100\,mmHg$ (achieved when breathing high-concentration oxygen), ventilation is only slightly reduced.

Unlike central chemoreceptors, peripheral chemoreceptors are directly stimulated by blood pH. Although peripheral chemoreceptors are stimulated by P_aCO_2, their response is much less than that of central chemoreceptors (less than 10% of the effect).

In summary:

- Lowered P_aO_2 (especially below $50\,mmHg$) increases ventilation.
- Increased P_aCO_2 increases ventilation (but this is < 10% of the effect of central receptors).
- Raised hydrogen ion concentration increases ventilation (however, aortic bodies do not respond).

It is the peripheral chemoreceptors that are responsible for the ventilatory response to hypoxaemia that occurs at high altitude (see p. 111).

- The response of these receptors is very fast and can oscillate within a respiratory cycle.

Receptors in the lung

Afferent impulses arising from receptors in the lung travel via the vagal nerve to the respiratory centres of the brain where they influence the control of breathing. There are three main types of afferent receptor:

- Rapidly adapting receptors.
- Slowly adapting receptors.
- C-fibre receptors – formerly juxtapulmonary or J receptors.

Their characteristics are described in Figure 6.10 and their function discussed below.

Rapidly adapting receptors

Rapidly adapting receptors are involved in lung defence and form part of the cough reflex. This is reflected in their location in the upper airways. They produce only transitory responses and may be sensitized by inflammatory mediators, making them more sensitive to stimulation.

Slowly adapting receptors

Slowly adapting receptors are important in the control of breathing, not the cough reflex, and produce sustained responses. They are stimulated by inflation (which stretches the lungs):

- Inflation leads to decreased respiration (inflation reflex or Hering–Breuer reflex).
- Deflation leads to increased respiration (deflation reflex).

These reflexes are active in the first year of life, but are weak in adults. Therefore, they are not thought to determine the rate and depth of breathing in adults. However, these reflexes are seen to be more active if the tidal volume increases above $1.0\,L$ and therefore might have a role in exercise.

Afferent fibres travel to the respiratory centres through the vagus nerve. The functions of these receptors are:

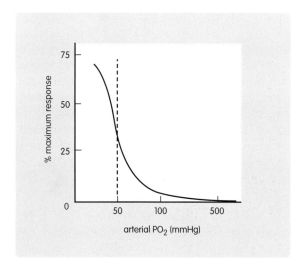

Fig. 6.9 Response of ventilation to P_aO_2. The response to a lowered P_aO_2 is small until the P_aO_2 falls below a value of $50\,mmHg$, after which point the response increases dramatically.

Fig. 6.10 Characteristics of the three principal types of afferent receptors in the lung

Receptor type	Stretch receptors		C-fibres receptors
	Rapidly adapting stretch receptor (RAR)	Slowly adapting stretch receptor (SAR)	
Location in airway	Primarily upper airways – nasopharynx, larynx, trachea, carina	Trachea and main bronchus	Throughout airways
Location in airway wall	Just below epithelium	Airway smooth muscle	Alveolar wall and bronchial mucosa
Structure	Small myelinated fibres	Small myelinated fibres	Free nerve endings
Conduction speed	Fast	Fast	Slower
Stimuli	Mechanical deformation Chemical irritants and noxious gases Inflammatory stimuli	Inflation	Chemical mediators – histamine and capsaicin (an extract of chilli peppers and the 'C' that gives 'C-fibres' their name Inflation and forced deflation Pulmonary vascular congestion Oedema – interstitial fluid in the alveolar wall

- The termination of inspiration.
- Regulation of the work of breathing.
- Reinforcement of respiratory rhythm in the first year of life.

However, if the nerve is blocked by anaesthesia there is no change seen in the rate and depth of breathing.

C-fibres
Stimulation of C-fibres results in:

- Closure of the larynx.
- Rapid, shallow breathing.
- Bradycardia.
- Hypotension.

C-fibres also contribute to the breathlessness of heart failure, and although they are afferent nerve endings, C-fibres are able to release inflammatory mediators (neurokinins and substance P).

Receptors in the chest wall

Receptors in the chest wall consist of:

- Joint receptors – measure the velocity of rib movement.
- Golgi tendon organs – found within the muscles of respiration (e.g. diaphragm and intercostals) and detect the strength of muscle contraction.
- Muscle spindles – monitor the length of muscle fibres both statically and dynamically (i.e. detect muscle length and velocity).

These receptors help to minimize changes to ventilation imposed by an external load (e.g. lateral flexion of the trunk). They achieve this by modifying motor neuron output to the respiratory muscles. The aim is to achieve the most efficient respiration in terms of tidal volume and frequency.

Mrs Roberts, a middle-aged woman, presented to her GP with a 4-week history of cough and sinusitis. The GP believed the cough to be caused by constant irritation and stimulation of pulmonary nerve receptors by postnasal drip originating from the sinusitis.

It is thought that stimulation of mechanoreceptors in the chest wall, along with hypercapnia and hypoxaemia, leads to increased respiratory effort in a patient with sleep apnoea. It is this sudden respiratory effort that then wakes the patient up.

Thus, reflexes from muscles and joints stabilize ventilation in the face of changing mechanical conditions.

Arterial baroreceptors

Hypertension stimulates arterial baroreceptors, which inhibit ventilation. Hypotension has the opposite effect.

Pain receptors

Stimulation of pain receptors causes a brief apnoea, followed by a period of hyperventilation.

COORDINATED RESPONSES OF THE RESPIRATORY SYSTEM

Response to carbon dioxide

Carbon dioxide is the most important factor in the control of ventilation. Under normal conditions P_aCO_2 is held within very tight limits and ventilatory response is very sensitive to small changes in P_aCO_2.

The response of ventilation to carbon dioxide has been measured by inhalation of mixtures of carbon dioxide, raising the P_aCO_2 and observing the increase in ventilation (Fig. 6.11).

Note that a small increase in P_ACO_2 causes a significant increase in ventilation. The response to P_ACO_2 is also dependent upon the arterial oxygen tension. At lower values of P_aO_2 the ventilatory response is more sensitive to changes in P_aCO_2 (steeper slope) and ventilation is greater for a given P_aCO_2. If the P_aCO_2 is reduced, this causes a significant reduction in ventilation.

Factors that affect ventilatory response to P_aCO_2 are:

- P_aO_2.
- Blood pH.
- Genetics.
- Age.
- Psychiatric state.
- Fitness.
- Drugs (e.g. opiates, such as morphine and diamorphine, reduce respiratory and cardiovascular drive).

Response to oxygen

As mentioned above, the response to reduced P_aO_2 is by stimulation of the peripheral chemoreceptors. This response, however, is not significant until the P_aO_2 drops to around 50 mmHg. The relationship between P_aO_2 and ventilation has been studied by measuring changes in ventilation while a subject breathes hypoxic mixtures (Fig. 6.12). It is assumed that end expiratory P_AO_2 and P_ACO_2 are equivalent to arterial gas tensions.

The response to P_AO_2 is also seen to change with different levels of P_ACO_2.

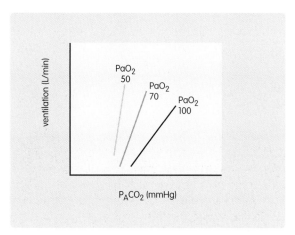

Fig. 6.11 The response of ventilation to CO_2. *Note that at higher levels of P_aO_2 an increase in P_ACO_2 has less effect on ventilation (the curve is less steep).*

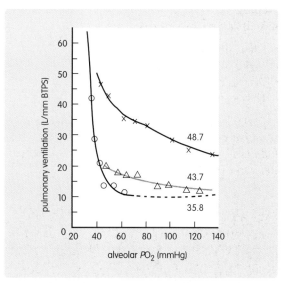

Fig. 6.12 The response of ventilation to P_AO_2 at three values of P_ACO_2. Lowered P_AO_2 has a much greater effect on ventilation when increased values of P_ACO_2 are present.

- The greater the carbon dioxide tension, the earlier the response to low oxygen tension.
- Therefore, at high P_aCO_2, a decrease in oxygen tension below 100 mmHg causes an increase in ventilation.

Under normal conditions, P_aO_2 does not fall to values of around 50 mmHg and, therefore, daily control of ventilation does not rely on hypoxic drive. However, under conditions of severe lung disease, or at high altitude, hypoxic drive becomes increasingly important. A patient with COPD may rely almost entirely on hypoxic drive alone, having lost ventilatory response to carbon dioxide (described above). Central chemoreceptors have become unresponsive to carbon dioxide; in addition, ventilatory drive from the effects of reduced pH on peripheral chemoreceptors is also lessened by renal compensation for the acid–base abnormality. Administration of high-concentration oxygen therapy (e.g. 100% O_2) may abolish any hypoxic drive that the patient was previously relying upon, depressing ventilation and worsening the patient's condition.

Response to pH

From earlier in the chapter you should remember that hydrogen ions do not cross the blood–brain barrier and therefore affect only peripheral chemoreceptors. It is difficult to separate the response from increased P_aCO_2 and decreased pH. Any change in pH may be compensated in the long term by the kidneys and therefore has less effect on ventilation than might be expected.

An example of how pH may drive ventilation is seen in the case of metabolic acidosis. The patient will try to achieve a reduction in hydrogen ion concentration by blowing off more carbon dioxide from the lungs. This is achieved by increasing ventilation.

Response to exercise

As human beings, we are capable of a huge increase in ventilation in response to exercise: approximately 15 times the resting level. In moderate exercise, the carbon dioxide output and oxygen uptake are well matched. The increase in respiratory rate and tidal volume do not cause hyperventilation, and the subject is said to be hyperpnoeic:

- P_aCO_2 does not increase, but may fall slightly.
- P_aO_2 does not decrease.
- In moderate exercise, arterial pH varies very little.

Hyperpnoea is an increased depth of breathing and occurs in exercise. Tachypnoea is an abnormally high respiratory rate (over 20 breaths per minute) often seen in patients with pneumonia. Both are responses to increased metabolic demand, and are therefore different from hyperventilation (defined as ventilation that is too great for metabolic needs).

So where does the drive for ventilation come from? Many causes have been suggested for the increase in ventilation seen during exercise, but none is completely satisfactory:

- Carbon dioxide load within venous blood returning to the lungs affects ventilation.
- Change in pattern of oscillations of P_aCO_2 (Fig. 6.13).
- Central control of P_aCO_2 is reset to a lower value and held constant during exercise.
- Movement of limbs activates joint receptors, which contribute to increased ventilation.
- Increase in body temperature during exercise may also stimulate ventilation.
- The motor cortex stimulates respiratory centres.
- Adrenaline released in exercise also stimulates respiration.

The possible role of oscillations of P_aCO_2

It is suggested that there are cyclical changes of P_aCO_2, with inspiration and expiration. Although mean P_aCO_2 does not change during moderate exercise, the amplitude of these oscillations may increase, providing the stimulus for ventilation.

In heavy exercise, there can be measurable changes in P_aO_2 and P_aCO_2, which stimulate respiration. In addition, the pH falls because anaerobic metabolism leads to production of lactic acid (blood lactate levels increase 10-fold). This lactic acid is not oxidized because the oxygen supply cannot keep up with the demands of the exercising muscles (i.e. an 'oxygen debt' is incurred). Rises in potassium ion concentration and temperature may also contribute to the increase in ventilation.

When exercise stops, respiration does not immediately return to basal levels. It remains elevated to provide an increased supply of oxygen to

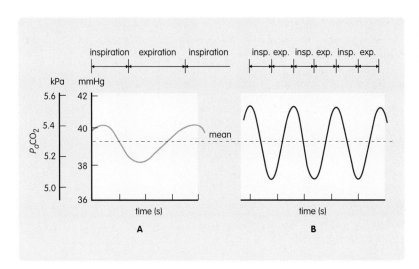

Fig. 6.13 Cyclical changes of P_aCO_2 with inspiration and expiration: (A) at rest; (B) during exercise. Larger oscillations are thought to alter ventilation.

the tissues to oxidize the products of anaerobic metabolism ('repaying the oxygen debt').

Abnormalities of ventilatory control

Cheyne–Stokes respiration

In Cheyne–Stokes respiration, ventilation alternates between progressively deeper breaths and then progressively shallower breaths, in a cyclical manner. Ventilatory control is not achieved and the respiratory system appears to become unstable:

- Arterial carbon dioxide and oxygen tensions vary significantly.
- Tidal volumes wax and wane (Fig. 6.14).
- There are short periods of apnoea separated by periods of hyperventilation.

Cheyne–Stokes breathing is observed at various times:

- At altitude – often when asleep.
- During sleep.

Mr Campbell, an inpatient with heart failure, was noted by nursing staff to develop an abnormal pattern of respiration. The nurses described Mr Campbell's breathing as swinging from very shallow to very heavy. He was also noted to appear pale and uncomfortable at rest. The medical staff were alerted to this Cheyne–Stokes pattern of breathing, a result of Mr Campbell's heart failure.

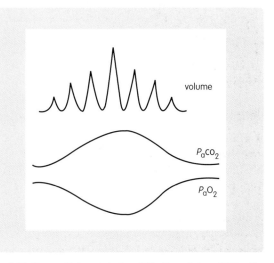

Fig. 6.14 Cheyne–Stokes respiration. (After Berne & Levy 1993, with permission of Mosby.)

- During periods of hypoxia.
- After voluntary hyperventilation.
- During disease, particularly with combined right and left heart failure and uraemia.
- Secondary to brainstem lesions or compression.

RESPIRATORY RESPONSE TO EXTREME ENVIRONMENTS

Response to high altitude

At high altitude, the barometric pressure is much lower than at sea level; for example, at the top of

Mount Everest (8848 m), the barometric pressure is only 250 mmHg compared with 760 mmHg at sea level. Hence, the partial pressure of oxygen is lower. Dalton's law of partial pressures states that 'The pressure exerted by a mixture of non-reacting gases is equal to the sum of the partial pressures of the separate components.' Thus:

$$P_{atm} = PO_2 + PN_2 + PCO_2 + PH_2O$$

In addition, the partial pressure of water vapour is constant, because inspired air is saturated at body temperature. Therefore, the partial pressure of oxygen in the alveoli (and in the blood) is significantly lower than at sea level.

The carriage of oxygen in the blood is dependent on:

- Partial pressure of oxygen in the blood.
- Haemoglobin concentration.
- The oxyhaemoglobin dissociation curve.

At altitude the partial pressure of oxygen in the blood is lowered. This would tend to limit the amount of oxygen carriage. To combat this problem the body can:

- Hyperventilate in an attempt to decrease the partial pressure of carbon dioxide in the alveoli and therefore increase the partial pressure of oxygen.
- Increase the amount of haemoglobin in the blood, thereby increasing oxygen carriage (oxygen capacity).
- Shift the oxygen dissociation curve.
- Alter the circulation.
- Increase anaerobic metabolism in tissues, increase cytochrome oxidase activity, and increase myoglobin in muscle tissue.

Hyperventilation

It can be seen by looking at the alveolar gas equation that if we hyperventilate, thereby reducing P_ACO_2, it is possible to bring the partial pressure of oxygen in the alveolar gas much closer to the partial pressure of inspired gas.

$$P_AO_2 = P_iO_2 - (P_ACO_2/R) + K$$

This is very advantageous at altitude – at 5000 ft, the partial pressure of oxygen is about 130 mmHg. Thus, for saturated air entering the lungs:

$$P_iO_2 = 130 - 47 = 93 \, mmHg$$

If a subject's P_ACO_2 was 40 mmHg and $R = 0.8$, then from the alveolar gas equation:

$$P_AO_2 = 93 - (40/0.8) = 43 \, mmHg$$

If the P_ACO_2 were reduced to 10 mmHg, then the P_AO_2 would be 80.5 mmHg.

At higher altitudes, because of the shape of the oxyhaemoglobin dissociation curve, the effect on oxygen carriage in the blood is more dramatic.

Hyperventilation is stimulated by the effect of hypoxia on peripheral chemoreceptors.

Polycythaemia

The function of the polycythaemia that is experienced by those living at altitude is not to give a rosy-cheeked complexion, but to increase the haemoglobin concentration and therefore the oxygen-carrying capacity of the blood. The P_aO_2 and oxygen saturation of the haemoglobin are unchanged, but the total amount of oxygen per unit volume of blood is increased towards normal levels.

Hypoxaemia stimulates the kidney to release the hormone erythropoietin, which increases red-cell production. This leads to a higher oxygen capacity, but has the adverse effect of increasing blood viscosity and therefore increasing the tendency for thrombus formation.

Shifting of the oxyhaemoglobin dissociation curve

It would be extremely advantageous if we as humans could significantly shift the oxyhaemoglobin dissociation curve to the left when loading haemoglobin with oxygen, and to the right when unloading oxygen. At altitude, there is a shift to the right, which aids unloading. This is caused by an increase in 2,3-diphosphoglycerate as a result of respiratory alkalosis.

Adverse effects of altitude

Low oxygen tensions in the alveoli cause vasoconstriction of the pulmonary vasculature. This leads to hydrodynamic pulmonary hypertension and increased work for the right heart. Because this alters the Starling forces affecting the pulmonary vessels, pulmonary oedema may occur (reducing gaseous exchange). The permeability of capillaries is increased and a high-protein transudate forms.

Diving

Increased pressure applies in underwater situations. When diving, pressure increases because of the weight of the column of water above. The pressure rises by 1 atm (760 mmHg) for every 10 m descended. Solids and liquids are incompressible, and any increased pressure has little effect on these. Gases, however, are compressible and gas contained within a cavity or in solution (Henry's law) is affected by pressure changes.

Thus, on descent, the pressure increases and a gas is:

- Compressed.
- Forced into solution.

On ascent, gas may:

- Expand (which if enclosed in a cavity or sinus could rupture the surrounding structure).
- Come out of solution.

The different types of dive are discussed briefly below.

Single-breath dive

A single-breath dive is short enough to be accomplished on the air inhaled at the surface. The diver holds his breath and submerges. The air in the diver's lung is subjected to increased pressure, increasing the PO_2 and PCO_2. Oxygen supply is increased, but so is carbon dioxide, stimulating the chemoreceptors: the diver soon must return to the surface. The dive can be prolonged by hyperventilation before submerging, but this can be dangerous on ascent because, as the ambient pressure falls, so the PO_2 falls to levels at which the diver may become unconscious. Standard advice is that four maximum breaths are allowed.

The ratio of total lung volume to residual volume limits the depth of the dive (6.0/1.5 = 4 atm – i.e. 40 m).

Snorkel dive

A snorkel dive is carried out at a shallow depth, so that connection with the air can be maintained by a tube. The maximum lung pressure that the inspiratory muscles can generate is about 100 mmHg, equivalent to a depth of about 1.2 m. This pressure cannot be maintained for more than a few minutes; thus the length of the snorkel is reduced to approximately 40 cm, reducing the dead space in the tube.

Conventional and SCUBA dives

Conventional dives involve being enclosed within a chamber while breathing compressed gases.

During SCUBA (self-contained underwater breathing apparatus) dives, gas is breathed through a regulated valve system from a pressure tank carried by the diver. The pressure of gas breathed is ambient, eliminating problems of lung mechanics. There are problems with conventional and SCUBA dives at depths over 50 m (5 atm) because of:

- Increased density of the inhaled gas, increasing the work of breathing.
- Nitrogen narcosis.
- Decompression sickness.

Nitrogen narcosis

Nitrogen has high solubility in fat and this solubility increases with increasing pressure. Nitrogen acts like a general anaesthetic, expanding the lipid components of cell membranes, leading to the destruction of membrane proteins, including ion channels that are responsible for neural signalling. It is believed this property leads to narcosis. Symptoms of nitrogen narcosis include:

- Euphoria.
- Mental confusion.
- Impaired neuromuscular coordination (clumsiness).
- Loss of consciousness.

Effects are detectable at 4 atm; serious impairment of performance occurs at 10 atm; full surgical anaesthesia occurs at 30 atm.

Decompression sickness

Under normal atmospheric pressure, the solubility of nitrogen is low and body tissues contain little nitrogen in solution: 9 mL nitrogen dissolved per litre of body water; 50 mL of nitrogen dissolved per litre of body fat. As we descend during a dive, ambient pressure increases, thus increasing the partial pressure of nitrogen and forcing nitrogen into solution (especially in adipose tissue).

On ascending, the nitrogen comes out of solution. If ascent is rapid, there is inadequate time for the nitrogen to reach the lungs and be blown off.

Instead it comes out of solution and forms bubbles (like formation of bubbles on opening a bottle of lemonade). Bubbles obstruct the circulation, especially in tissues with a high fat content, leading to bends (bubble formation in the joints) and chokes (bubble formation in the pulmonary vessels).

A student in a university diving club made too quick an ascent during a dive in open water. Within 30 minutes of surfacing, he began to complain of shortness of breath, cough and joint pains. Friends noticed that his skin appeared mottled. He was diagnosed with decompression sickness and treated with oxygen while being taken to the nearest recompression chamber.

Disorders of the lungs

Objectives

By the end of this chapter you should be able to:

- Describe the two main ways in which atelectasis can occur.
- Classify and give examples of the causes of atelectasis.
- List the causes of pulmonary oedema.
- List the multifactorial aetiology of adult respiratory distress syndrome.
- List the investigations required to diagnose pulmonary embolism.
- Describe the consequences of pulmonary hypertension.
- Define chronic bronchitis and emphysema.
- Describe the management of patients with COPD.
- Describe the management of a patient with bronchial asthma.
- Describe the pathology of bronchiectasis.
- List the complications of cystic fibrosis.
- Describe the management of a patient with pneumonia.
- Describe the pathogenesis of tuberculosis.
- List the common causes of pneumonia in the immunocompromised patient.
- Describe the pathogenesis of pulmonary fibrosis.
- Describe the different forms of pneumoconioses.
- Describe the relationship between cigarette smoking and bronchogenic carcinomas.
- Describe the differences between small-cell and non-small-cell carcinomas.
- Describe the endocrine manifestations of bronchogenic carcinomas.
- Describe the relationship between asbestos and pleural disease.

INTRODUCTION

A large number of lung disorders are covered in this chapter; they are grouped mainly according to the 'surgical sieve' approach, that is in categories reflecting the type of disorder (e.g. congenital) or underlying pathology (e.g. infection). The aim is to provide a clear structure for revision, allowing the disorders to be worked through in a logical fashion.

The surgical sieve can be a tool for formulating a differential diagnosis, making sure that no possible cause has been forgotten. A number of mnemonics exist for the categories. One is: TIN CAN BED PAN. This is short for:
Trauma Inflammatory Neoplastic Congenital Arteriovenous Neurological Blood Endocrine Drugs Psychogenic Allergic Not known.

CONGENITAL ABNORMALITIES

Congenital cysts

The respiratory system is an outgrowth of the ventral wall of the foregut. Bronchogenic cysts may result from abnormal budding of the tracheobronchial tree. Cysts are classified according to position:

- Central (mediastinal) – 85%.
- Peripheral (intrapulmonary) – 15%.

Cysts are usually single, spherical or oval, unilocular masses. They are mainly asymptomatic and can present at any age, although they are more common in men. Surgical excision is recommended. Radiologically, it is impossible to differentiate between a bronchogenic cyst and malignancy (Fig. 7.1).

Lobar sequestrations

Lobar sequestrations are masses of pulmonary tissue that do not communicate anatomically with the tracheobronchial tree (Fig. 7.2).

Vascular abnormalities

Vascular abnormalities include absent pulmonary artery trunk, absent unilateral pulmonary artery, pulmonary artery stenosis, pulmonary arteriovenous malformations, anomalous origin of the left pulmonary artery and anomalous pulmonary venous drainage.

Congenital lobar emphysema

Lobar emphysema is an overdistension of a lobe (usually an upper lobe) caused by intermittent bronchial obstruction. Symptoms in early life are caused by pressure effects. Pathogenesis includes defects in the bronchial cartilage, mechanical causes of bronchial obstruction and idiopathic causes. Prognosis is good.

Agenesis and hypoplasia

Agenesis

Agenesis is a complete absence of one or both lungs with no trace of bronchial or vascular supply.

Hypoplasia

In hypoplasia, the bronchus is fully formed, but reduced in size; there is failure of alveolar development. Hypoplasia is associated with other congenital abnormalities such as Potter's syndrome and diaphragmatic hernia.

Abnormalities of trachea or bronchi

Abnormalities of the trachea or bronchi include tracheal agenesis, tracheo-oesophageal fistula, tracheal stenosis, tracheal narrowing caused by extrinsic pressure, tracheomalacia and tracheobronchomegaly.

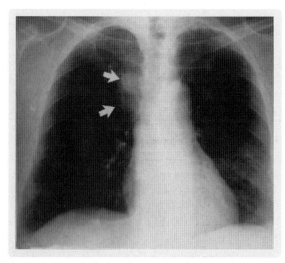

Fig. 7.1 Radiograph of a bronchogenic cyst. There is a right paratracheal mass (arrows). (Courtesy of Dr D Sutton and Dr JWR Young.)

Fig. 7.2A Differences between extralobular and intralobular sequestrations

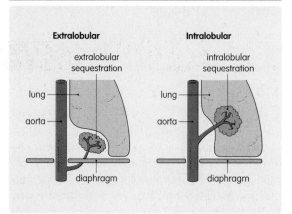

Fig. 7.2B Comparison between intralobular and extralobular sequestrations

	Intralobular	Extralobular
incidence	more common	less common
male-to-female ratio	1 : 1	4 : 1
side of thorax	60% left	90% left
arterial supply	70% thoracic aorta	40% thoracic aorta
venous drainage	pulmonary veins	systemic
position	within normal lung and its pleural covering	separate from normal lung in its own pleural cover
other congenital defects	uncommon	frequent

Fig. 7.7 Atypical pneumonias found in the immunocompromised

Organism		Presentation	Pathology	Diagnosis	Treatment
Pneumocystis carinii	fungus	Insidious or abrupt onset of dry cough, fever and dyspnoea. Pleural effusions are rare	Interstitial infiltrate of mononuclear cells. Alveolar air spaces filled with eosinophilic material	Giemsa, methanamine-silver papanicolaou or Gram–Weigert stains with monoclonal antibodies Chest X-ray: bilateral alveolar and interstitial shadowing spreading out in a butterfly pattern	High dose co-trimoxazole May be given prophylactically if low CD4$^+$ counts or if previous infection 100% mortality if untreated. 20–50% mortality in treated patients
Cytomegalovirus	DNA virus (part of herpes family)	90% of AIDS patients are infected with CMV, but only rarely does it cause pneumonia (non-productive cough, dyspnoea, fever). Disseminated CMV can occur, causing, for example, encephalitis	Interstitial infiltrate of mononuclear cells, scattered alveolar hyaline membranes, protein-rich fluid in alveoli and intranuclear inclusion bodies in alveolar epithelial cells	Characteristic 'owl's eyes' intranuclear inclusions in tissues on histology Can also be detected by direct immunofluorescence	Ganciclovir
Aspergillus fumingatus	fungus	Invasive aspergillosis can cause necrotizing pneumonia, abscesses or solitary granulomas		Microabscesses show characteristic fungal filaments	Amphotericin Poor prognosis

and antivirals may be of use. The overall mortality is ~ 11%.

Lung abscess

Lung abscess is a localized area of infected parenchyma, with necrosis and suppuration.

Aetiology

A lung abscess may occur due to:

- Aspiration of infected material (e.g. in alcoholism, unconscious patients).
- Complications of pneumonia.
- Infection of cavities in bronchiectasis or TB.
- Bronchial obstructions (e.g. tumours or foreign body).
- Pulmonary infarction.

Clinical features

Onset may be acute or insidious, depending on the cause of the abscess. Acute symptoms include malaise, anorexia, fever and a productive cough. Copious foul-smelling sputum is present, caused by the growth of anaerobic organisms.

In large abscesses there may be dullness to percussion. Pallor is common, caused by anaemia. Clubbing is a late sign.

Complications

Abscesses can heal completely leaving a small fibrous scar. Complications include empyema, bronchopleural fistula, pyopneumothorax, pneumatoceles, haemorrhage caused by erosion of a bronchial or pulmonary artery, meningitis and cerebral abscess.

Investigations

- Investigations must exclude necrosis in a malignant tumour or cavitation caused by tuberculosis; bronchoscopy may be indicated to sample cells or exclude an obstruction. Chest radiography shows a walled cavity with fluid level.
- Sputum culture may identify a causative organism.
- Blood culture and full blood count show that the patient is often anaemic with high erythrocyte sedimentation rate. Patients usually have mild to moderate leucocytosis.

Treatment

Follow disease carefully with regular chest radiographs and sputum collections. Resolution of disease is prompt after institution of appropriate antibiotics. Postural drainage should be used. Surgery is not usually indicated.

Tuberculosis

Tuberculosis is the world's leading cause of death from a single infectious disease. It is a notifiable disease and the prevalence is on the increase, primarily due to the arrival of the Human Immunodeficiency Virus (HIV). In the UK, 6000 new cases occur per year, with the highest incidence among immigrants, who are 40 times more likely to develop the disease than the native Caucasian population. Their UK-born children are regarded as being at high risk and as such are immunized soon after birth. Other risk factors for tuberculosis are homelessness, drug or alcohol abuse and immunodeficiency, notably HIV.

The causative agent in tuberculosis is *Mycobacterium tuberculosis*. Patients with pre-existing lung disease or the immunosuppressed may also be infected by opportunistic mycobacteria. These are also known as atypical mycobacteria or non-tuberculous mycobacteria and include:

- *Mycobacterium kansasii.*
- *Mycobacterium avium* complex (MAC).

Transmission and dissemination

Transmission is through the air or from direct contact. The pulmonary or bronchial focus ulcerates into an airway. A cough, sneeze or exhalation then discharges droplets of viable mycobacteria. The droplet nuclei are then inhaled by an uninfected person and can lodge anywhere in the lungs or airways. Initial infection usually occurs in childhood.

Primary tuberculosis

The initial lesion is usually solitary, 1–2 cm in diameter, and subpleural in the middle or upper zones of the lung. The focus of primary infection is called a Ghon complex. The primary infection has two components:

- The initial inflammatory reaction.
- Resultant inflammation in lymph nodes draining the area.

Within 3–8 weeks, the process becomes a tubercle, a granulomatous form of inflammation. The granulomatous lesion commonly undergoes necrosis in a process called caseation and is surrounded by multinucleated giant cells and epithelioid cells (both derived from macrophages). The caseous tissue may liquefy, empty into an airway, and be transmitted to other parts of the lung. Lymphatic spread of mycobacteria occurs. The combination of tuberculous lymphadenitis and the Ghon complex is termed the primary complex.

In most cases, the primary foci will organize and form a fibrocalcific nodule in the lung with no clinical sequelae.

Secondary tuberculosis (post-primary tuberculosis)

Secondary tuberculosis results from reactivation of a primary infection or reinfection. Any form of immunocompromise may allow reactivation. The common sites are posterior or apical segments of the upper lobe or the superior segment of the lower lobe. Tubercle follicles develop and lesions enlarge by formation of new tubercles. Infection spreads by lymphatics and a delayed hypersensitivity reaction occurs.

In secondary tuberculosis, the lesions are often bilateral and usually cavitated. Most lesions are connected to fibrocalcific scars.

Progressive tuberculosis

Progressive tuberculosis may arise from a primary lesion or may be caused by reactivation of an incompletely healed primary lesion or reinfection. Tuberculosis progresses to widespread cavitation, pneumonitis and lung fibrosis. Early symptoms are seldom diagnostic.

Miliary tuberculosis

In miliary tuberculosis, an acute diffuse dissemination of tubercle bacilli occurs through the bloodstream. Numerous small granulomas form in many organs, with the highest numbers found in the lungs. These form a characteristic pattern on chest X-ray. These granulomas often contain numerous mycobacteria and are usually the result of a delay in diagnosis or commencement of treatment.

Miliary tuberculosis may be a consequence of either primary or secondary tuberculosis and is universally fatal without treatment.

The pathology of tuberculosis is shown in Figure 7.8; complications are shown in Figure 7.9.

Clinical features

Primary tuberculosis is usually asymptomatic but may cause a mild febrile illness, with or without erythema nodosum. If the illness follows the progressive course, other symptoms then appear either immediately or gradually over weeks or months. Symptoms range from tiredness, anorexia and malaise to bronchopneumonia with fever, cough, dyspnoea and respiratory distress. Sputum is purulent, mucoid or blood-stained.

Fig. 7.9 Early and late complications of tuberculosis

Early	Late
pneumonia	bronchiectasis
empyema	mycetomas in cavities
haemoptysis	colonization of fibrotic lung with a non-tuberculous mycobacterium
laryngitis	extra-pulmonary disease
pneumothorax	

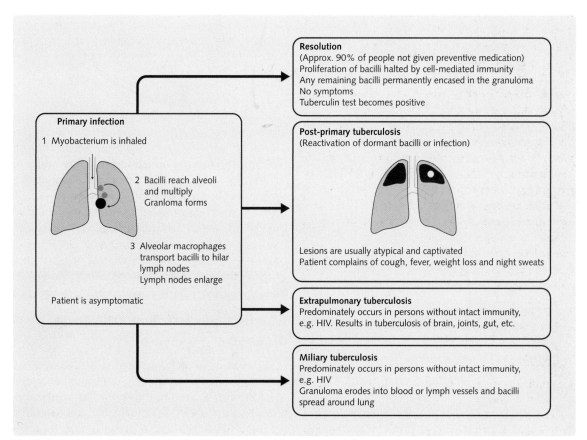

Resolution
(Approx. 90% of people not given preventive medication)
Proliferation of bacilli halted by cell-mediated immunity
Any remaining bacilli permanently encased in the granuloma
No symptoms
Tuberculin test becomes positive

Primary infection
1 Myobacterium is inhaled
2 Bacilli reach alveoli and multiply Granloma forms
3 Alveolar macrophages transport bacilli to hilar lymph nodes Lymph nodes enlarge
Patient is asymptomatic

Post-primary tuberculosis
(Reactivation of dormant bacilli or infection)
Lesions are usually atypical and captivated
Patient complains of cough, fever, weight loss and night sweats

Extrapulmonary tuberculosis
Predominately occurs in persons without intact immunity, e.g. HIV. Results in tuberculosis of brain, joints, gut, etc.

Miliary tuberculosis
Predominately occurs in persons without intact immunity, e.g. HIV
Granuloma erodes into blood or lymph vessels and bacilli spread around lung

Fig. 7.8 The pathogenesis of tuberculosis with different outcomes following primary infection.

A pleural effusion or pneumonia may be the presenting complaint; often the disease is discovered due to an abnormal chest radiograph in an asymptomatic patient.

Tuberculosis in HIV

In early HIV, tuberculosis appears similar to in non-infected individuals; however, as CD4$^+$ counts fall, presentation becomes atypical. Classical chest X-ray changes may not be present and extra-pulmonary involvement becomes more common. Tuberculosis at any site in an HIV patient is an AIDS-defining illness.

Extra-pulmonary tuberculosis

Tuberculosis can occur in most organs, including gut, skin, kidney, genital tract and bone, commonly causing vertebral collapse. In the brain, tuberculosis can cause chronic meningitis or a space-occupying lesion (tuberculoma), and though tuberculosis of the adrenal glands is now rare in the UK, it is a historically important cause of Addison's disease.

Diagnosis

Tuberculosis may be suspected on chest radiographs showing upper zone shadows and fibrosis; however, it is essential to confirm suspicions with microbiology. Sequential sputum samples are taken on 3 consecutive days:

- Staining and microscopy: bacilli appear red on a blue background using the Ziehl–Neelsen stain, or bright luminous yellow against a dark background using the more modern auramine-phenol stain. Bacilli are acid- and alcohol-fast.
- Culture: use Lowenstein–Jensen medium or a broth. Culture is important because it is more sensitive than staining and allows bacilli to be tested for drug sensitivity, but takes up to 8 weeks on Lowenstein–Jensen medium.
- RNA/DNA amplification: a new technique used in specialist centres. Advantage is that it is as sensitive as culture but faster (days).

If no sputum is available, other clinical samples can be used, e.g. pleural fluid from chest drain or lung tissue from bronchoscopy.

Prevention

BCG (bacille Calmette–Guérin) vaccine is made from non-virulent tubercle bacilli. The BCG vaccination is offered to schoolchildren at 12–13 years in the UK and to newborns of high-risk groups (e.g. Asians). It is given to individuals who are tuberculin negative. A positive tuberculin test indicates prior infection and those testing positive are screened with a chest X-ray. A 0.1 mL intradermal dose of the vaccine (chosen dilution is usually 1 : 1000) is given to children and adults either as a subcutaneous injection (Mantoux test) or using a multipuncture device (Heaf test). Immunization decreases the risk of developing tuberculosis by up to 70%. Once an individual has been vaccinated, subsequent tuberculin tests are positive.

Treatment

Most patients are treated on an outpatient basis with combination therapy, involving four drugs: isoniazid, rifampicin, pyrazinamide and ethambutol.

Treatment lasts 6 months and is in two phases:

- Initial phase lasting 2 months (rifampicin, isoniazid, pyrazinamide plus streptomycin or ethambutol).
- Continuation phase lasting 4 months (isoniazid and rifampicin).

The fourth drug (streptomycin or ethambutol) may be omitted in the initial phase except in drug-resistant strains. In adults the daily doses in the initial phase are: rifampicin 600 mg (taken 30 min before breakfast), isoniazid 300 mg, pyrazinamide 1.5–2.0 g. Patients should be warned that rifampicin will turn their tears, sweat and urine orange.

Patients should be regularly followed up because lack of compliance is a major reason for treatment failure. Directly observed therapy short course (DOTS) can be used to improve compliance by offering an incentive, e.g. a free meal, for attending a daily clinic where medications are taken under supervision.

DISORDERS OF THE AIRWAYS

Chronic obstructive pulmonary disease

COPD is an inflammatory lung disease characterized by infiltration of neutrophils and resulting in airway obstruction. The airway obstruction is unlike that seen in asthma, being progressive and only partially reversed by bronchodilators. Unfortunately, because of progressive decline in lung function, COPD is a significant cause of disability and death in smokers and it has been predicted that, by the year 2020, COPD will be the third commonest cause of death worldwide.

COPD is an umbrella term for different disease processes – the most important being chronic bronchitis and emphysema, which differ in pathology and site and are dealt with separately below.

Aetiology

In both emphysema and chronic bronchitis, cigarette smoke is the most important aetiological factor, although only 15% of smokers develop the disease. The general effects of cigarette smoke in COPD are:

- Inflammation resulting from inflammatory cell activation (Fig. 7.10). Cigarette smoke stimulates epithelial cells, macrophages and neutrophils to release inflammatory mediators and proteases, in particular neutrophil elastase, that are capable of destroying lung tissue. In heath, proteases are neutralized by antiproteases, but in COPD so many proteases are produced that they overwhelm the antiproteases resulting in digestion of lung tissue. This is termed the 'protease–antiprotease imbalance' and is believed to be particularly important in the development of emphysema.
- Inflammation resulting from the direct effect of oxidants in cigarette smoke.

Inflammatory cell activation and oxidative stress cause alveolar destruction (especially important in the emphysematous patient) and mucus hypersecretion (especially important in the bronchitic patient). Mucus may be further accumulated when cigarette smoke impairs ciliary movement, so reducing clearance of mucus and debris.

The specific pathogenesis of emphysema and bronchitis are discussed below.

Atmospheric pollution, occupational exposure and recurrent bronchial infections are also implicated. Recurrent bronchial infections are frequent causes of acute exacerbations.

2% of COPD patients have a genetic deficiency of a serum acute phase-protein produced in the liver called α_1-antitrypsin. α_1-Antitrypsin acts as an antiprotease in the lung and inhibits neutrophil elastase, so deficiency creates a protease–antiprotease imbalance, resulting in early-onset emphysema (less than 40 years of age) and death. Deficiency is autosomal dominant with equal distribution between sexes. The homozygous state has an incidence of $1:3630$ in Caucasians, but is rarer in dark-skinned people.

Emphysema

Emphysema is a permanent enlargement of the air spaces distal to the terminal bronchiole as a result of alveolar septal destruction due to a protease–antiprotease imbalance. Because distal airways are

Fig. 7.10 The overall pathogenesis of COPD.

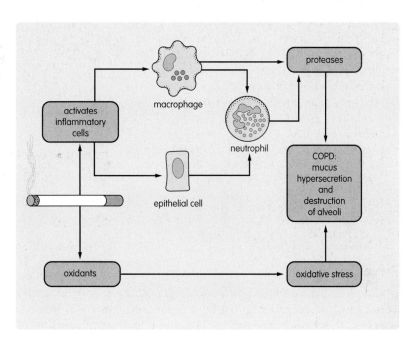

held open by the alveolar septa, destruction of alveoli causes the airways to collapse, resulting in airway obstruction (see Fig. 7.11).

As alveolar walls are destroyed, bullae form which may rupture causing pneumothorax. Destruction of the parenchyma increases compliance of the lung and causes a mismatch in ventilation : perfusion.

Classification of emphysema is based on anatomical distribution (Fig. 7.12). The two main types are centriacinar and panacinar.

Centriacinar (centrilobular) emphysema

Septal destruction and dilatation is limited to the centre of the acinus, around the terminal bronchiole and predominantly affects upper lobes (Fig. 7.12B). This pattern of emphysema is associated with smoking and therefore also seen in chronic bronchitis.

Panacinar (panlobular) emphysema

The whole of the acinus is involved distal to the terminal bronchioles, and lower lobes are predominantly affected. This is the characteristic of α_1-antitrypsin deficiency and not of smoking; therefore it is not usually associated with chronic bronchitis (Fig. 7.12C).

Irregular emphysema

Irregular emphysema is associated with scarring and damage affecting lung parenchyma, commonly found around old healed tuberculosis scars in the lung apices. Air trapping caused by fibrosis is thought to be the pathogenesis.

Irregular emphysema overlaps clinically with paraseptal emphysema (Fig. 7.12D).

Paraseptal (distal acinar) emphysema

In paraseptal (distal acinar) emphysema, alveolar wall destruction is restricted to the periphery of the acinus, with the upper lobes more frequently

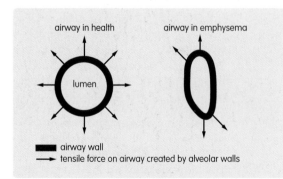

Fig. 7.11 The mechanism underlying airway obstruction in emphysema.

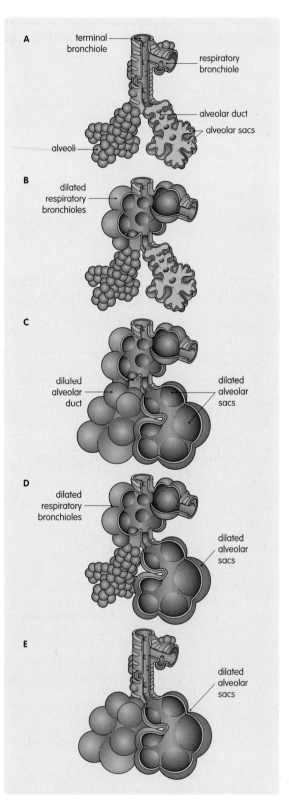

Fig. 7.12 Main types of emphysema. (A) Normal distal lung acinus; (B) centriacinar emphysema; (C) panacinar emphysema; (D) irregular emphysema; (E) paraseptal emphysema.

affected. If dilated air space measures more than 10 mm in diameter, the condition is termed bullous (Fig. 7.12E).

Chronic bronchitis

Chronic bronchitis is defined clinically as a persistent cough with sputum production for at least 3 months of the year for 2 consecutive years. Cigarette smoke causes hyperplasia and hypertrophy of mucus-secreting glands found in the submucosa of the large cartilaginous airways. Mucous gland hypertrophy is expressed as gland–wall ratio or by the Reid index (normally <0.4). Hyperplasia of the intraepithelial goblet cells occurs at the expense of ciliated cells in the lining epithelium. Regions of epithelium may undergo squamous metaplasia.

Small airways become obstructed by intraluminal mucus plugs, mucosal oedema, smooth muscle hypertrophy and peribronchial fibrosis. Secondary bacterial colonization of retained products occurs (Fig. 7.13).

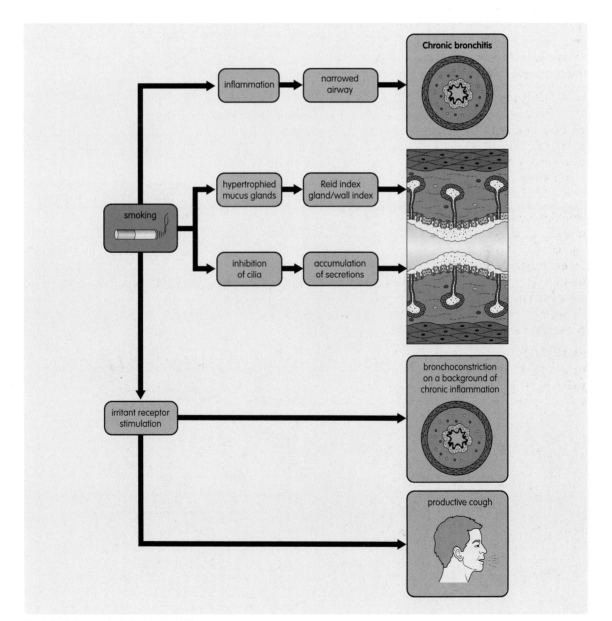

Fig. 7.13 Pathogenesis of chronic bronchitis.

The effect of these changes is to cause obstruction, increasing resistance to airflow. A mismatch in ventilation : perfusion occurs, impairing gas exchange.

Clinical features

The clinical presentation of COPD varies widely, depending on which of the two diseases predominates; two clinical groups of patients can be identified, although these represent the two ends of a spectrum of illness and in practice most patients will fall between the two (Fig. 7.14). Patients predominantly complain of shortness of breath and cough, with sputum production in chronic bronchitis. Weight loss and peripheral muscle weakness/wasting may be present because of systemic inflammation.

Typical signs found on examination are shown in Figure 7.15.

Complications of COPD

Exacerbations

An acute worsening of the patient's condition is usually due to infection, which can be viral (e.g. influenza) or bacterial (commonly *H. influenzae*). A mild exacerbation may only require an increase in medication at home. If the exacerbation is severe, the patient may deteriorate rapidly and require hospitalization.

Respiratory failure

In severe exacerbations the patient may be unable to maintain normal blood gases. This state is known as respiratory failure and is discussed in more detail elsewhere. Respiratory failure is the leading cause of death in patients with COPD and is often hypercapnic (type II).

Cor pulmonale

Mortality increases in those patients with COPD who develop cor pulmonale, or right ventricular enlargement secondary to disorders affecting the lungs. In COPD it is pulmonary hypertension that causes the right ventricle to hypertrophy and eventually fail. Further details are found under pulmonary hypertension below.

Investigations

Spirometry is the gold standard diagnostic test, showing an obstructive pattern with a reduced FEV_1/FVC ratio. A diagnosis of COPD can be made if the ratio is < 70% while the reduction in FEV_1 is used to classify the disease as mild (Stage 1), moderate (Stage 2), severe (Stage 3) or very severe (Stage 4):

- Mild = FEV_1 > 80% predicted.
- Moderate = FEV_1 < 80% but ≥ 50% predicted.

> Bob, a 71-year-old man, presented to his GP with a 12-month history of shortness of breath and reduced exercise tolerance. He was noted to have smoked 30 cigarettes a day for the last 25 years. Examination revealed him to be cachectic and breathing through pursed lips. A diagnosis of COPD was made on spirometry.

Fig. 7.14 'Pink puffers' and 'blue bloaters'

	Pink puffer	Blue bloater
body size	thin	obese
chest hyperinflation	marked	present
predominant disease	emphysema	chronic bronchitis
postmortem finding	panacinar emphysema	centrilobular emphysema
cor pulmonale	absent	present
secondary polycythaemia	absent	present
cyanosis	absent	centrally
blood gases	low P_aCO_2	raised P_aCO_2

Fig. 7.15 Signs of COPD

on inspection	central cyanosis
	barrel chest
	use of accessory muscles
	intercostal indrawing
	pursed-lip breathing
	flapping tremor
	tachypnoea
on palpation	tachycardia
	tracheal tug
	reduced expansion
on percussion	hyperresonant lung fields
on auscultation	wheeze
	prolongation of expiration

- Severe= $FEV_1 < 50\%$ but $\geq 30\%$ predicted.
- Very severe = $FEV_1 < 30\%$ predicted.

Lung function tests show an obstructive pattern. Transfer factor/diffusing capacity is low (note that it is normal in asthma). Exercise testing assesses the extent of disability. Bronchodilator reversibility should be assessed to exclude asthma.

Chest radiography typically shows hyperinflation or flat hemidiaphragms, reduced peripheral vascular markings, and bullae. Alternatively, radiographs may appear normal.

Full blood counts may show secondary polycythaemia, and though arterial blood gas tests are often normal they are important in monitoring the need for oxygen therapy in severe disease. Serum α_1-antitrypsin levels should be measured.

Treatment

No intervention can halt or reverse lung function decline in COPD, but smoking cessation slows deterioration and may increase a patient's life expectancy by years, even in late stages of the disease. Therefore, smoking cessation is a key intervention and encouraged by offering counselling and the drugs described in Chapter 8 (p. 173).

Treatment options are summarized in Figure 7.16 and include:

- Bronchodilators – anticholinergics, β_2 agonists and theophylline offer symptomatic relief. Combining drugs may be useful (NB: anticholinergics are more effective than β_2 agonists).
- Inhaled corticosteroids – not all patients will respond, so only prescribe these if there is a documented spirometric response after a corticosteroid trial, or if FEV_1 is < 50% of predicted and patient suffers from repeated exacerbations. Combination therapies may again be more useful.
- Antibiotics – shorten exacerbations and should always be given in acute episodes.
- Vaccine – annual flu vaccine.

Fig 7.16 Clinical features and management of COPD. (From Clinical features and management of COPD, 1997, with permission of the British Thoracic Society.)

FEV$_1$	Clinical features signs and symptoms	Improve function bronchodilator therapy
80%	**Mild** No abnormal signs 'Smoker's cough'. Little or no breathlessness.	• Short acting β_2-agonist or inhaled anticholinergic as required depending upon symptomatic response
60% 40%	**Moderate** Breathlessness (± wheeze) on moderate exertion. Cough (± sputum). Variable abnormal signs – general reduction in breath sounds, presence of wheezes.	• As for mild disease but regular therapy with either drug or a combination of the two may be needed. • Consider steroid trial
FEV$_1$	**Severe** Breathlessness on any exertion/ at rest. Wheeze and cough often prominent. Lung overinflation usual; cyanosis, peripheral oedema, and polycythaemia in advanced disease, especially during exacerbations.	• Combination therapy with regular β_2-agonist and anticholinergic • Consider addition of other agents • Perform steroid trial • Assess for home nebulizer

Lung function (% Predicted)

- Long-term domiciliary oxygen therapy – if necessary, administer for 19 hours per day at a flow rate of 1–3 L/min. Arterial oxygen saturation needs to be above 90%.
- Surgery – may be indicated to remove emphysematous lung.
- α_1-Antitrypsin replacement therapy – only for those with the genetic defect, and should not be routinely administered.
- Pulmonary rehabilitation (see Ch. 8).

The interventions above are described in more detail in Chapter 8 (p. 171) for management of COPD exacerbations.

Asthma

Asthma is a chronic inflammatory disorder of the lung airways characterized by air flow obstruction, which is usually reversible (either spontaneously or with treatment), airway hyperresponsiveness and inflamed bronchi.

Prevalence

Of the adult population, 5% are receiving therapy for asthma at any one time. Prevalence of asthma in the western world is rising, particularly in children; up to 20% have symptoms at some time in their childhood.

Classification

Bronchial asthma may be categorized into two groups on the basis of atopy: extrinsic or intrinsic (Fig. 7.17). Precipitating factors are described in Figure 7.18.

Occupational asthma is increasing; currently there are over 200 materials encountered at the workplace that are implicated (Fig. 7.19). Occupational asthma may be classified as:

- Allergic (immunologically mediated with a latent period between exposure and symptoms).
- Non-allergic (immediate response after exposure, e.g. to toxic gases).

Pathogenesis of asthma

The pathogenesis of asthma is very complex. Airway inflammation (Fig. 7.20) causes:

- Smooth muscle constriction.

Take a full history, including occupational history. Do symptoms improve at the weekend or on holiday? If so, there may be an occupational cause.

Fig. 7.17 Classification of asthma		
	Extrinsic asthma	**Intrinsic asthma**
underlying abnormality	immune reaction (atopic)	abnormal autonomic regulation of airways
onset	childhood	adulthood
distribution	60%	40%
allergens	recognized	none identified
family history	present	absent
predisposition to form IgE antibodies	present	absent
association with chronic obstructive pulmonary disease	none	chronic bronchitis
natural progression	improves	worsens
eosinophilia	sputum and blood	sputum
drug hypersensitivity	absent	present

- Thickening of the airway wall (smooth muscle hypertrophy and oedema).
- Basement membrane thickening.
- Mucus and exudate in the airway lumen.

Microscopically, the viscid mucus contains:

- Desquamated epithelial cells.
- Whorls of shed epithelium (Curschmann's whorls).

- Charcot–Leyden crystal (eosinophil cell membranes).
- Infiltration of inflammatory cells, particularly CD4$^+$ T lymphocytes.

Inflammatory mediators

Inflammatory mediators play a vital role in the pathogenesis of asthma. Inflammatory stimuli activate mast cells, epithelial cells, alveolar macrophages

Fig. 7.18 Precipitating factors for asthma

Allergens	Occupational sensitizers	Viral infections	Atmospheric factors	Drugs	Other factors
house dust mite (*Dermatophagoides pteronyssinus*)	colophony fumes (from soldering)	para influenza	cigarette smoke	β-blockers	cold air
flour	isocyanates (from polyurethane varnishes)	respiratory syncytial virus	ozone	nonsteroidal anti-inflammatory drugs	emotion
animal danders	acid anhydrides (from industrial coatings)	rhinovirus	sulphur dioxide		fumes
grain					exercise

Fig. 7.19 Factors implicated in occupational asthma

Agents	Workers at risk include:
High-molecular weight agents	
cereals	bakers, millers
animal-derived allergens	animal handlers
enzymes	detergent users, pharmaceutical workers, bakers
gums	carpet makers, pharmaceutical workers
latex	health professionals
seafoods	seafood processors
Low-molecular weight agents	
isocynates	spray painters, insulation installers etc.
wood dusts	forest workers, carpenters
anhydrides	users of plastics, expoxy resins
fluxes	electronic workers
chloramine	janitors, cleaners
acrylate	adhesive handlers
drugs	pharmaceutical workers, health professionals
metals	solderers, refiners

(After Criner & D'Alonzo 1999, by permission of Fence Creek Publishing.)

131

Fig. 7.20 Mechanisms of airway narrowing in asthma. (From Criner & D'Alonzo 1999, by permission of Fence Creek Publishing.)

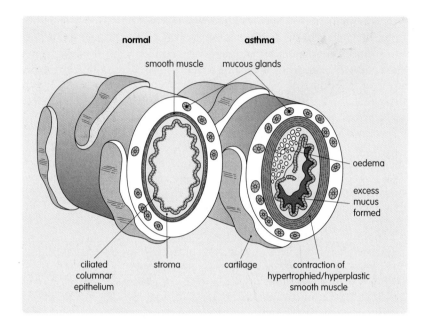

Fig. 7.21 Pathogenesis of asthma. IL-4 = interleukin 4; IL-5 = interleukin 5; MBP = major basic protein; ECP = eosinophil cationic protein; PGD_2 = prostaglandin D_2; LTC_4 = leukotriene C_4; IgE = immunoglobulin E.

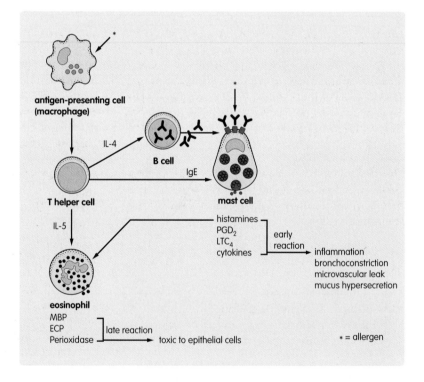

and dendritic cells resident within the airways, causing the release of mediators that are chemotactic for cells derived from the circulation – secondary effector cells (eosinophils, neutrophils and platelets).

Mediators that are thought to be involved in asthma include (Fig. 7.21):

- Preformed mediators – present in cytoplasmic granules ready for release. Associated with human lung mast cells and include histamine, neutral proteases and chemotactic factors for eosinophils.
- Newly generated mediators – manufactured secondary to the initial triggering stimulus after

release of preformed mediators. Some of these mediators are derived from the membrane phospholipids and are associated with the metabolism of arachidonic acid (e.g. prostaglandins and leukotrienes). The production of inflammatory cytokines and chemokines is important in the activation and recruitment of inflammatory cells.

Early and late responses

Two patterns of response can be considered; in practice most asthmatics show evidence of both responses, although either may be absent.

Immediate (early) reaction. The release of preformed mediators (predominantly from mast cells) causes vascular leakage and smooth muscle contraction within 10–15 minutes of challenge, with a return to baseline within 1–2 hours. The mast cells are activated by allergens that cross-link with the IgE molecules that are bound to high-affinity receptors on the mast cell membrane.

Late reaction. The influx of inflammatory cells (predominantly eosinophils) and the release of their inflammatory mediators cause airway narrowing after 3–4 hours which is maximal after 6–12 hours. This is much more difficult to reverse than the immediate reaction and there is an increase in the level of airway hyperreactivity.

Airway remodelling

This is a term used to describe the specific structural changes that occur in long-standing asthma with severe airway inflammation. The characteristic features include:

- Increased vascular permeability.
- Loss of surface epithelial cells and hypertrophy of goblet cells.
- Hypertrophy of smooth muscle.
- Myofibroblast accumulation and increased collagen deposition, hence causing basement membrane thickening.

Airway remodelling may cause a fixed airway obstruction which may not be reversible with anti-inflammatory agents or bronchodilators.

Clinical features

Symptoms (breathlessness, chest tightness, cough, wheeze) classically show a diurnal variation, often being worse at night. For example, nocturnal coughing is a common presenting symptom, especially in children.

Clinical features vary according to the severity of asthma (classified from mild to severe and either intermittent or persistent). Acute severe asthma in adults is diagnosed if:

- Patient cannot complete sentences in one breath.
- Respiration rate ≥25 breaths/min.
- Pulse ≥ 110 beats/min.
- PEFR ≤ 50% of predicted or best.

Life-threatening asthma is characterized by the following:

- PEFR < 33% of predicted or best.
- Silent chest and cyanosis.
- Bradycardia or hypotension.
- Exhaustion, confusion or coma.
- $P_aO_2 < 8\,\mathrm{kPa}$.

Investigations

- Lung function tests – FEV_1/FVC is reduced, RV may be increased; tests demonstrate an improvement in FEV_1 of more than 15% after bronchodilator administration.
- Peak expiratory flow rate – morning and evening measurements. Useful in the long-term assessment of asthma; a characteristic morning dipping pattern is seen in poorly controlled asthma.
- If PEFR < 50%, arterial blood gases should be tested.
- Exercise laboratory tests.
- Bronchial provocation tests – performed rarely in normal clinical practice, using histamine or methacholine to demonstrate bronchial hyperreactivity.
- Chest radiography – no diagnostic features of asthma on chest radiograph; used to rule out a diagnosis of allergic bronchopulmonary aspergillosis and pneumothorax in the emergency setting.
- Skin prick tests – allergen injections into the epidermis of the forearm, which are used to identify extrinsic causes. Look for weal development in sensitive patients.

Treatment

Identify and avoid extrinsic factors. Follow the British Thoracic Society (BTS) guidelines with a stepwise approach to drug treatment as illustrated by Figure 7.22. Each step up the treatment ladder is carried out if the patient's symptoms are not sufficiently controlled. The key point to remember about the stepwise management of asthma is to step down the treatment once the patient has good symptom control. Education with inhaler technique and drug compliance can also contribute to the management of asthma.

The pharmacology of the drugs used in treating asthma is discussed in Chapter 8.

Comparison of asthma and COPD is often asked in exam questions. Figure 7.23 summarizes the main differences between asthma and COPD.

Bronchiectasis

Bronchiectasis is defined as an abnormal and permanent dilatation of the bronchi and is associated with chronic infection. Most cases arise in childhood.

Aetiology

Bronchiectasis can either be acquired or, less commonly, has a congenital cause. However, about 50–60% of cases are idiopathic.

Acquired bronchiectasis
Bronchiectasis is usually caused by a severe childhood infection (e.g. bronchopneumonia, measles or whooping cough). Inflammation can damage and weaken the bronchial wall, leading to dilatation. It may also be caused by bronchial obstruction (e.g. by a foreign body, tuberculous lymph nodes or tumour) followed by infection in the lung distal to the obstruction. Other conditions associated which bronchiectasis include allergic

Fig 7.22 The stepwise management of asthma (adults and children over 5).

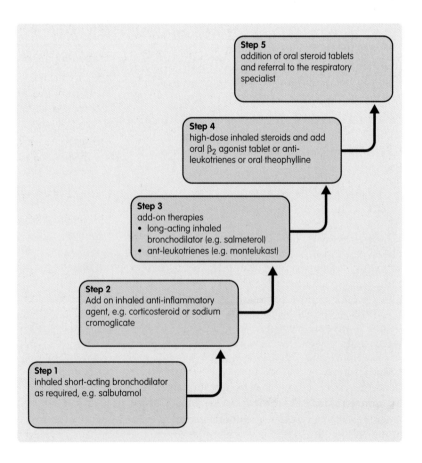

Step 5
addition of oral steroid tablets and referral to the respiratory specialist

Step 4
high-dose inhaled steroids and add oral β_2 agonist tablet or anti-leukotrienes or oral theophylline

Step 3
add-on therapies
• long-acting inhaled bronchodilator (e.g. salmeterol)
• ant-leukotrienes (e.g. montelukast)

Step 2
Add on inhaled anti-inflammatory agent, e.g. corticosteroid or sodium cromoglicate

Step 1
inhaled short-acting bronchodilator as required, e.g. salbutamol

Fig. 7.23 Comparison table: asthma vs. COPD

	Asthma	COPD
Genetic components	polygenetic	fewer genes involved, e.g. α1-antitrypsin
Age of onset	can occur at any age but more common during childhood	mainly affects the adult population
Inflammatory cells involved	eosinophils and mast cells are the main culprits	mainly neutrophils
Symptoms	variable – wheeze, cough	persistent – SOB on exertion, cough
Investigations	diurnal variation in FEV_1	progressive decline in FEV_1 over time
Reversibility	marked	sometimes
Most effective bronchodilator	β2-adrenoceptor agonist, e.g. salbutamol	anticholinergics, e.g. ipratropium bromide
Steroid treatment	beneficial	not very beneficial but useful in acute exacerbations

bronchopulmonary aspergillosis, inflammatory bowel disease and rheumatoid arthritis.

Congenital bronchiectasis

Congenital abnormalities that interfere with ciliary function (e.g. primary ciliary dyskinesia, Kartagener's syndrome and Young's syndrome) impair the transport of mucus and cause recurrent infection. Kartagener's syndrome, which is a rare cause, is also associated with dextrocardia and sinusitis. The viscous mucus and recurrent infections of cystic fibrosis may also lead to bronchiectasis. Recurrent infections are also a feature of immunoglobulin deficiencies (e.g. of IgA); therefore these are also associated with bronchiectasis.

Pathology

Infection leads to obstruction, dilatation of bronchi and often loss of cilia. Destruction of the alveolar walls and fibrosis of lung parenchyma occur and pulmonary haemodynamic changes can take place. The dependent portions of the lungs, usually the lower lobes, are affected most commonly.

Symptoms

Cough is the most common symptom; this is often persistent and accompanied by sputum which may be mucopurulent or copious, purulent and foul-smelling. Systemic features of infection such as fever and malaise also occur.

Haemoptysis may be present and can be massive. Clubbing occurs and coarse inspiratory crackles are heard on auscultation in the infected areas.

Complications

Complications of bronchiectasis include:

- Pneumonia.
- Pneumothorax.
- Empyema.
- Meningitis.
- Metastatic abscess (e.g. in brain).
- Amyloid formation (e.g. in kidney).

Investigations

Bronchiectasis can be investigated through:

- Radiology – chest radiograph may be normal or show bronchial wall thickening. If disease is advanced, cystic spaces may be seen.
- High-resolution CT – the investigation of choice to detect bronchial wall thickening.
- Sputum tests – Gram stain, anaerobic and aerobic culture, and sensitivity testing are vital during an infective exacerbation. Major pathogens include *Staphylococcus aureus*, *Pseudomonas aeruginosa*, *Haemophilus influenzae* and anaerobes.
- Tests for cystic fibrosis where appropriate (cystic fibrosis sweat test).

- Lung function spirometry (may show an obstructive pattern).
- Immunoglobulin levels – may demonstrate a specific deficiency.

Treatment

Aims of treatment are twofold:

- Control of infection.
- Removal of secretions.

Infections should be eradicated with antibiotics if progression of the disease is to be halted. Treatment regimens depend on infecting organism (e.g. flucloxacillin 500 mg 6-hourly to treat *Staphylococcus aureus* infection). If there is no improvement with treatment, the patient is likely to be infected with *Pseudomonas aeruginosa*: treat with ceftazidime aerosol or parenterally. Secretions are removed by postural drainage for 10–20 minutes, three times a day. Patients are trained in the method by physiotherapists.

Bronchodilators are useful if demonstrable air flow limitation exists. Surgery is of limited value but may be indicated in a young patient with adequate lung function, if disease is localized to one lung or segment.

Cystic fibrosis

Cystic fibrosis is a disorder characterized by the production of abnormally viscid secretions by exocrine glands and mucus-secreting glands, such as those in the pancreas and respiratory tract. Impaired mucociliary clearance in the airways leads to recurrent infections and bronchiectasis.

Cystic fibrosis is the commonest genetically transmitted disease in Caucasians. It is an autosomal recessive condition occurring in 1 : 2000 live births. The gene has been identified on the long arm of chromosome 7. Prevalence of heterozygous carriers is 4%.

Aetiology

The commonest mutation is a specific gene deletion in the codon for phenylalanine at position 508 in the amino-acid sequence (ΔF508). This results in a defect in a transmembrane regulator protein known as the cystic fibrosis transmembrane conductive regulator (CFTR). Mutation causes a failure of opening of the chloride channels in response to elevated cAMP in epithelial cells, leading to:

- Decreased excretion of chloride into the airway lumen.
- Increased reabsorption of sodium into the epithelial cells.
- Increased viscosity of secretions.

Pathology

The thick secretions produced by the epithelial cells cause:

- Small airway obstruction, leading to recurrent infection and ultimately bronchiectasis.
- Pancreatic duct obstruction, causing pancreatic fibrosis and ultimately pancreatic insufficiency.

Clinical features

Presentation depends on age. Usually, the condition presents in infancy with gastrointestinal manifestations (Fig. 7.24).

Stools are bulky, greasy, and offensive in smell. Respiratory signs are normal and symptoms are non-specific:

- Lungs are normal at birth.
- Frequent infections with cough and wheeze as the child gets older.
- Clubbing and dyspnoea occur.

Almost all men with cystic fibrosis are infertile; females may be subfertile.

CF patients are prone to respiratory infections especially *Pseudomonas aeruginosa*. It is thought that the naturally occurring antibiotic peptides (defensins) become inactive in CF patients, as these peptides are salt-sensitive.

Fig. 7.24 Manifestations of cystic fibrosis

Respiratory manifestations	Gastrointestinal manifestations
recurrent bronchopulmonary infection bronchiectasis	meconium ileus rectal prolapse diarrhoea failure to thrive malabsorption

Investigations

Family history is sought (e.g. affected siblings). Genetic screening is available for couples with a family history.

Prenatal diagnosis is available by chorionic villous sampling or amniocentesis.

Tests include:

- Guthrie test – heel prick test.
- Immunoreactive trypsin test (IRT) – positive test shows low levels.
- Sweat test – raised levels of sodium and chloride in sweat. It is thought that because of the CFTR mutation the sweat ducts are unable to reabsorb Cl^- from the ductal lumen into the interstitium resulting in sweat having an increased salt content.
- Chest X-ray – may show accentuated bronchial markings and small ring shadows.

The complications of cystic fibrosis are described in Figure 7.25.

Treatment

Treatment (Fig. 7.26) is based on:

- Physiotherapy.
- Antibiotics (see below).
- DNase (see below).
- Anti-inflammatory drugs (steroids).
- Nutritional support.

Intravenous antibiotics may be given at home (e.g. through implantable venous access devices) to reduce hospital admissions and improve patient independence.

DNA fragments from decaying neutrophils can accumulate within the lung lining fluid in CF patients. This makes the sputum more viscous and more difficult to expectorate. Human DNase has been cloned, sequenced and expressed by recombinant techniques. When DNase is given in a nebulized form it is capable of degrading the DNA and has been shown to improve the FEV_1. This treatment is expensive but very effective in combination with regular physiotherapy.

Heart–lung and liver transplantations are possible in severely affected patients.

Research into replacing the CFTR gene by using viral vectors and liposomes has been trialled in patients but gene therapy is extremely far from being an effective treatment for CF.

Prognosis

Prognosis is improving: currently, mean survival is 29 years. Death is mainly caused by respiratory complications.

Cough

Cough is a normal defensive reflex which can be elicited by either physical (e.g. foreign bodies) or chemical (e.g. cigarette smoke) factors acting in the upper respiratory tract, or a cough reflex can be elicited via a central stimulus. Cough is the third most common symptom presented to the GP. Coughing can be quite a minor, short-lasting symptom for most people but when chronic it can be a distressing and exhausting (physically and psychologically) symptom for some patients. Thus, the cause of the cough must be addressed.

Aetiology

Cough can be said to be acute (cough that persists for <3 weeks) or chronic (cough that persists for

Fig. 7.25 Complications of cystic fibrosis	
Respiratory complications	**Other complications**
allergic aspergillosus	abdominal pain
bronchiectasis	biliary cirrhosis
cor pulmonale	delayed puberty
haemoptysis	diabetes mellitus
lobar collapse	gall stones
nasal polyps	growth failure
pneumothorax	male infertility
sinusitis	portal hypertension
wheezing	rectal prolapse

Fig. 7.26 Summary of treatment of cystic fibrosis	
Respiratory	**Gastrointestinal**
drain secretions, postural drainage	pancreatic enzyme supplements with all meals and snacks
prevent infection where possible	high-energy, high-protein diet
exercise encouraged	do not restrict fat in diet
regular sputum cultures	vitamin A, D, and E supplements
immunization against measles and influenza	

> 3 weeks). The underlying cause can be pulmonary or extra-pulmonary related. Figure 7.27 outlines the main causes of cough.

Investigations

- History and examination findings usually pinpoint the diagnosis.
- Imaging techniques such as chest X-ray and CT scanning (especially for smokers) to help diagnose lung cancer and interstitial lung disease.

Further specific diagnostic investigations are used to support initial findings:

- ENT examination and CT of sinuses for postnasal drip syndrome.
- Peak flow diary, lung function tests and histamine or methacholine bronchoprovocation test to confirm asthma.
- 24-hour pH monitoring and barium swallow studies for GORD.
- $\dot{V}/\dot{Q}$ scanning for pulmonary embolism.

Treatment

The aims are usually to give either antitussive or protussive therapy, depending on the cause of the cough.

Antitussive therapy
- Treating the underlying cause, e.g.:
  - Bronchodilators and anti-inflammatory agents for asthma
  - Antibiotic therapy for pneumonia and postnasal drip syndrome
  - Histamine antagonist or proton pump inhibitors for GORD
  - Discontinuing the ACE inhibitor in exchange for an angiotensin II receptor antagonist.
- Treating the cough symptom, e.g.:
  - Simple linctus for acute cough caused by a viral infection
  - Opiates, which work centrally to suppress cough.

Protussive therapy
This aims to enhance cough effectiveness, therefore helping the patient cough up sputum to relieve breathlessness. CF and COPD patients benefit from expectorants, mucolytics and physiotherapy treatments to help with expectoration.

The pharmacology of antitussives and protussives is further explored in Chapter 8.

DISORDERS OF THE PULMONARY VESSELS

Pulmonary congestion and oedema

Pulmonary oedema is defined as an abnormal increase in the amount of interstitial fluid in the lung. The two main causes are:

- Increased venous hydrostatic pressures.
- Injury to alveolar capillary walls or vessels, leading to increased permeability.

Less common causes are blockage of lymphatic drainage and lowered plasma oncotic pressure.

Fig. 7.27 Causes of cough

	Acute (< 3 weeks)	Chronic (> 3 weeks)
Pulmonary	viral/bacterial – upper respiratory tract infection pneumonia TB PE	asthma COPD bronchiectasis cystic fibrosis lung tumours interstitial lung disease
Extra-pulmonary	inhaled foreign body congestive heart failure	Gastro-oesophageal reflux disease (GORD) postnasal drip syndrome middle ear disease iatrogenic, e.g. ACE inhibitors psychogenic/habit

High-pressure pulmonary oedema

High-pressure or haemodynamic pulmonary oedema is cardiogenic; it may occur acutely as a result of a myocardial infarction or chronically in aortic and mitral valve disease.

Fluid movement between intravascular and extra-vascular compartments is governed by Starling forces (see Fig. 5.11, p. 79). Net fluid flow through a capillary wall (out of the blood) is governed by:

- Hydrostatic pressure (arterial blood pressure) at the arteriolar end of the capillary bed.
- Capillary permeability.
- Opposing oncotic pressure exerted by serum proteins (mainly albumin); interstitial oncotic pressure may also contribute to the outflow.

Reabsorption of interstitial fluid is governed by:

- Plasma oncotic pressure (pulling pressure).
- Hydrostatic pressure in the interstitial space (tissue pressure).
- Fall in hydrostatic pressure at venous end of capillary.

Imbalances in Starling forces and a reduced plasma oncotic pressure will cause expansion of the interstitial spaces.

No pathological conditions cause a local reduction of plasma protein concentration within the lung capillaries. However, many conditions (e.g. left ventricular failure) cause an elevation of hydrostatic pressure. If left arterial pressure rises, so do pulmonary venous and capillary pressures, thereby raising hydrostatic pressure and causing oedema formation. Pulmonary oedema occurs only after the lymphatic drainage capacity has been exceeded. Lymphatic drainage can increase 10-fold without oedema formation. However, if lymphatic drainage is blocked (e.g. in cancer), oedema occurs more readily.

Oedema due to haemodynamic causes has a low protein content.

Oedema caused by microvascular injury

This is the non-cardiogenic form of pulmonary oedema.

Capillary blood is separated from alveolar air by three anatomical layers:

- Capillary endothelium.
- Narrow interstitial layer.
- Alveolar epithelium.

Damage to capillary endothelium

Normal alveolar capillary endothelial cells are joined by tight junctions containing narrow constrictions. Many conditions can damage the pulmonary capillary endothelium, resulting in movement of fluid and a transcapillary leak of proteins. Interstitial oncotic pressure rises; thus, a natural defence against oedema formation is disabled.

After damage, fibrinogen enters and coagulates within the interstitium. Interstitial fibrosis subsequently occurs, leading to impaired lymphatic drainage. Oedema caused by microvascular damage characteristically has a high protein content.

Progression of pulmonary oedema

Fluid first accumulates in loose connective tissue around the bronchi and large vessels. Fluid then distends the thick, collagen-containing portions of the alveolar wall. The final stage of pulmonary oedema is accumulation of fluid within the alveolar spaces. If pulmonary oedema is chronic, recurrent alveolar haemorrhages lead to the accumulation of haemosiderin-laden macrophages along with interstitial fibrosis.

Clinical features

Clinical features of oedema are as follows:

- Acute breathlessness.
- Wheezing.
- Anxiety.
- Tachypnoea.
- Profuse perspiration.
- Production of pink sputum while coughing.
- Peripheral circulatory shutdown.
- Tachycardia.
- Basal crackles and wheezes heard on auscultation.
- Respiratory impairment with hypoxaemia.
- Overloaded lungs, predisposing to secondary infection.

Treatment

The patient should be placed in a sitting position and 60% O_2 administered. Intravenous diuretics give an immediate response. Morphine sedates the patient and causes systemic vasodilatation: if systemic arterial pressure falls below 90 mmHg do not use morphine. Aminophylline can be infused over 10 minutes, but should be used only when bronchospasm is present.

Adult respiratory distress syndrome (ARDS)

Adult respiratory distress syndrome (ARDS) is non-cardiogenic pulmonary oedema defined as diffuse pulmonary infiltrates, refractory hypoxaemia, stiff lungs and respiratory distress (Fig. 7.28). ARDS forms part of a systemic inflammatory reaction.

Aetiology

Causes are as follows:

- Pulmonary:
  - Trauma or shock
  - Infection (e.g. pneumonia)
  - Gas inhalation (e.g. smoke)
  - Gastric contents aspiration
  - Near drowning.
- Extra-pulmonary
  - Gram-negative septicaemia
  - Pancreatitis
  - Burns
  - Cardiopulmonary bypass
  - Perforated viscus
  - Disseminated intravascular coagulation
  - Oxygen toxicity
  - Drug overdose (e.g. opiate).

The underlying insult is damage to the alveolar capillary wall, leading to diffuse alveolar damage.

Precipitating mechanisms of ARDS

Mechanisms include pulmonary capillary hypoxaemia, microembolism and loss of surfactant caused by pulmonary epithelium damage.

Pathology

As noted above, the key feature of ARDS is non-cardiogenic pulmonary oedema. Pulmonary venous and capillary engorgement occurs, leading to interstitial oedema. Pulmonary epithelium damage also occurs.

Pulmonary hypertension is common; hypoxic vasoconstriction redirects blood to better areas of oxygenation.

A protein-rich intra-alveolar haemorrhagic exudate promotes formation of hyaline membranes that line alveolar ducts and alveoli.

In long-standing cases, pulmonary fibrosis ensues and the alveolar walls become lined by metaplastic cuboidal epithelium (Fig. 7.28).

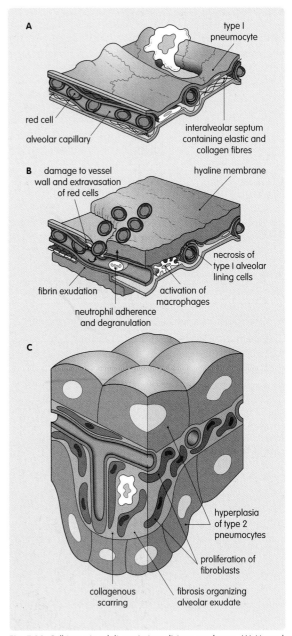

Fig. 7.28 Cell types in adult respiratory distress syndrome. (A) Normal alveolar wall; (B) acute phase of ARDS; (C) organization phase of ARDS.

Resolution

Resolution occurs as follows:

- Resorption of oedema.
- Ingestion of red cells and hyaline membranes by alveolar macrophages.
- Regeneration of type II pneumocytes.

rtension

ular lesion

pillary (e.g. left-to-right shunt)

lary (e.g. hypoxia)

apillary (e.g. left ventricular
e)

scular resistance is of most
medicine. This can occur due

onary vessels.

ruction or living at high
ronic hypoxia. This is also
yndrome where pulmonary
 by poor respiration associ-
Because insignificant intimal
dition is largely reversible.

ary vessels
 pulmonary hypertension, a
wn aetiology, predominantly
20–30 years. The condition

nary vasculature are initially
versible. Obliterative fibrosis
 and arterioles occurs later,
ases in pulmonary vascular

f pulmonary hypertension
 pulmonary venous pressure
ry blood flow) are primarily
sidered here.

ypertension include:

ulmonary arteries.
ertrophy.
ion.

Clinical features

Clinical features are as follows:

- Symptoms of the underlying cause.
- Chest pain and exertional dyspnoea.
- Syncope and fatigue.
- Prominent a-wave in jugular venous pulse.
- Right ventricular heave.
- Loud pulmonary component to second heart sound.
- Midsystolic ejection murmur.

Investigations

When investigating pulmonary hypertension, a possible cause should be sought.

A full blood count may show secondary polycythaemia. Chest radiography may reveal right ventricular enlargement, pulmonary artery dilatation, or oligaemic peripheral lung fields.

Electrocardiography may indicate right ventricular hypertrophy, right-axis deviation, a prominent R wave in V_1, or inverted T waves in the right precordial leads.

Radioisotope lung scans and echocardiography may also be useful.

Treatment

Treatment is dependent upon cause. Primary pulmonary hypertension is treated with anticoagulation therapy.

If the underlying cause of hypertension is untreatable, the patient will progress to cor pulmonale and death. Continuous oxygen therapy is beneficial in patients with cor pulmonale. Diuretics are used to treat fluid overload.

Heart–lung transplantation is recommended in young patients.

Prognosis is poor: 5-year survival rate is 40%.

Cor pulmonale

Cor pulmonale is a major complication of pulmonary hypertension. It is defined as right heart failure secondary to lung disease and occurs as a result of any disorder that leads to pulmonary hypertension. Of most interest here is its presence in lung disease. As noted above, lung disease that causes chronic hypoxia may lead to pulmonary hypertension and therefore cor pulmonale. The main respiratory diseases associated with cor pulmonale are:

- COPD.
- Severe, chronic asthma.
- Bronchiectasis.

Clinical features

Features change during the progression of ARDS. Patients with ARDS present with:

- Tachypnoea, often unexplained.
- Dyspnoea.
- Pulmonary oedema – fine crackles throughout both lung fields.
- Arterial hypoxaemia, refractory to oxygen therapy.

Chest radiography shows bilateral diffuse shadowing.

Management

- Treat underlying condition and provide supportive measures.
- Treat as for pulmonary oedema: the aim is to achieve a negative fluid balance.
- Provide cardiovascular support and mechanical ventilation (e.g. positive end-expiratory pressure (PEEP)).
- PEEP prevents the alveolae from collapsing during expiration. However, low tidal volume ventilation is used to prevent overstretching the alveoli, which can worsen the lung injury. Also, ventilation in the prone position has been shown to be beneficial to ARDS patients, as ventilation is more evenly distributed throughout the lung.
- Non-ventilatory management such as the use of inhaled vasodilators (e.g. nitric oxide, prostacyclin) have been shown to improve the $\dot{V}/\dot{Q}$ matching in ARDS patients. Steroids have also been shown to be beneficial, especially in the late stages of ARDS as they can dampen down the inflammation and also have antifibrotic properties.
- The use of surfactant is highly beneficial in infant respiratory distress syndrome but there is no clear evidence of any benefit in ARDS.

Prognosis

Prognosis is dependent upon the cause, but the overall mortality is greater than 50%. Of that 50%, 9/10 will die from septic shock and the remaining 1/10 from a fat embolism.

Prognosis is poor in the elderly.

Death is caused by cardiac arrhythmias with sepsis, usually from Gram-negative organisms.

Embolism, haemorrhage and infarction

Vascular disease of the lungs can be caused by:

- Vessel obstruction.
- Vessel wall damage.
- Intravascular pressure variations.

Obstruction: pulmonary embolism (PE)

An embolus is an abnormal mass of material that is transported in the bloodstream from one part of the circulation to another and which impacts finally in the lumen of a vessel that has a calibre too small to allow passage. The end result of an embolus derived from venous thrombus is impaction in the pulmonary arterial tree. Most thrombi originate in the deep veins of the calf or pelvis.

This is a common condition: incidence of pulmonary emboli at autopsy has been reported to be 12%. Pulmonary emboli rarely have a cardiac cause and are very rare in children.

Predisposing factors

Predisposing factors are:

- Immobilization (e.g. prolonged bed rest, long-haul flights).
- In women, the oral contraceptive pill – minor risk factor, increased by cigarette smoking.
- Malignancy, especially of pancreas, uterus, breast and stomach.
- Cardiac failure.
- Chronic pulmonary disease.
- Postoperative recovery.
- Fractures of the pelvis or lower limb.
- Hypercoagulable states (e.g. pregnancy).

Clinical features

Common symptoms are:

- Dyspnoea.
- Tachypnoea.

Mrs Clarke complained of sudden-onset chest pain following total hip replacement surgery. In light of her recent surgery, pulmonary embolism was suspected. A plain chest X-ray showed no abnormality; however, a ventilation : perfusion scan showed a perfusion defect in her right lung consistent with a pulmonary embolism.

- Pleuritic pain.
- Apprehension.
- Tachycardia.
- Cough.
- Haemoptysis.
- Leg pain/clinical DVT.

Symptoms are related to the size of the embolus and the corresponding volume of lung tissue deprived of blood in addition to the presence or absence of congestion in the pulmonary circulation at the time of impaction.

Pulmonary embolism can be classified as massive, moderate or small.

Massive pulmonary embolism

A massive pulmonary embolism is a clinical emergency. The embolus is typically derived from a thrombus that occludes a long venous segment in the lower limb. The calibre of the main pulmonary arteries is greater than the iliac and femoral veins; therefore, thrombi must loosely bundle together to block the pulmonary arteries (as seen in a saddle embolus, which occurs at the bifurcation of the left and right pulmonary arteries).

Within normal human lung, occlusion of more than 50% of the pulmonary vascular bed is necessary for a massive pulmonary embolism to prove fatal.

Clinical features

This is a clinical emergency presenting as sudden-onset severe chest pain and dyspnoea. Often onset occurs when straining during defecation. Classically, a massive pulmonary embolism occurs a week or more after operation.

There are signs of shock: tachycardia, low blood pressure. Right ventricular heave, gallop rhythm and a prominent a-wave in the jugular venous pulse may also be noted.

Sudden death can occur.

Small or medium-sized pulmonary embolism

Moderate pulmonary embolism is caused by occlusion of a lobar or segmental artery. Perfusion of a segment may be reduced, producing an area of localized necrosis.

An area of necrosis secondary to ischaemia is known as an infarct.

Clinical features

Pulmonary infarction presents with sudden-onset pleuritic chest pain. Cough with haemoptysis and dyspnoea are other symptoms.

Multiple microemboli

Multiple small emboli can occlude arterioles but this process is usually clinically silent. Gradual occlusion of the pulmonary arterial bed leads to pulmonary hypertension.

This is a rare condition characterized by exertional dyspnoea, tiredness and syncope. Basal crackles are heard on auscultation.

Other forms of emboli

Fat embolism

Fat embolism results from massive injury to subcutaneous fat or fracture of bones containing fatty marrow. Globules of lipid enter the torn vessels.

Air embolism

Air embolism arises during childbirth or abortion or after chest wall injury. These microemboli can cause tiny infarcts in several organs.

Tumour embolism

Tumour cells, like other particulate matter, become trapped in the pulmonary capillary bed. This is an important mechanism in the development of metastases.

Amniotic fluid embolism

Amniotic fluid embolism can occur during childbirth or abortion, and may be fatal. Small fragments of trophoblast are commonly found in lungs of pregnant women at autopsy, but do not cause any symptoms.

Investigations in suspected pulmonary emboli

- Chest radiography is usually unremarkable, but valuable in excluding other causes.
- Electrocardiography may show signs of right ventricular strain (deep S waves in lead I, Q waves in lead III, and inverted T waves in lead III).
- Arterial blood gases show arterial hypoxaemia and hypocapnia.
- D-dimers are degradation products of cross-linked fibrin, and are released into the circulation when a thrombus begins to dissolve. Detection of D-dimers in the blood is not diagnostic for a PE as D-dimers can be elevated in infection, malignancy and post-surgery. However, a negative test result makes the presence of an acute PE unlikely and therefore further investigation in low-risk patients may be unnecessary.
- Radioisotope ventilation: perfusion scans demonstrate ventilated areas of lung and filling defects on the corresponding perfusion scans; these are assessed on the basis of probability of pulmonary embolism (see Ch. 11). In non-diagnostic scans, pulmonary angiography should be performed in the acutely ill patient or leg ultrasound if the patient is stable.

Treatment

Treatment is based on:

- Supportive measures (analgesia, oxygen, etc.).
- Anticoagulation.
- Thrombolysis.

Anticoagulation

Further emboli should be prevented (patients with a pulmonary embolism have a 30% chance of developing further emboli). Intravenous heparin is administered:

- Bolus: 10 000 IU.
- Continuous infusion: 400–600 IU/kg daily.

Oral anticoagulants are given after 48 hours, and heparin is reduced. Oral anticoagulants are continued for between 6 weeks and 6 months.

Thrombolysis

Thrombolysis is indicated in patients who are haemodynamically unstable (e.g. hypotensive). It is possible to break down thrombi by:

- Intravenous streptokinase 250 000 IU infusion over 30 minutes.
- Intravenous streptokinase 100 000 IU hourly for up to 24 hours.

Surgery is performed only on massive pulmonary emboli in patients who fail to respond to thrombolysis.

Prevention

This is by avoidance of deep vein thromboses:

- Early mobilization of patients after operation.
- Use of tight elastic stockings.

Fig. 7.29 Pulmonary hyp

Aetiology	Vas
Cardiac disease	Pre
Hypoxia	Cap
Fibrosis	Pos fail
Miscellaneous	
Idiopathic (primary)	

The increase in va interest in respiratory to:

- Chronic hypoxia.
- Obstruction of pul
- Pulmonary fibrosis

Chronic hypoxia

Chronic airflow obs altitude can lead to seen in Pickwickian hypertension is cause ated with gross obesity fibrosis occurs, the co

Obstruction of pulmo

This is seen in primar rare condition of unkn seen in women aged may be familial.

Pulmonary fibrosis

Early changes of pulm muscular in type and of pulmonary arterie with irreversible incr resistance.

The other causes (those due to increase and increased pulmo cardiac and are not co

Pathology

Effects of pulmonary

- Enlarged proximal
- Right ventricular h
- Right arterial dilata
- Necrotizing arteriti

Clinical features

Features change during the progression of ARDS. Patients with ARDS present with:

- Tachypnoea, often unexplained.
- Dyspnoea.
- Pulmonary oedema – fine crackles throughout both lung fields.
- Arterial hypoxaemia, refractory to oxygen therapy.

Chest radiography shows bilateral diffuse shadowing.

Management

- Treat underlying condition and provide supportive measures.
- Treat as for pulmonary oedema: the aim is to achieve a negative fluid balance.
- Provide cardiovascular support and mechanical ventilation (e.g. positive end-expiratory pressure (PEEP)).
- PEEP prevents the alveolae from collapsing during expiration. However, low tidal volume ventilation is used to prevent overstretching the alveoli, which can worsen the lung injury. Also, ventilation in the prone position has been shown to be beneficial to ARDS patients, as ventilation is more evenly distributed throughout the lung.
- Non-ventilatory management such as the use of inhaled vasodilators (e.g. nitric oxide, prostacyclin) have been shown to improve the $\dot{V}/\dot{Q}$ matching in ARDS patients. Steroids have also been shown to be beneficial, especially in the late stages of ARDS as they can dampen down the inflammation and also have antifibrotic properties.
- The use of surfactant is highly beneficial in infant respiratory distress syndrome but there is no clear evidence of any benefit in ARDS.

Prognosis

Prognosis is dependent upon the cause, but the overall mortality is greater than 50%. Of that 50%, 9/10 will die from septic shock and the remaining 1/10 from a fat embolism.

Prognosis is poor in the elderly.

Death is caused by cardiac arrhythmias with sepsis, usually from Gram-negative organisms.

Embolism, haemorrhage and infarction

Vascular disease of the lungs can be caused by:

- Vessel obstruction.
- Vessel wall damage.
- Intravascular pressure variations.

Obstruction: pulmonary embolism (PE)

An embolus is an abnormal mass of material that is transported in the bloodstream from one part of the circulation to another and which impacts finally in the lumen of a vessel that has a calibre too small to allow passage. The end result of an embolus derived from venous thrombus is impaction in the pulmonary arterial tree. Most thrombi originate in the deep veins of the calf or pelvis.

This is a common condition: incidence of pulmonary emboli at autopsy has been reported to be 12%. Pulmonary emboli rarely have a cardiac cause and are very rare in children.

Predisposing factors

Predisposing factors are:

- Immobilization (e.g. prolonged bed rest, long-haul flights).
- In women, the oral contraceptive pill – minor risk factor, increased by cigarette smoking.
- Malignancy, especially of pancreas, uterus, breast and stomach.
- Cardiac failure.
- Chronic pulmonary disease.
- Postoperative recovery.
- Fractures of the pelvis or lower limb.
- Hypercoagulable states (e.g. pregnancy).

Clinical features

Common symptoms are:

- Dyspnoea.
- Tachypnoea.

Mrs Clarke complained of sudden-onset chest pain following total hip replacement surgery. In light of her recent surgery, pulmonary embolism was suspected. A plain chest X-ray showed no abnormality; however, a ventilation : perfusion scan showed a perfusion defect in her right lung consistent with a pulmonary embolism.

- Pleuritic pain.
- Apprehension.
- Tachycardia.
- Cough.
- Haemoptysis.
- Leg pain/clinical DVT.

Symptoms are related to the size of the embolus and the corresponding volume of lung tissue deprived of blood in addition to the presence or absence of congestion in the pulmonary circulation at the time of impaction.

Pulmonary embolism can be classified as massive, moderate or small.

Massive pulmonary embolism

A massive pulmonary embolism is a clinical emergency. The embolus is typically derived from a thrombus that occludes a long venous segment in the lower limb. The calibre of the main pulmonary arteries is greater than the iliac and femoral veins; therefore, thrombi must loosely bundle together to block the pulmonary arteries (as seen in a saddle embolus, which occurs at the bifurcation of the left and right pulmonary arteries).

Within normal human lung, occlusion of more than 50% of the pulmonary vascular bed is necessary for a massive pulmonary embolism to prove fatal.

Clinical features

This is a clinical emergency presenting as sudden-onset severe chest pain and dyspnoea. Often onset occurs when straining during defecation. Classically, a massive pulmonary embolism occurs a week or more after operation.

There are signs of shock: tachycardia, low blood pressure. Right ventricular heave, gallop rhythm and a prominent a-wave in the jugular venous pulse may also be noted.

Sudden death can occur.

Small or medium-sized pulmonary embolism

Moderate pulmonary embolism is caused by occlusion of a lobar or segmental artery. Perfusion of a segment may be reduced, producing an area of localized necrosis.

An area of necrosis secondary to ischaemia is known as an infarct.

Clinical features

Pulmonary infarction presents with sudden-onset pleuritic chest pain. Cough with haemoptysis and dyspnoea are other symptoms.

Multiple microemboli

Multiple small emboli can occlude arterioles but this process is usually clinically silent. Gradual occlusion of the pulmonary arterial bed leads to pulmonary hypertension.

This is a rare condition characterized by exertional dyspnoea, tiredness and syncope. Basal crackles are heard on auscultation.

Other forms of emboli

Fat embolism

Fat embolism results from massive injury to subcutaneous fat or fracture of bones containing fatty marrow. Globules of lipid enter the torn vessels.

Air embolism

Air embolism arises during childbirth or abortion or after chest wall injury. These microemboli can cause tiny infarcts in several organs.

Tumour embolism

Tumour cells, like other particulate matter, become trapped in the pulmonary capillary bed. This is an important mechanism in the development of metastases.

Amniotic fluid embolism

Amniotic fluid embolism can occur during childbirth or abortion, and may be fatal. Small fragments of trophoblast are commonly found in lungs of pregnant women at autopsy, but do not cause any symptoms.

Investigations in suspected pulmonary emboli

- Chest radiography is usually unremarkable, but valuable in excluding other causes.
- Electrocardiography may show signs of right ventricular strain (deep S waves in lead I, Q waves in lead III, and inverted T waves in lead III).
- Arterial blood gases show arterial hypoxaemia and hypocapnia.
- D-dimers are degradation products of cross-linked fibrin, and are released into the circulation when a thrombus begins to dissolve. Detection of

D-dimers in the blood is not diagnostic for a PE as D-dimers can be elevated in infection, malignancy and post-surgery. However, a negative test result makes the presence of an acute PE unlikely and therefore further investigation in low-risk patients may be unnecessary.

- Radioisotope ventilation : perfusion scans demonstrate ventilated areas of lung and filling defects on the corresponding perfusion scans; these are assessed on the basis of probability of pulmonary embolism (see Ch. 11). In non-diagnostic scans, pulmonary angiography should be performed in the acutely ill patient or leg ultrasound if the patient is stable.

Treatment

Treatment is based on:

- Supportive measures (analgesia, oxygen, etc.).
- Anticoagulation.
- Thrombolysis.

Anticoagulation

Further emboli should be prevented (patients with a pulmonary embolism have a 30% chance of developing further emboli). Intravenous heparin is administered:

- Bolus: 10 000 IU.
- Continuous infusion: 400–600 IU/kg daily.

Oral anticoagulants are given after 48 hours, and heparin is reduced. Oral anticoagulants are continued for between 6 weeks and 6 months.

Thrombolysis

Thrombolysis is indicated in patients who are haemodynamically unstable (e.g. hypotensive). It is possible to break down thrombi by:

- Intravenous streptokinase 250 000 IU infusion over 30 minutes.
- Intravenous streptokinase 100 000 IU hourly for up to 24 hours.

Surgery is performed only on massive pulmonary emboli in patients who fail to respond to thrombolysis.

Prevention

This is by avoidance of deep vein thromboses:

- Early mobilization of patients after operation.
- Use of tight elastic stockings.
- Leg exercises.
- Prophylactic anticoagulation.

Pulmonary infarction

Less than 10% of pulmonary emboli cause infarction within the lung. Lung infarcts are more common in the lower lobes; infarction is less common in the lungs than in other organs because of the lungs' dual blood supply.

Pulmonary infarction is usually a consequence of a moderate pulmonary embolism. Pulmonary infarction is rare in young people.

Predisposing factors

Predisposing factors for infarction include:

- Rise in pulmonary venous pressure.
- Mitral stenosis or left ventricular failure.
- Bronchial occlusion.
- Pleural effusion.
- Infection.

Pathology

A wedge-shaped section of the lung downstream from the blockage becomes necrotic. The base of the wedge is situated toward the pleural aspect of the lung. Pleural inflammation over the infarcted area is common. Organization of pulmonary infarcts proceeds rapidly.

Clinical features

Clinical features include sudden-onset pleuritic chest pain and dyspnoea.

Investigations

Blood tests show increases in erythrocyte sedimentation rate and lactate dehydrogenase (LDH) levels. Polymorphonuclear leucocytosis is present.

Arterial blood gas measurement reveals hypoxaemia, but normal PCO_2.

Ventilation : perfusion scans show mismatching.

Pulmonary hypertension and vascular sclerosis

Pulmonary hypertension occurs when blood pressure in the pulmonary circulation exceeds 30 mmHg (Fig. 7.29).

Pulmonary hypertension can be caused by:

- Increased vascular resistance in the pulmonary circulation.
- Increased pulmonary venous pressure.
- Increased pulmonary blood flow.

Fig. 7.29 Pulmonary hypertension

Aetiology	Vascular lesion
Cardiac disease	Precapillary (e.g. left-to-right shunt)
Hypoxia	Capillary (e.g. hypoxia)
Fibrosis	Postcapillary (e.g. left ventricular failure)
Miscellaneous	
Idiopathic (primary)	

The increase in vascular resistance is of most interest in respiratory medicine. This can occur due to:

- Chronic hypoxia.
- Obstruction of pulmonary vessels.
- Pulmonary fibrosis.

Chronic hypoxia

Chronic airflow obstruction or living at high altitude can lead to chronic hypoxia. This is also seen in Pickwickian syndrome where pulmonary hypertension is caused by poor respiration associated with gross obesity. Because insignificant intimal fibrosis occurs, the condition is largely reversible.

Obstruction of pulmonary vessels

This is seen in primary pulmonary hypertension, a rare condition of unknown aetiology, predominantly seen in women aged 20–30 years. The condition may be familial.

Pulmonary fibrosis

Early changes of pulmonary vasculature are initially muscular in type and reversible. Obliterative fibrosis of pulmonary arteries and arterioles occurs later, with irreversible increases in pulmonary vascular resistance.

The other causes of pulmonary hypertension (those due to increased pulmonary venous pressure and increased pulmonary blood flow) are primarily cardiac and are not considered here.

Pathology

Effects of pulmonary hypertension include:

- Enlarged proximal pulmonary arteries.
- Right ventricular hypertrophy.
- Right arterial dilatation.
- Necrotizing arteritis.

Clinical features

Clinical features are as follows:

- Symptoms of the underlying cause.
- Chest pain and exertional dyspnoea.
- Syncope and fatigue.
- Prominent a-wave in jugular venous pulse.
- Right ventricular heave.
- Loud pulmonary component to second heart sound.
- Midsystolic ejection murmur.

Investigations

When investigating pulmonary hypertension, a possible cause should be sought.

A full blood count may show secondary polycythaemia. Chest radiography may reveal right ventricular enlargement, pulmonary artery dilatation, or oligaemic peripheral lung fields.

Electrocardiography may indicate right ventricular hypertrophy, right-axis deviation, a prominent R wave in V_1, or inverted T waves in the right precordial leads.

Radioisotope lung scans and echocardiography may also be useful.

Treatment

Treatment is dependent upon cause. Primary pulmonary hypertension is treated with anticoagulation therapy.

If the underlying cause of hypertension is untreatable, the patient will progress to cor pulmonale and death. Continuous oxygen therapy is beneficial in patients with cor pulmonale. Diuretics are used to treat fluid overload.

Heart–lung transplantation is recommended in young patients.

Prognosis is poor: 5-year survival rate is 40%.

Cor pulmonale

Cor pulmonale is a major complication of pulmonary hypertension. It is defined as right heart failure secondary to lung disease and occurs as a result of any disorder that leads to pulmonary hypertension. Of most interest here is its presence in lung disease. As noted above, lung disease that causes chronic hypoxia may lead to pulmonary hypertension and therefore cor pulmonale. The main respiratory diseases associated with cor pulmonale are:

- COPD.
- Severe, chronic asthma.
- Bronchiectasis.

- Pulmonary emboli.
- Pulmonary fibrosis.

The principal signs are those of the underlying disease in addition to oedema, raised JVP and atrial gallop rhythm. Arterial blood gases show hypoxaemia with or without hypercapnia.

DISORDERS OF THE LUNG INTERSTITIUM

The interstitial lung diseases are a diverse group of over 200 different lung diseases. They all affect the lung interstitium, i.e. the space between the alveolar epithelium and capillary endothelium (see Fig. 3.12, p. 31) and their pathology can be broadly classed as either granulomatous (e.g. sarcoid) or fibrosis (e.g. idiopathic fibrosing lung disease). Aetiology is variable but they all present in a similar fashion, typically with shortness of breath and chest X-ray shadows. Though separately each disease is rare, collectively they affect 1/2000 of the population. Outcome varies between patients and disease, but pulmonary fibrosis represents the common, irreversible end stage of interstitial lung disease.

Confusion may arise over terminology. To clarify, the term Diffuse Parenchymal Lung Disease (DPLD) may be used interchangeably with interstitial lung disease but not with fibrosing or granulomatous lung disease. This is because fibrosis and granulomas can occur in conditions other than interstitial lung disease. Additional synonyms are mentioned under each condition.

Some of the most important of the interstitial lung diseases are discussed below.

Pulmonary fibrosis

Pulmonary fibrosis is the end result of many respiratory diseases (Fig. 7.30) and is characterized by scar tissue in the lungs which decreases lung compliance, i.e. the lungs become stiffer.

The pathogenesis of pulmonary fibrosis is complex, involving many factors (Fig. 7.31). The main features are:

- A lesion affecting the alveolar-capillary basement membrane.
- Cellular infiltration and thickening by collagen of the interstitium of the alveolar wall.
- Fibroblasts proliferate leading to further collagen deposition.

The end stage is characterized by a honeycomb lung, a non-specific condition in which cystic spaces develop in fibrotic lungs with compensatory dilatation of unaffected neighbouring bronchioles.

Note from Figure 7.31 that the initial injury to the alveolar-capillary basement membrane may be caused by several different mechanisms. Some (e.g. dusts) are considered below.

Clinical features

Patients become progressively breathless and develop a dry, non-productive cough. On examination, lung

The end stage of chronic interstitial lung disease is termed honeycomb lung.

Fig. 7.30 Causes of pulmonary fibrosis

Dusts		Inhalants	Infection	Iatrogenic causes	Other causes
Mineral	Biological				
coal	avian protein	oxygen	postpneumonic infection	cytotoxic drugs	sarcoidosis
silica	*Actinomyces*	sulphur dioxide	tuberculosis	non-cytotoxics	connective-tissue disease
asbestos	*Aspergillus*	nitrogen dioxide	—	radiation	chronic pulmonary oedema

Fig. 7.31 Pathogenesis of pulmonary fibrosis. Macrophages can be activated by several factors (e.g. soluble immune complexes and sensitized T lymphocytes), resulting in the release of various cytokines leading to fibrosis. (From Kumar & Clark 1994, with permission of Baillière Tindall.)

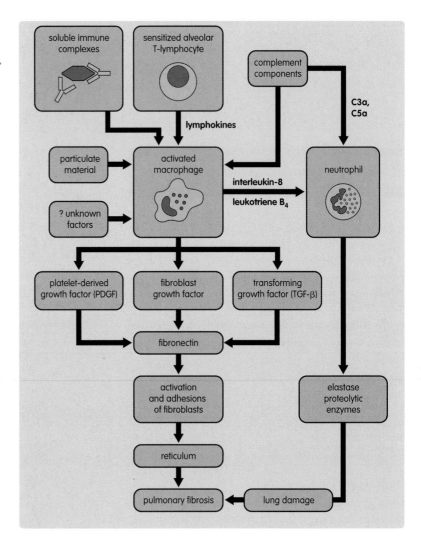

expansion is reduced and end-inspiratory crackles are heard.

Investigations

Chest X-ray may show fine reticular, nodular or reticulonodular infiltration in the basal areas. High-resolution CT (HRCT) or biopsy may be used to aid diagnosis. Lung function tests demonstrate a restrictive pattern along with a decreased transfer factor.

The pneumoconioses

The pneumoconioses are a group of disorders caused by inhalation of mineral or biological dusts. The incidence is decreasing as working conditions continue to improve.

Four types of reaction occur:

- Inert (e.g. simple coal-worker's pneumoconiosis).
- Fibrous (e.g. asbestosis).
- Allergic (e.g. extrinsic allergic alveolitis).
- Neoplastic (e.g. mesothelioma).

Distribution of lung disease depends on the dust involved: particles measuring less than 2–3 μm in diameter reach the distal alveoli.

Coal-worker's pneumoconiosis

The incidence of coal-worker's pneumoconiosis is related to total dust exposure: it is highest in men who work at the coal face. Two syndromes exist: simple pneumoconiosis and an advanced form, progressive massive fibrosis.

Simple pneumoconiosis

Simple pneumoconiosis is the commonest type of pneumoconiosis, reflecting coal dust deposition within the lung. It is asymptomatic and diagnosis is made on the basis of small round opacities in the upper zone on chest X-rays. Those with severe disease may go on to develop progressive massive fibrosis.

Progressive massive fibrosis

In progressive massive fibrosis, large, round fibrotic nodules measuring more than 10 mm in diameter are seen, usually in the upper lobes. Scarring is present. Nodules may show central liquefaction and become infected by tuberculosis. The associated emphysema is always severe.

Symptoms include dyspnoea, cough and sputum production (which may be black as cavitating lesions rupture). Lung function tests show a mixed restrictive and obstructive pattern.

The disease may progress once exposure has ceased (unlike simple coal-worker's pneumoconiosis) and there is no specific treatment.

Caplan's syndrome

Caplan's syndrome is the association of coal-worker's pneumoconiosis and rheumatoid arthritis.

Rounded lesions, measuring 0.5–5.0 cm in diameter, are seen on X-ray.

Asbestosis

Asbestosis is diffuse pulmonary fibrosis caused by the inhalation of asbestos, a mixture of silicates of iron, nickel, magnesium, aluminium and cadmium mined from the ground. In the UK exposure is most likely to occur during building renovations as in the past asbestos was used in housing materials such as insulation. Therefore occupations such as plumbers, electricians and builders are at high risk of exposure.

Several types of asbestos exist: serpentine fibres which do not cause pulmonary disease and amphibole fibres that do. The most important type of amphibole asbestos is crocidolite (blue asbestos), a straight fibre 50 μm long and 1–2 μm wide that cannot be cleared by the immune system. Fibres remain in the lung indefinitely and become coated in iron (haemosiderin) to form the classical drumstick shaped asbestos bodies.

Histology shows asbestos bodies and features of pulmonary fibrosis, affecting the lower lobes more commonly.

You might be forgiven for thinking that asbestosis is yet another synonym. But it does not simply mean exposure to asbestos (this in itself may not cause symptoms), nor is it a synonym for pleural plaques (you can have asbestosis with or without plaques), and mesothelioma is different again (see below).

A considerable time lag, sometimes as long as 20–40 years, exists between exposure and disease development. The first clinical symptoms are dyspnoea and a dry cough; signs include clubbing. Bilateral end-inspiratory crackles indicate significant diffuse pulmonary fibrosis. No treatment is available.

Exposure to asbestos is a risk factor for mesothelioma.

Extrinsic allergic alveolitis

Hypersensitivity pneumonitis is also known as extrinsic allergic alveolitis. The condition is a widespread diffuse inflammatory reaction caused by a type III hypersensitivity reaction and results from the individual being already sensitized to the inhaled antigen. Antigens that can cause allergic lung disease include:

- Mouldy hay (e.g. farmer's lung).
- Bird faeces (e.g. in bird fancier's lung).
- Cotton fibres (e.g. byssinosis).
- Sugar cane fibres (e.g. bagassosis).

Neutrophils infiltrate small airways and alveolar walls after antigen exposure. Lymphocytes and macrophages then infiltrate, leading to the development of non-caseating granulomas, which may resolve or organize leading to pulmonary fibrosis.

Clinical features consist of cough, shortness of breath, fever and malaise that occur acutely several hours after exposure to antigen. Onset is more insidious in long-term exposure to small amounts. Coarse end-inspiratory crackles can be heard on auscultation.

Investigations include polymorphonuclear leucocyte count, precipitating antibodies (evidence of exposure not disease), nodular shadowing on chest X-ray, lung function tests showing a restrictive pattern and bronchoalveolar lavage.

A 32-year-old pigeon fancier presented with a long-standing history of cough and flu-like symptoms, starting a few hours after tending his pigeons. Although chest X-ray was normal, a high-resolution CT scan showed changes consistent with extrinsic allergic alveolitis caused by inhalation of pigeon faeces. The chest physician had to use forceful persuasion to convince the pigeon fancier to give up his hobby, but after selling his pigeons his symptoms resolved.

History taking in these diseases should include a detailed evaluation of systemic features such as fever, rashes, eye signs, etc.

Most diseases will regress once the patient is prevented from further exposure to the antigen. Corticosteroids may speed recovery but do not alter the ultimate level of lung function. High-resolution CT scans can detect disease in patients with normal chest X-rays.

Sarcoidosis

Sarcoidosis is a multisystem granulomatous disorder of unknown aetiology. Pulmonary involvement is common in sarcoidosis where non-caseating granulomas form in the lung. Granulomas show infiltration of Th1 lymphocytes and monocytes/macrophages which fuse to form multinucleated epithelioid cells. These usually heal, leading to spontaneous remission, but in 10–20% the disease progresses to interstitial fibrosis.

Women are more likely to develop the condition, which has a peak incidence in patients aged 20–40 years. Prevalence in the UK is 19 : 100 000. A geographical distribution shows that it is common in the USA and rare in Japan. The course of the disease is more severe in American blacks.

Clinical features

The presentation of sarcoidosis depends on the organ involved, but greater than 90% of patients have pulmonary involvement causing dyspnoea, dry cough and chest pain. Non-specific signs include lymphadenopathy, fever, fatigue and weight loss. Involvement of other systems may cause rash (erythema nodosum or lupus pernio), arthralgia and uveitis. More infrequently, involvement of the central nervous system may cause cranial nerve palsies, and involvement of the heart, cor pulmonale.

Signs and symptoms of hypercalcaemia may be present.

If asymptomatic (30% of patients), sarcoidosis may be first detected on a routine chest X-ray.

Investigations

Chest X-ray shows:

- Bilateral hilar lymphadenopathy.
- Reticular shadows typically in upper lobes.

Chest radiographs are used to stage the disease (see Fig. 7.32), which reflects prognosis. Staging does not necessarily reflect disease progression; for example, stage III can develop without a patient ever having stage I disease. CT reveals granulomas but is not required if typical chest X-ray changes are present.

Biopsy of lung lesions by bronchoscopy shows non-caseating epitheliod cell granulomas. Granulomas are seen on biopsy of other affected sites such as lymph nodes.

Full blood count can show mild normochromic normocytic anaemia and raised erythrocyte sedimentation rate. Cells in the granuloma secrete vitamin D_3 (causing hypercalcaemia) and angiotensin-converting enzyme. Though serum angiotensin-converting enzyme (ACE) can be twice the upper limit of normal it is of no diagnostic value because it may be raised in other diseases. Serum ACE may be used to monitor the response to treatment.

In the Kveim test an intradermal injection of sarcoid lymph node tissue is given to the patient. A small papule, 3–8 mm in diameter seen 2–3 days after the injection, is diagnostic of sarcoidosis. The Kveim test is no longer performed because of infection risk.

Treatment

If the patient has hilar lymphadenopathy and no lung involvement, then no treatment is required.

Staging of sarcoidosis by chest radiographs					
Stage	0	I	II	III	IV
Chest radiograph					
Chest X-ray changes	normal chest X-ray	bilateral hilar lymphadenopathy	bilateral hilar lymphadenopathy and pulmonary infiltration	pulmonary infiltration without bilateral hilar lymphadenopathy	pulmonary fibrosis
% of patients entering spontaneous remission		55–90%	40–70%	10–20%	0%

Fig. 7.32 The staging of sarcoidosis by chest radiographs.

If infiltration has occurred for more than 6 weeks, treat with corticosteroids (20–40 mg per day for 4–6 weeks, then reduced dose for up to 1 year).

Prognosis

Prognosis is dependent on disease stage. Mortality is less than 5% in UK Caucasians and approximately 10% in Afro-Americans. If shadowing is present on chest radiographs for more than 2 years, the risk of fibrosis increases.

Idiopathic pulmonary fibrosis

Also known as fibrosing alveolitis or cryptogenic fibrosing alveolitis, idiopathic pulmonary fibrosis is a rare, progressive chronic pulmonary fibrosis of unknown aetiology. It has a peak incidence in patients aged 45–65 years.

Clinical features

Clinical features of idiopathic pulmonary fibrosis include progressive breathlessness and a dry cough. Fatigue and considerable weight loss can occur. There is progression to cyanosis, respiratory failure, pulmonary hypertension and cor pulmonale over time.

Clubbing occurs in two-thirds of patients; chest expansion is reduced and bilateral, fine, end-inspiratory crackles are heard on auscultation.

> Interstitial lung diseases provide an opportunity for the examiner's favourite – questions about clubbing. Note that clubbing occurs in idiopathic fibrosing alveolitis and asbestosis but not in other interstitial diseases.

Pathology

The alveolar walls are thickened because of fibrosis, predominantly in the subpleural regions of the lower lobes. An increased number of chronic inflammatory cells are in the alveoli and interstitium. This pattern is termed 'usual interstitial pneumonitis' and is a progressive condition.

Patterns of disease also include:

- Desquamative interstitial pneumonitis.
- Bronchiolitis obliterans.

Idiopathic pulmonary fibrosis has been reported with a number of other conditions: connective-tissue disorders, coeliac disease, ulcerative colitis and renal tubular acidosis.

Investigations

Several investigations are made:

- Transbronchial or open lung biopsy to confirm histological diagnosis.
- CT scan.
- Blood gases may show arterial hypoxaemia.
- Full blood count may show raised erythrocyte sedimentation rate.
- Lung function test shows a restrictive pattern.
- Bronchoalveolar lavage shows increased numbers of neutrophils.
- Autoantibody tests.
- Antinuclear factor is positive in one-third of patients. Rheumatoid factor is positive in one-half of patients.

Prognosis

Of patients with the condition, 50% die within 4–5 years.

Treatment

About 50% of patients respond to immunosuppression. Combined therapy is recommended with:

- Prednisolone 0.5 mg/kg daily for 1 month and then tapered.
- Azathioprine (2–3 mg/kg).

Cyclophosphamide may be substituted for azathioprine.

Single lung transplantation may be attempted where necessary.

Supportive treatment includes oxygen therapy.

Diffuse pulmonary haemorrhage syndromes

Goodpasture's syndrome

Goodpasture's syndrome is characterized by glomerulonephritis and respiratory symptoms. The syndrome is driven by a type II hypersensitivity reaction whereby IgG autoantibodies to glomerular basement membrane attach to the glomerulus to cause glomerulonephritis, but can also cross-react with alveolar basement membrane to cause pulmonary haemorrhage. The patient complains of haemoptysis, haematuria and anaemia. Treatment is by corticosteroids or plasmapheresis to remove anti-bodies. The course of the disease is variable: some patients resolve completely, others proceed to renal failure.

Idiopathic pulmonary haemosiderosis

Idiopathic pulmonary haemosiderosis is a rare condition, typically occurring in children aged under 7 years, causing haemoptysis, cough and dyspnoea. An association with sensitivity to cow's milk has been suggested. Treatment is by corticosteroids and azathioprine. Prognosis is poor.

Pulmonary eosinophilia

Pulmonary eosinophilia is a group of syndromes characterized by abnormally high levels of eosinophils in the blood, or in the case of acute eosinophilic pneumonia, in lung lavage fluid. The severity of these diseases can range from mild to fatal (Fig. 7.33).

Bronchiolitis obliterans

In bronchiolitis obliterans, characteristic histological appearance shows:

- Polypoid masses of organizing inflammatory exudate.
- Granulation tissue extending from alveoli to bronchioles.

Aetiology is unknown, although an association with a number of clinical conditions exists:

- Viral infections (e.g. respiratory syncytial virus).
- Aspiration.
- Inhalation of toxic fumes.
- Extrinsic allergic alveolitis.
- Pulmonary fibrosis.
- Collagen or vascular disorders.

Bronchiolitis obliterans is sensitive to corticosteroid treatment.

Collagen disorders and vascular disorders

Rheumatoid diseases

The respiratory system is affected in 10–15% of patients with rheumatoid disease. Patients characteristically have severe seropositive rheumatoid disease. Diffuse pulmonary fibrosis may occur as can bronchiolitis obliterans, follicular bronchiolitis,

Fig. 7.33 The causes of pulmonary eosinophilia

Disease	Aetiology	Symptoms	Blood eosinophils (%)	Multisystem involvement	Duration	Outcome
simple	passage of parasitic larvae through lung	mild	10	none	<1 month	good
prolonged	unknown	mild/moderate	<20	none	>1 month	good
asthmatic	often type 1 hypersensitivity to *Aspergillus*	moderate/severe	5-20	none	years	fair
tropical	hypersensitivity reaction to filarial infestation	moderate/severe	>20	none	years	fair
hyper-eosinophilic syndrome	unknown	severe	>20	always	months/years	poor
Churg–Strauss syndrome	possibly immune complex vasculitis	severe	>20	always	months/years	poor/fair

pleural fibrosis and small plural effusions. Rheumatoid nodules are rare in the lung.

Caplan's syndrome is discussed above (p. 147).

Wegener's granulomatosis

Wegener's granulomatosis is a rare, necrotizing vasculitis of unknown aetiology affecting small arteries and veins. It classically involves the upper and lower respiratory tract and the kidneys (glomerulonephritis). Mucosal thickening and ulceration occur, producing the clinical features of rhinorrhoea, cough, haemoptysis and dyspnoea.

If untreated, mortality after 2 years is 93%, but the disease responds well to high-dose prednisolone and cyclophosphamide.

Systemic lupus erythematosus

In patients with systemic lupus erythematosus (SLE), respiratory involvement is usually in the form of pleurisy, with or without an effusion, and pulmonary fibrosis is rare.

Desquamative interstitial pneumonitis

Desquamative interstitial pneumonitis is found in patients with fibrosing alveolitis. It is more diffuse than usual interstitial pneumonitis. A proliferation of macrophages in the alveolar air spaces occurs, along with interstitial thickening by mononuclear inflammatory cells. Lymphoid tissue and a small amount of collagen are sometimes present.

Desquamative interstitial pneumonitis has a distinctly uniform histological pattern. The alveolar walls show relatively little fibrosis.

Corticosteroids may be beneficial, and prognosis is good.

Alveolar proteinosis

Alveolar proteinosis, also known as alveolar lipoproteinosis, is a rare condition of unknown aetiology and pathogenesis. Clinically dyspnoea and cough, and rarely haemoptysis and chest pain, result. Alveolar proteinosis is associated with a high incidence of concomitant fungal infections and may complicate other interstitial disease.

The course of the disease is variable, but the majority of patients enjoy spontaneous remission.

NEOPLASTIC DISEASE OF THE LUNG

Bronchial carcinoma

Bronchial carcinoma accounts for 95% of all primary tumours of the lung and is the commonest malignant tumour in the western world. Bronchogenic carcinoma affects men more than women (M : F ratio, 3.5 : 1) but incidence is rising in women and it is now the commonest cancer in both sexes. Typically patients are aged 40–70 years at presentation; only 2–3% occur in younger patients.

Aetiology

Risk factors are summarized in Figure 7.34. Cigarette smoking is the largest contributory factor:

- It is related to the amount smoked, duration and tar content. 20% of smokers will develop lung cancer.
- The rise in incidence of lung cancer correlates closely to the increase in smoking over the past century.
- In non-smokers, the incidence is 3–5 cases per 100 000. In the UK, there are 100 deaths per 100 000 smokers per year.

Fig. 7.34 Risk factors in lung cancer	
Factor	Relative risk
non-smoker	1
smoker, 1–2 packs/day	42
ex-smoker	2 to 10
passive smoke exposure	1.5 to 2
asbestos exposure	5
asbestos plus tobacco	90

(After Criner & D'Alonzo 1999, by permission of Fence Creek Publishing.)

- The risk in those who give up smoking decreases with time.
- Passive smoking also increases risk.

Environmental and occupational factors include:

- Radon released from granite rock.
- Asbestos.
- Air pollution (e.g. beryllium emissions).

Histological types

There are four main histological types of bronchogenic carcinoma:

- Non-small-cell carcinomas (70%):
  - Squamous cell carcinoma (52%)
  - Adenocarcinoma (13%)
  - Large-cell carcinoma (5%).
- Small-cell carcinomas (30%).

The different types of tumour are summarized in Figure 7.35.

Tumours may occur as discrete or mixed histological patterns; the development from the initial malignant change to presentation is variable:

- Squamous cell carcinoma: 8 years.
- Adenocarcinoma: 15 years.
- Small-cell carcinoma: 3 years.

Squamous cell carcinoma

Squamous cell carcinoma arises from squamous epithelium in the large bronchi. A strong association

Fig. 7.35 Summary of tumour types				
	Non-small-cell tumours			Small cell
	Squamous cell tumour	Adeno-carcinoma	Large cell	
incidence (%)	52	13	5	30
male/female incidence	M>F	F>M	M>F	M>F
location	hilar	peripheral	peripheral/central	hilar
histological stain	keratin	mucin	–	–
relationship to smoking	high	low	high	high
growth rate	slow	medium	rapid	very rapid
metastasis	late	intermediate	early	very early
treatment		surgery		chemotherapy
prognosis		2-year survival = 50%		3 months if untreated; 1 year if treated

between cigarette smoking and squamous cell carcinoma exists. Males are affected most commonly, with a mean age at diagnosis of 57 years.

Squamous cell carcinomas are histologically well differentiated and are associated with keratinization. The cancer commonly produces a substance similar to parathyroid hormone (PTH) which leads to hypercalcaemia and bone destruction (see Fig. 7.37).

The major mass of the tumour may occur outside the bronchial cartilage and encircle the bronchial lumen, producing obstructive phenomena. The tumours are almost always hilar and are prone to massive necrosis and cavitation, with upper lobe lesions more likely to cavitate. Of squamous cell carcinomas, 13% show cavitation on chest radiographs. Peripheral lesions tend to be larger than those seen in adenocarcinomas.

If squamous carcinoma occurs in the apical portion of the lung, it may produce Pancoast's syndrome (see below).

Squamous cell carcinoma is the least likely type to metastasize and untreated it has the longest patient survival of any of the bronchogenic carcinomas.

Adenocarcinoma

Adenocarcinomas are most common in:

- Non-smoking elderly women.
- The Far East.

Adenocarcinomas are associated with diffuse pulmonary fibrosis and honeycomb lung. Bronchogenic tumours associated with occupational factors are mainly adenocarcinomas. 90% of adenocarcinomas occur between 40–69 years of age, with the mean age for diagnosis being 53.3 years. Two-thirds of adenocarcinomas are found peripherally. Usually, tumours measure more than 4 cm in diameter.

Adenocarcinoma arises from glandular cells such as mucus goblet cells, type II pneumocytes and Clara cells. Histologically, they are differentiated from other bronchogenic tumours by their glandular configuration and mucin production. The gland structure may be acinar or papillary.

Clinically, two growth patterns are seen:

- Discrete nodule in the periphery with pleural tethering (most common).
- Multifocal and bilateral diffuse tumour (so-called bronchoalveolar cell carcinoma).

As the tumour is commonly in the periphery, obstructive symptoms are rare, so the tumour tends to be clinically silent. Symptoms include coughing, haemoptysis, chest pain and weight loss. A wide range of paraneoplastic syndromes are seen (see below). Malignant cells are detected in the sputum in 50% of patients, and the commonest radiological presentation is a solitary peripheral pulmonary nodule, close to the pleural surface.

Resection is possible in a small proportion of cases; 5-year survival rate is less than 10%. Invasion of the pleura and mediastinal lymph nodes is common, as too is metastasis to the brain and bones.

Metastasis in the gastrointestinal tract, pancreas or ovaries must be excluded after having made a diagnosis.

Large-cell anaplastic tumour

Large-cell anaplastic tumours are diagnosed by a process of elimination. No clear-cut pattern of clinical or radiological presentation distinguishes them from other malignant lung tumours.

Under light microscopy, findings include:

- Pleomorphic cells with large, darkly staining nuclei.
- Prominent nucleoli, abundant cytoplasm and well-defined cell borders.
- Abundant mitoses.

Large-cell anaplastic tumours are variable in location, but are usually centrally located. Peripherally located lesions are larger than adenocarcinomas. The point of origin of the carcinoma influences symptomatic presentation of the disease: central lesions present earlier than peripheral lesions as they cause obstruction.

The tumour causes coughing, sputum production and haemoptysis. When a tumour occurs in a major airway, obstructive pneumonia can occur. Sputum

Adenocarcinoma of the lung is usually a peripheral tumour.

Large-cell anaplastic carcinomas lack features of differentiation.

Mr Thomas, a 54-year-old man who had smoked since his early teens, complained of a 4-week history of cough. Within the last week he had developed severe backache. A chest X-ray revealed a solitary mass near his right main bronchus from which a biopsy was taken on bronchoscopy. Squamous cell carcinoma was diagnosed on histology. Unfortunately, a bone scan revealed that the cancer had spread to Mr Thomas' spine and so only palliative care could be offered.

A middle-aged woman with small-cell carcinoma was noted to have hyponatraemia, resulting in fatigue, anorexia and headache. On investigation, this was found to be due to inappropriate production of vasopressin by her cancer, a typical endocrine disturbance in small-cell lung cancers.

cytology and bronchoscopy with bronchial biopsy make the diagnosis.

On electron microscopy, these tumours turn out to be poorly differentiated variants of squamous cell carcinoma and adenocarcinoma; they are extremely aggressive and destructive lesions. Early invasion of blood vessels and lymphatics occurs, and treatment is by surgical resection whenever possible.

Small-cell carcinoma

Small-cell carcinomas arise from endocrine cells – Kulchitsky cells, members of the amine precursor uptake decarboxylase (APUD) system.

The incidence of this carcinoma is directly related to cigarette consumption and it is considered to be a systemic disease. Small-cell carcinomas are the most aggressive malignancy of all the bronchogenic tumours.

Most small-cell anaplastic tumours originate in the large bronchi, and obstructive pneumonitis is frequently seen. Several histological subgroups of this carcinoma exist and all have:

- Cell size: 6–8 μm.
- High nucleus : cytoplasm ratio.
- Hyperchromatism of the nuclei.

When almost no cytoplasm is present, and the cells are compressed into an ovoid form, the neoplasm is called an oat-cell carcinoma. On radiography, the oat-cell carcinoma does not cavitate.

There is a high occurrence of paraneoplastic syndromes associated with this type of tumour, so presentation may be varied. The most frequent presenting complaint is coughing. Spread is rapid, and metastatic lesions may be the presenting sign. Small-cell carcinomas metastasize through the lymphatic route.

Chest radiography may help in diagnosis, although the diagnosis must be confirmed by histological or cytological means.

Prognosis is very poor, with a mean survival time for untreated patients with small-cell carcinoma of 7 weeks after diagnosis. Death is generally caused by metastatic disease.

Small-cell carcinoma is the only bronchial carcinoma that responds to chemotherapy.

Mixed tumours

A number of mixed tumour types exist that are commonly seen in resection material at autopsy.

Many pathologists base their diagnosis on the prominent cell type present because the predominant cell type predicts prognosis of the condition.

Clinical features

Features specific to the histological types have already been introduced above. There are no specific signs of bronchogenic carcinoma. Diagnosis always needs to be excluded in cigarette smokers who present with recurrent respiratory symptoms:

- Persistent cough – commonest presentation; may be productive if obstruction leads to infection.
- Haemoptysis – occurs at some stage in disease in 50%.
- Dyspnoea – rarely at presentation but occurs as disease progresses.
- Chest pain – often pleuritic, caused by obstructive changes.
- Wheezing – monophonic, due to obstruction.

Unexplained weight loss is also a common presenting complaint. Other symptoms may be present due to complications described below.

In 10–30% of patients finger clubbing is present on examination.

Complications

Local complications
Symptoms may be caused by:

- Ulceration of bronchus; occurs in up to 50% of patients and produces haemoptysis in varying degrees.
- Bronchial obstruction. The lumen of the bronchus becomes occluded; distal collapse and retention of secretions subsequently occur. This clinically causes dyspnoea, secondary infection and lung abscesses.
- Central necrosis. Carcinomas can outgrow their blood supply, leading to central necrosis. The main complication is then the development of a lung abscess.

Figure 7.36 summarizes the effects of local spread.

Pancoast's syndrome

Pancoast's syndrome can be caused by all types of bronchogenic carcinoma, although two-thirds originate from squamous cells. As the tumour grows outward from the pulmonary parenchymal apex, it encroaches on anatomical structures, including:

- Chest wall.
- Subpleural lymphatics.
- Sympathetic chain.

As noted above, Pancoast's tumour can affect the sympathetic chain, resulting in loss of sympathetic tone and an ipsilateral Horner's syndrome (mild ptosis, pupil constricted with no reaction to shading, and reduced sweating on ipsilateral side of the head and neck). Intractable shoulder pain occurs when the upper rib is involved. The subclavian artery and vein may become compressed. Destruction of the inferior trunk of the brachial plexus leads to pain in the ulnar nerve distribution and may lead to small-muscle wasting of the hand.

Pancoast's tumour is diagnosed by percutaneous needle aspiration of the tumour.

Metastatic complications

Local metastases to lymph nodes, bone, liver and adrenal glands occur.

Metastases to the brain present as:

- Change in personality.
- Epilepsy.
- Focal neurological lesion.

Paraneoplastic syndromes

Paraneoplastic syndromes (Fig. 7.37) cannot be explained by direct invasion of the tumour. They are caused by production by tumour cells of polypeptides

Fig. 7.36 Effects and symptoms of local spread

Site of spread	Symptoms
pleura/ribs	pain on respiration/pathological fractures
brachial plexus	shoulder pain and small muscle wasting of the hand
sympathetic ganglia	ipsilateral Horner's syndrome
recurrent laryngeal nerve	hoarse voice and bovine cough
superior vena cava	facial congestion; distended neck veins

Fig. 7.37 Paraneoplastic disorders associated with lung cancer

	Mechanism	Clinical features	Lung cancer association
SIADH	excess scretion of ADH	headache, nausea, muscle weakness, drowsiness, confusion, eventually coma	small cell
ectopic ACTH	adrenal hyperplasia and secretion of large amounts of cortisol	Cushings: polyuria, oedema, hypokalaemia, hypertension, increased pigmentation	small cell or carcinoid
hypercalcaemia	ectopic PTH secretion	lethargy, nausea, polyuria, eventually coma	squamous cell (but may be due to bone metastases)
hypertrophic pulmonary osteoarthropathy	unknown	digital clubbing and periosteal inflammation	adenocarcinoma, squamous cell
gonadotrophins	ectopic secretion	gynaecomastia, testicular atrophy	large cell

ACTH = adrenocorticotrophic hormone; ADH = antidiuretic hormone (vasopressin); PTH = parathyroid hormone; SIADH = syndrome of inappropriate antidiuretic hormone.

that mimic various hormones. Paraneoplastic syndromes are commonly associated with small-cell lung cancer.

Investigations

Investigations are performed to confirm diagnosis and assess tumour histology and spread.

Chest radiography

Good posteroanterior and lateral views are required. 70% of bronchial carcinomas arise centrally, and chest radiography demonstrates over 90% of carcinomas. The mass needs to be between 1–2 cm in size to be recognized reliably. Lobar collapse and pleural effusions may be present.

CT scan

CT scanning gives good visualization of the mediastinum and is good at identifying small lesions. Valuable to assess extent of tumour and the operability of the mass. Lymph nodes < 1.5 cm are pathological.

Scan should include brain, liver and adrenals to identify distant metastases.

Fibreoptic bronchoscopy

Confirms central lesion, assesses operability, and allows accurate cell type to be determined. Used to obtain cytological specimens. Mucus secretions plus sputum can be examined for presence of malignant cells.

If carcinoma involves the first 2 cm of either main bronchus the tumour is inoperable.

Transthoracic fine-needle aspiration biopsy

In transthoracic fine-needle aspiration biopsy, the needle is guided by X-ray or CT. Direct aspiration of peripheral lung lesions takes place through the chest wall; 25% of patients suffer pneumothorax due to the procedure.

Implantation metastases do not occur.

Staging

Small-cell and non-small-cell cancers are staged differently. Small-cell is staged as either limited or extensive whilst the TNM system (Fig. 7.38) is used for non-small-cell cancer.

Treatment

Surgery

The only treatment of any value in non-small-cell carcinoma is surgery; however, only 15% of cases are operable at diagnosis.

Surgery can only be performed after:

- Lung function tests show the patient has sufficient respiratory reserve.
- CT scan shows no evidence of metastases.

Radiation therapy

Treatment of choice if the tumour is inoperable. Good for slowly growing squamous carcinoma.

Radiation pneumonitis develops in 10–15% and radiation fibrosis occurs to some degree in all cases.

Chemotherapy

Only effective treatment for small-cell carcinoma, but is not undertaken with intent to cure. Platinum compounds can achieve good results.

Terminal care

Endoscopic therapy and transbronchial stenting are used to provide symptomatic relief in patients with terminal disease. Daily prednisolone (maximum

Fig. 7.38 Staging in non-small-cell lung cancer	
T1	<3 cm – no evidence of invasion proximal to a lobar brochus
T2	≥3 cm or any site involving pleura or hilum; within a lobar bronchus or at least 2 cm distal to the carina
T3	any size extending into the chest wall, diaphragm, pericardium (not involving great vessels etc.)
T4	inoperable tumour of any size with invasion of the mediastium or involving heart great vessels, trachea, oesophagus, vertebral body or carina or malignant pleural effusion

Regional lymph nodes		Distant metastases	
N0	no nodal involvement	M0	no metastases
N1	peribronchial and/or ipsilateral hilar nodes	M1	distant metastases
N2	ipsilateral mediastinal and sub-carinal lymph nodes		
N3	inoperable contralateral node involvement		

dose: 15 mg) may improve appetite. Opioid analgesia is given to control pain and laxatives should be prescribed to counteract the opioid side-effects. Candidiasis is a common treatable problem.

Both patient and relatives require counselling.

Prognosis

Overall prognosis is poor; only 6–8% survive 5 years and mean survival is less than 6 months.

Rarer types of lung tumours

Malignant tumours

Bronchoalveolar cell carcinoma

A distinctive type of adenocarcinoma occurring in the distal portions of the pulmonary parenchyma accounting for 3% of all primary neoplasms of lung. The carcinoma affects males and females equally and the incidence is not related to cigarette consumption.

Unifocal point of origin is within the lung with the major bulk of the tumour seen in the alveoli rather than the bronchi. The lesion grows very slowly and spreads by the bronchial route to implant on other portions of the respiratory epithelium. The lesion may be stable for 5–10 years.

Associated with profuse mucoid sputum production.

In the early stage, radiography may show a non-specific peripheral coin lesion. Diagnosis of the disease is based on histological examination of tissue obtained by transbronchial or open lung biopsy.

Surgical resection may be curative, although surgical intervention is useless once dissemination has occurred.

Bronchial carcinoid

Low-grade malignant tumour accounting for 1% of tumours found in the lungs. It affects males and females equally and presents < 40 years.

Bronchial carcinoids are locally invasive, highly vascular tumours that cause recurrent haemoptysis. The tumour grows slowly, eventually blocking a bronchus.

Rarely gives rise to the carcinoid syndrome and the 5-year survival is > 80%.

Malignant mesenchymal tumours (sarcomas) are extremely rare.

Primary pulmonary lymphomas

Rare tumours composed of small B lymphocytes arising from the bronchus- and bronchiole-associated lymphoid tissue. Monotypic immunoglobulin may be secreted into the blood.

Benign tumours

Adenomas

Arise from bronchial mucous glands. They present as polypoid or sessile lesions and symptoms are related to obstruction.

Benign mesenchymal tumours

Arise anywhere that mesenchyme occurs. The lesion is probably a hamartoma, which is a well-circumscribed round lesion (1–2 cm in diameter), composed of cartilage and found in the periphery of the lung. Rarely, the tumour arises from a major bronchus and presents as an isolated coin lesion on radiographs.

Metastatic malignancy to the lung

Metastases to the lung are a common clinical and radiological finding. Metastases are more likely to be multiple than solitary. Most haematogenous metastases are sharply circumscribed with smooth edges, and the appearance of multiple smoothly circumscribed nodules is highly suggestive of metastatic disease. Cavitation is unusual in metastatic lesions.

Solitary pulmonary metastases do occur as sarcomas of soft tissue or bone, carcinoma of the breast, colon and kidney.

Multinodular lung metastases may be of varying sizes (Fig. 7.39):

- Very large dimensions – cannonball pattern.
- Many small nodules – snowstorm pattern.

Fig. 7.39 Metastatic malignancy of lung and the resulting radiological appearance

Multinodular patterns		Solitary nodule
Cannonball	Snowstorm	
salivary gland	breast	breast
kidney	kidney	kidney
bowel	bladder	bowel
uterus/ovarian	thyroid	
testis	prostate	

DISEASES OF IATROGENIC ORIGIN

Drug-induced lung disease

Pulmonary disease caused by medication is a growing problem. The mechanisms of drug-induced lung damage are either immunological or cytotoxic and the type of adverse reaction can be either:

- Predictable if caused by a dose-related effect.
- Unpredictable if caused by the development of hypersensitivity reactions.

There are no specific clinical, functional or radiological findings in drug-induced pulmonary disease. The commonest symptoms include dyspnoea and cough (Fig. 7.40).

Examples of drug-induced lung diseases include:

- Bleomycin – the development of bleomycin-induced pulmonary disease is dose-dependent. Bleomycin causes oxygen-radical-induced lung damage. Incidence is approximately 3%, with a mortality rate of 1–2%.
- Amiodarone – a class III antiarrhythmic drug, which can cause fatal interstitial pneumonitis. Lung damage has its onset several months after commencement of amiodarone treatment. Incidence of toxicity is 1–2%. The condition responds well to corticosteroid treatment.

Fig. 7.40 Summary of pulmonary manifestations of adverse drug reactions

Adverse reaction	Examples
diffuse alveolar damage	bleomycin, methotrexate, amiodarone, radiotherapy
interstitial pneumonitis	methotrexate, busulfan, amiodarone, gold
eosinophilic pneumonia	bleomycin, naproxen, sulfasalazine
bronchiolitis obliterans	methotrexate, gold, mitomycin
pulmonary haemorrhage	amphotericin B, anticoagulants, hydralazine
pulmonary oedema	codeine, methadone, naloxone, salicylates
pleural effusions and fibrosis	amiodarone, hydralazine, bleomycin, bromocriptine

- β-blockers – are contraindicated in patients with asthma as they also block airway β receptors, thus precipitating bronchoconstriction.
- Aspirin – may induce asthma, either through decreased prostaglandin production or by increased leukotriene production. Recovery is usual on discontinuation of the drug.

Complications of radiotherapy

The lungs are very sensitive to radiation. Clinical effects depend on the dose given, volume of lung irradiated, and length of treatment. Pulmonary response to radiation is characterized by:

- Acute phase of radiation pneumonitis.
- Chronic phase of healing or fibrosis.

Acute radiation pneumonitis

Acute radiation pneumonitis is defined as an acute infiltrate precisely confined to the radiation area and occurring within 3 months of radiotherapy. Acute radiation pneumonitis rarely produces symptoms within the first month after therapy. Symptoms have an insidious onset and include non-productive cough, shortness of breath on exertion, and low-grade fever.

Diffuse alveolar damage occurs, consisting of a proteinaceous exudate of material in the alveolar air spaces associated with hyaline membranes, especially in alveolar ducts. Endothelial damage, loss of normal respiratory epithelium, and hyperplasia of type II pneumocytes also occur.

Radiation pneumonitis results in a restrictive lung defect, and corticosteroids should be given in the acute phase.

Chronic fibrosis

Acute radiation pneumonitis can resolve spontaneously or progress to pulmonary fibrosis. The chronic fibrosing state is usually asymptomatic. Proliferation and fragmentation of elastic fibres occurs and bronchiolitis obliterans and bronchial fibrosis may be present.

Chronic fibrosis is not precisely confined to irradiated areas.

Lung transplantation

Single lung transplantation is preferred to double transplantation because of donor availability.

Bilateral lung transplantation is required in infective conditions to prevent bacterial spill-over from a diseased lung to a single lung transplant.

Patients must have end-stage lung or pulmonary vascular disease with no other treatment options (Fig. 7.41).

Complications

The complications of lung transplantation are described in Figure 7.42.

Strategies for avoiding rejection

Lung transplantation does not require any significant degree of matching based on tissue type. The main criteria are compatibility of blood group and size match between organ and recipient.

Suppression of the immune system

All transplant patients require immunosuppression for life. This begins immediately before transplantation; drugs used include:

- Prednisolone.
- Azathioprine.
- Ciclosporin.

Large doses are given in the initial postoperative period. Lower maintenance doses are achieved after a few months. Rejection episodes are treated with high-dose intravenous corticosteroids.

Prognosis

1-year survival rates are 60–70%.

DISEASES OF THE PLEURA

Pleural effusions

A pleural effusion is the presence of fluid between the visceral and parietal pleura. Effusions can be categorized as transudative or exudative, depending on the protein concentration (Fig. 7.43). Transudative pleural effusions ($<30\,g/L$) occur as a result of an imbalance between hydrostatic and osmotic forces, for example in congestive cardiac failure (hydrothorax). Exudative pleural effusions ($>30\,g/L$) occur when local factors influencing pleural fluid formation and reabsorption are altered, specifically through injury or inflammation. Causes of each type of effusion are shown in Figure 7.44. Exudative effusions often occur as a complication of pneumonia; these are termed parapneumonic effusions.

Gross appearance

On examination, the pleural fluid may be clear and straw-coloured, turbid (signifying infection) or haemorrhagic. If a haemorrhagic effusion exists, neoplastic infiltration, pulmonary infarction and TB need to be excluded. Leading malignancies that have

Fig. 7.41 Indications and diseases treated by lung transplantation

Indications	Diseases treated by transplantation
age <60 years	pulmonary fibrosis
life expectancy <18 months without transplantation	primary pulmonary hypertension
no underlying cancer	bronchiectasis and cystic fibrosis
no serious systemic disease	emphysema including α_1-antitrypsin deficiency

Fig. 7.42 Summary of the complications of lung transplantation

Complication	Time
hyperacute rejection	seconds/minutes
pulmonary oedema	12–72 hours
bacterial lower respiratory tract infection: donor-acquired recipient-acquired	hours/days days/years
acute rejection	day 5/years
airway complications	week 1/months
opportunistic infection	week 4/years
chronic rejection (e.g. bronchiolitis obliterans)	week 6/years

Fig. 7.43 Classification of pleural effusions

Transudate		Exudate	
protein	<30 g/L	protein	>30 g/L
lactate dehydrogenase	<200 IU/L	lactate dehydrogenase	>200 IU/L
usually bilateral		unilateral in focal disease; bilateral in systemic disease	

Fig. 7.44 Causes of transudates and exudates

Transudate	Exudate
left heart failure	bacterial pneumonia
hypoproteinaemia	carcinoma bronchus
constrictive pericarditis	pulmonary infarction
hypothyroidism	tuberculosis
cirrhosis	connective-tissue disease

Fig. 7.45 Haemothorax

Degree	Management
minimal (<350 mL)	blood usually reabsorbs spontaneously with conservative treatment
moderate (300–1500 mL)	thoracentesis and tube drainage with underwater seal drainage
massive (>1500 mL)	two drainage tubes inserted; immediate or early thoracotomy may be necessary to arrest bleeding

associated pleural effusions are breast carcinoma, bronchial carcinoma and lymphomas/leukaemia.

Clinical features

Pleural effusions are typically asymptomatic until > 500 mL of fluid is present. Pleuritic chest pain may develop in addition to dyspnoea, which is dependent on the size of effusion.

Signs on examination include a stony dull percussion note; see Chapter 10.

Investigations

Features on a chest radiograph include blunting of costophrenic angles. Ultrasound is used to detect small effusions not seen on CXR and for guiding aspiration, which is performed for microbiological examination or therapeutically.

A pleural biopsy with Abrams' needle may be necessary if the aspiration is inconclusive.

Treatment

Treat the underlying disease. If the patient is symptomatic, drain the effusion. Drain fluid slowly. Malignant effusions – chemical pleurodesis can provide temporary relief. Use bleomycin/tetracycline.

Empyema

Also known as a pyothorax, this is a collection of pus within the pleural cavity caused by:

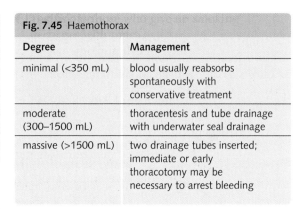

Questions on the cause of exudative and transudative pleural effusions are common in clinical examinations.

- Complication of thoracic surgery.
- Rupture of lung abscess into the pleural space.
- Perforation of oesophagus.
- Mediastinitis.
- Bacterial spread of pneumonia.

The empyema cavity can become infected by anaerobes. The patients are pyrexial and ill. The pus must be drained and appropriate antibiotic treatment should be initiated immediately.

Haemothorax

Blood in the pleural cavity. Common in both penetrating and non-penetrating injuries of the chest and may cause hypovolaemic shock and reduce vital capacity through compression. Due to the defibrinating action that occurs with motions of respiration and the presence of an anticoagulant enzyme, the clot may be defibrinated and leave fluid radiologically indistinguishable from effusions of another cause.

Blood may originate from lung, internal mammary artery, thoracoacromial artery, lateral thoracic artery, mediastinal great vessels, heart, or abdominal structures via the diaphragm. See Figure 7.45 for the management of haemothorax.

Chylothorax

Accumulation of lymph in the pleural space. Commonest causes are rupture or obstruction of the thoracic duct due to surgical trauma or neoplasm, e.g. lymphoma. A latent period between injury and onset of 2–10 days occurs. The pleural fluid is high in lipid content and is characteristically milky in appearance. The prognosis is generally good.

Chylous effusion

Caused by the escape of chyle into the pleural space from obstruction or laceration of the thoracic duct.

Chyliform effusion

Results from degeneration of malignant and other cells in pleural fluid.

Pneumothorax

Pneumothorax is the accumulation of air in the pleural space. It may occur spontaneously or following trauma.

Spontaneous

Results from rupture of a pleural bleb, which is a congenital defect of the alveolar wall connective tissue. Patients are typically tall, thin, young males. M : F ratio 6 : 1. Spontaneous pneumothoraces are usually apical, affecting both lungs with equal frequency.

Secondary causes of spontaneous pneumothorax occur in patients with underlying disease such as COPD, TB, pneumonia, bronchial carcinoma, sarcoidosis and cystic fibrosis.

Patients present with sudden onset of unilateral pleuritic pain and increasing breathlessness.

The main aim of treatment is to get the patient back to active life as soon as possible.

Investigations

Chest radiography may show an area devoid of lung markings. May be more clearly seen on the expiratory film.

Management

Small pneumothorax: no treatment, but review in 7–10 days. Moderate pneumothorax: admit for simple aspiration.

Tension pneumothorax

Medical emergency.
Commonest causes:

- Positive pressure ventilation.
- Stab wound or rib fracture.

Air escapes into pleural space and the rise above atmospheric pressure causes the lung to collapse. At each inspiration intrapleural pressure increases as the pleural tear acts as a ball valve that permits air to enter but not leave the pleural space. Venous return to the heart is impaired as pressure rises, and patients experience dyspnoea and chest pain. They may also be cyanotic.

Clinically:

- Mediastinum pushed over into contralateral hemithorax; tracheal deviation.
- Hyperresonance, absence of breath sounds.
- Intercostal spaces widened on ipsilateral side.

On ECG there is a rightward shift in mean frontal QRS complex, diminution in QRS amplitude, and inversion of precordial T waves.

Diagnosed on needle insertion.

Treat with immediate thoracostomy with underwater seal drainage, before requesting chest radiographs. See Figure 7.46 for a radiograph of a tension pneumothorax. Figure 7.47 gives a summary of non-inflammatory pleural effusions.

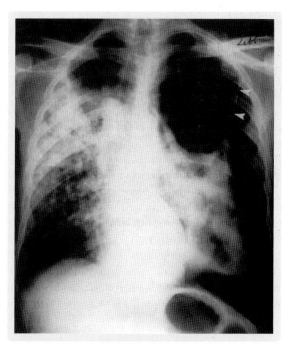

Fig. 7.46 Radiograph of a tension pneumothorax. Tension pneumothorax displacing mediastinum and depressing left hemidiaphragm. Extensive consolidation and cavitation in both lungs is due to tuberculosis. A pleural adhesion (arrowheads) is visible. (Courtesy of Dr D Sutton and Dr JWR Young.)

Fig. 7.47 Summary of non-inflammatory pleural effusions

Disorder	Collection	Cause
haemothorax	blood	chest trauma; rupture of aortic aneurysm
hydrothorax	proteinaceous fluid	congestive cardiac failure
chylothorax	lymph	neoplastic infiltration, trauma
pneumothorax	air	spontaneous; traumatic

A tension pneumothorax should never be diagnosed by chest radiography. It is a clinical diagnosis which requires treatment before requesting a chest radiograph.

NEOPLASMS OF THE PLEURA

Malignant mesothelioma

Malignant mesothelioma is a tumour of mesothelial cells most commonly affecting the visceral or parietal pleura. The incidence of mesothelioma is rising rapidly and has done so since the 1960s. Currently, there are approximately 1300 cases/year in the UK. In 90% of cases it is associated with occupational exposure to asbestos, especially fibres which are $<0.25\,\mu m$ diameter, e.g. crocidolite and amiosite. Workers bringing fibres home on their clothes expose family members to asbestos and an increased risk of mesothelioma. Wives who wash their husbands' overalls are especially at risk. The latent period between exposure and death is long, up to 40 years.

Two histological varieties exist – 50% of mesotheliomas have elements of both:

- Epithelial: tubular structure.
- Fibrous: solid structure with spindle-shaped cells.

The tumour begins as nodules in the pleura and goes on to obliterate the pleural cavity.

Clinical features

- Initial symptoms are very vague.
- Pain is the main complaint, often affecting sleep, and results from infiltration of the tumour into the chest wall with involvement of intercostal nerves and ribs.

Other features include:

- Dyspnoea.
- Weight loss.
- Finger clubbing.

Investigations

Features of chest radiograph are:

- Pleural effusions.
- Unilateral pleural thickening.
- Nodular appearance.

Mesothelioma should be considered in any patient with pleural thickening or pleural effusion, especially if pain is present. Open lung biopsy may be needed to confirm diagnosis.

Prognosis

No treatment is available and the condition is universally fatal. Pain responds poorly to therapy.

Metastases are common to hilar and abdominal lymph nodes with secondary deposits arising in lung, liver, thyroid, adrenals, bone, skeletal muscle and brain. The patient's symptoms become worse until death occurs, usually within 8–14 months of diagnosis; the cause of death is usually infection, vascular compromise or pulmonary embolus.

Patients eligible for industrial injuries benefit include those with mesothelioma, asbestosis, asbestos-related carcinoma of bronchus, and coalworker's pneumoconiosis.

Pleural fibroma

Rare neoplasm of the pleura not related to asbestos exposure, which consists of:

- Fibrous connective tissue.
- Mesothelial cells.

A solitary mass can grow to be very large and hypertrophic pulmonary osteoarthropathy is a frequent association. Affects females most commonly with the mean age at presentation 50 years.

Aetiology is unknown. Most patients are asymptomatic.

Tumours grow slowly and behave generally in a benign fashion, although malignant tumours do exist.

Surgical excision usually results in complete cure.

Up to 80% of localized fibrous tumours arise in relation to the visceral pleura.

Figure 7.48 is a radiograph showing pleural thickening.

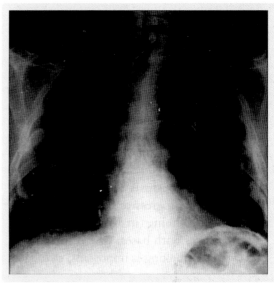

Fig. 7.48 Mesothelioma of the right pleura. The patient had a long history of asbestos exposure and has now developed a large pleural mass. (Courtesy of Professor CD Forbes and Dr WF Jackson.)

CLINICAL ASSESSMENT

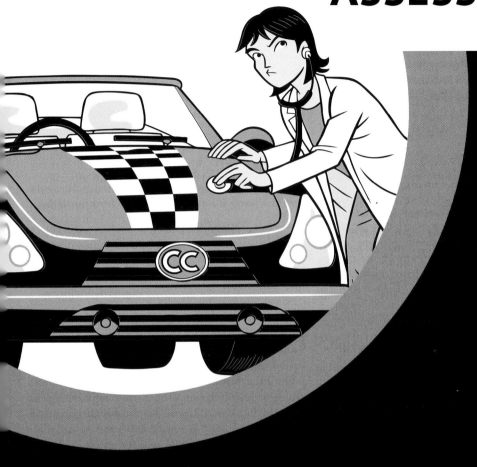

Pharmacological and non-pharmacological interventions

Objectives

By the end of this chapter you should be able to:

- Give examples of drugs used in the management of asthma and COPD, and describe their mechanism of action and side-effects.
- Describe indications for mucolytics and respiratory stimulants.
- Give examples of and describe the mechanism of action of drugs used in allergy.
- Describe pharmacological options in the management of cough.
- Describe pharmacological and non-pharmacological options in smoking cessation.
- Give examples of drugs which cause respiratory depression.
- Describe the management of oxygen therapy including invasive and non-invasive ventilation.
- Give examples of how physiotherapy can be used in respiratory medicine.
- Give an indication for surgery in COPD.

PHARMACOLOGICAL INTERVENTIONS

Overview

Many drugs are used to treat diseases of the respiratory system. Some are considered under the relevant diseases in Chapter 7; however, some important categories of drugs are introduced here. These categories are:

- Drugs used in asthma.
- Drugs used in COPD.
- Mucolytics.
- Respiratory stimulants.
- Drugs used in allergic disease.
- Cough preparations.
- Drugs used in smoking cessation.

We have not included a review of antibiotics here. You should ensure that you understand the mechanisms of action and main indications of common antibiotics used in respiratory medicine.

In addition, a number of drugs have side-effects upon the respiratory system; those drugs that cause respiratory depression are considered below.

Drugs used in the treatment of asthma

Drugs used in the treatment of asthma can be split into two main categories:

- Relievers (bronchodilators).
- Preventers (corticosteroids and less commonly leukotriene receptor antagonists or sodium cromoglicate).

The 'stepwise' approach to using these drugs to treat asthma is described in Chapter 7.

Relievers

Bronchodilators

Bronchodilators can be split into four groups:

- Short-acting β_2 agonists.
- Long-acting β_2 agonists (LABAs).
- Anticholinergics.
- Xanthines.

Short-acting β₂ agonists

Bronchial smooth muscle contains numerous β_2 receptors, which act through an adenylate cyclase/cAMP second-messenger system to cause smooth muscle relaxation and hence bronchodilatation (Fig. 8.1).

Examples of short-acting β_2 agonists are:

- Salbutamol.
- Terbutaline.

These drugs are usually inhaled, either as an aerosol, a powder, or as a nebulized solution. They can also be given intravenously, intramuscularly and subcutaneously. They are used for acute symptoms and act within minutes, producing effects lasting 4–5 hours.

The β_2 agonists are not completely specific and have some β_1 agonistic effects, especially in high doses.

Side-effects of β_2 agonists include:

- Tachycardia.
- Fine tremor.
- Nervous tension.
- Headache.

At the doses given by aerosol, these side-effects seldom occur. Tolerance may occur with high repeated doses.

Long-acting β₂ agonists (LABAs)

Like the short-acting β_2 agonists, these drugs also relax bronchial smooth muscle. They differ from the short-acting drugs in that their:

- Effect lasts for much longer (up to 12 hours).
- Full effect is only achieved after regular administration of several doses and generally less desensitization occurs.

For these reasons long-acting β_2 agonists should be used on a regular basis rather than to treat acute attacks.

The main long-acting β_2 agonists are:

- Salmeterol.
- Formoterol.
- Bambuterol.

Long acting β_2-agonists are also available in a combined preparation with a corticosteroid. Combination inhalers are more convenient that two separate inhalers and the drugs may act synergistically when administered together. They are used in asthma and COPD.

The main combination inhalers are:

- Seretide (salmeterol and fluticasone).
- Symbicort (formoterol and budesonide).

Xanthines

Xanthines (such as theophylline) appear to work by inhibiting phosphodiesterase, thereby preventing the breakdown of cAMP (Fig. 8.2). The amount of cAMP within the bronchial smooth muscle cells is therefore increased, which causes bronchodilatation in a similar way to β_2 agonists.

These drugs are metabolized in the liver and there is a considerable variation in half-life between individuals. This has important implications because

Tobacco shortens the half-life of theophylline (due to enzyme induction) and clearance can remain enhanced for up to 3 months after a patient has stopped smoking.

Fig. 8.1 Mechanisms of action of β_2 agonists – relaxation of bronchial muscle (which leads to bronchodilatation) and inhibition of mast-cell degranulation (β receptors on mast cell).

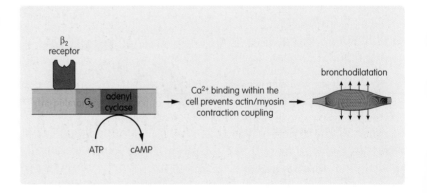

there is a small therapeutic window. Factors altering theophylline clearance are shown in Figure 8.3.

Theophylline can be given intravenously in the form of aminophylline (theophylline with ethylenediamine), but must be administered very slowly (over 20 minutes to administer dose). Aminophylline is given in cases of severe asthma attacks that do not respond to β_2 agonists and in acute asthma.

Preventers

Glucocorticosteroids

Steroids reduce the formation, release and action of many different mediators involved in inflammation. Their mode of action is complex and involves gene-modulation (Fig. 8.4) after binding to steroid receptors in the cytoplasm of cells and translocation of the active receptor into the nucleus. This has a number of effects including:

- Downregulation of pro-inflammatory cytokines and mediators, e.g. PLA_2.
- Production of anti-inflammatory proteins.

By reducing the activity and expression of phospholipase A_2, steroids can affect the production of arachidonic acid (Fig. 8.5).

Steroids in treatment of asthma may be topical (inhaled) or systemic (oral or parenteral).

Inhaled steroids

These include:

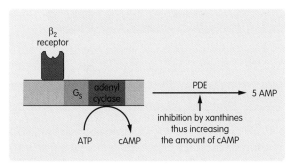

Fig. 8.2 Xanthines. The inhibition of phosphodiesterase (PDE) leads to an increase in cellular cyclic AMP which is believed to lead to bronchodilatation as in Figure 8.1.

| Fig. 8.3 Factors altering theophyiline clearance | |
Increased clearance	Decreased clearance
Smoking	Liver disease
Alcohol	Pneumonia
Rifampicin	Cimetidine
Childhood	Clarithromycin (erythromycin etc.)
	Old age
i.e. P450 enzyme induction	i.e. P450 enzyme inhibition

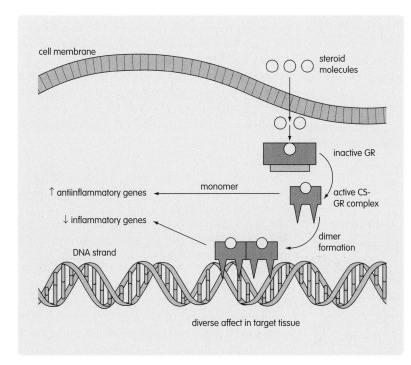

Fig. 8.4 Mechanism of action of steroids. Steroid molecules diffuse across cell membranes and bind to steroid receptors forming CS–GR complexes. These complexes may bind to DNA as dimers and increase the expression of many different anti-inflammatory gene products. Alternatively, CS–GR monomers may block induction of inflammatory genes by exogenous stimuli.

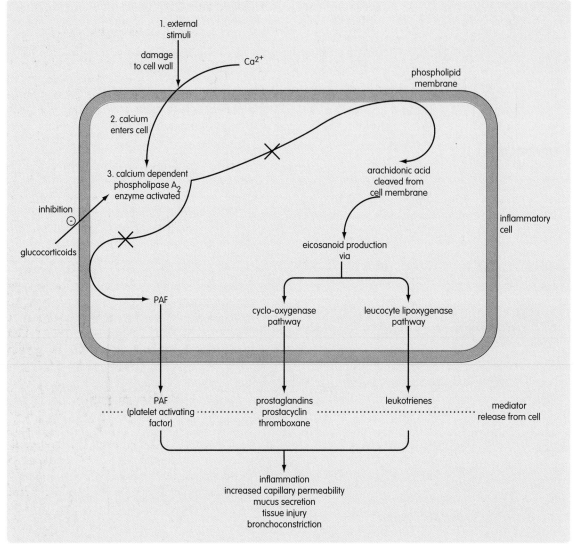

Fig. 8.5 Inhibition of inflammatory mediator cascade (i.e. cross through pathways to show that they are no longer active). (From Seaton D 2000, with permission of Blackwell Science.)

- Beclometasone.
- Budesonide.
- Fluticasone.
- Mometasone.

Side-effects of inhaled steroids in adults are relatively minor (primarily hoarseness and oral candidiasis). They may have a short-term effect on growth in children.

To prevent oral candidiasis, asthmatics are advised to wash their mouth out after taking their preventer inhaler.

Oral steroids

The primary oral steroid is prednisolone. Side-effects of systemic steroids include:

- Adrenal suppression.
- Effects on bones (including growth retardation in children and osteoporosis in adults).

A 66-year-old woman taking oral steroids for severe asthma was found to have osteoporosis on a DEXA scan of her bones. As her steroids could not be stopped she was prescribed a bisphosphonate to minimize further loss of bone density.

- Diabetes mellitus.
- Increased susceptibility to infection.
- Weight gain.
- Effects on skin (e.g. bruising and atrophy).
- Mood changes.

Because of these side-effects, regular oral steroids are avoided where possible.

Leukotriene receptor antagonists

Cysteinyl leukotrienes are eicosanoids that cause bronchoconstriction. Their pro-inflammatory actions (Fig. 8.6) centre on their ability to:

- Increase vascular permeability.
- Cause influx of eosinophils.

Leukotriene receptor antagonists (or 'leukotriene modifiers') therefore have anti-inflammatory and bronchodilatory effects.

The two key leukotriene receptor antagonists are montelukast and zafirlukast. Montelukast is used in prophylaxis of exercise-induced asthma and in patients with mild–moderate asthma whose symptoms are not well controlled by other asthma drugs.

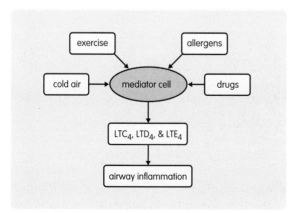

Fig. 8.6 Overview of cysteinyl leukotriene release.

Sodium cromoglicate

The mode of action of sodium cromoglicate is not completely understood. It is known to stabilize mast cells, possibly by blocking transport of calcium ions, and has no bronchodilator effect. It cannot be used to treat an acute attack, but is given for prophylaxis, especially in patients with atopy. The route of administration is by inhalation.

Its mechanism of action is to:

- Prevent mast-cell degranulation and hence mediator release.
- Reduce C-fibre response to irritants, therefore reducing bronchoconstriction.
- Inhibit platelet-activating factor (PAF)-induced bronchoconstriction.

In addition to its use in allergen-mediated asthma, sodium cromoglicate is effective in non-allergen-mediated bronchoconstriction (e.g. in exercise-induced asthma) and continued use results in reduced bronchial hyperactivity. It is often used in paediatrics. Nedocromil sodium is a drug with similar actions.

Drugs used in the management of COPD

In addition to the β_2 agonists and inhaled corticosteroids described above, anticholinergics are also used in the management of COPD.

The management of COPD is discussed in detail in Chapter 7.

Anticholinergics

Anticholinergics are competitive antagonists of muscarinic acetylcholine receptors. They therefore block the vagal control of bronchial smooth muscle tone in response to irritants and reduce the reflex bronchoconstriction. Ipratropium bromide and oxitropium bromide are both anticholinergics; they have two mechanisms of action:

- Reduction of reflex bronchoconstriction (e.g. from dust or pollen) by antagonizing muscarinic receptors on bronchial smooth muscle.
- Reduction of mucous secretions by antagonising muscarinic receptors on goblet cells.

These drugs reach their maximum effect within 60–90 minutes and act for between 4–6 hours. They are poorly absorbed orally; they must, therefore, be given by aerosol.

Anticholinergics are not the first-choice bronchodilator in asthma treatment because they only reduce the vagally mediated element of bronchoconstriction, having no effect on other important causes of bronchoconstriction such as inflammatory mediators. There is some evidence that anticholinergics are effective when given together with a β_2 agonist in severe asthma. In contrast, in COPD cholinergic hyperactivity significantly contributes to bronchoconstriction and therefore anticholinergics are more effective bronchodilators. The main use of anticholinergics is in COPD, which does not respond to β_2 agonists.

Side-effects are rare, but include:

- Dry mouth.
- Urinary retention.
- Constipation.

Mucolytics

Mucolytics (e.g. carbocisteine and methyl cysteine hydrochloride) are designed to reduce the viscosity of sputum, thereby aiding expectoration. The indications for use have been in:

- Chronic bronchitis.
- Chronic asthma.
- Cystic fibrosis.
- Bronchiectasis.

These drugs may be of benefit in treating acute exacerbations in COPD.

Respiratory stimulants

A respiratory stimulant (analeptic) such as doxapram can be used for patients with chronic obstructive pulmonary disease in type II respiratory failure. However, mechanical ventilation and a high incidence of side-effects have reduced their use. Doxapram stimulates carotid body chemoreceptors and must be given intravenously.

Side-effects of doxapram are:

- Tachycardia.
- Palpitations.
- Nausea.
- Sweating.
- Tremor.

Contraindications of doxapram are:

- Epilepsy.
- Hypertension.
- Hyperthyroidism.

Drugs used for allergies and anaphylaxis

H$_1$ histamine antagonists

These drugs are used in the treatment of allergies, such as hay fever. Examples of these drugs are:

- Promethazine.
- Trimeprazine.

The mechanism of action is to block H$_1$ receptors. These drugs cross the blood–brain barrier and have a general depressant action (sedative); in high doses, this action can cause respiratory depression.

Newer drugs such as terfenadine do not readily cross the blood–brain barrier and therefore do not cause respiratory depression.

Cough preparations

In the treatment of the common cold, simple linctus is an effective antitussive, partly due to a significant placebo effect, but other cough preparations are not indicated.

Cough arising from lung disease protects airways from mucus and particulate matter, and inhibition of cough could be dangerous, especially in chronic bronchitis and bronchiectasis. However, specific antitussive agents may be indicated for a chronic cough (>8 weeks) of unknown aetiology or cough in lung cancer.

Opiates acting centrally at the μ opioid receptor are effective antitussives. They have the adverse side-effects of respiratory depression and dependence, though morphine and diamorphine are used in terminally ill lung cancer patients in whom dependence is not an issue.

Weak opiates are more commonly used, posing a much reduced risk of dependence and causing respiratory depression only at high doses. Examples are:

- Codeine phosphate: side-effects include inhibition of ciliary activity, which reduces the clearance of secretions and constipation.
- Dextromethorphan: a synthetic, non-narcotic, non-analgesic and non-addictive opioid. It has a similar efficacy to codeine but does not have the side-effects.

Early on in their investigations and treatment, patients with chronic idiopathic cough should be warned that medications may not relieve their cough and that they might have to live with a persistent intractable cough.

Rarely, nebulized lidocaine (lignocaine) may be used to numb the back of the throat and inhibit the cough reflex in chronic cough.

Drugs used in smoking cessation

There are two main classes of drugs used in smoking cessation:

- Nicotine replacement therapy (NRT).
- Bupropion (amfebutamone).

NRT products (gums, patches and nasal sprays) are classified as over-the-counter medicines and have been shown to be effective in treating tobacco withdrawal and dependence. They should not be used in patients with severe cardiovascular disease (including immediately after myocardial infarction).

Bupropion is an antidepressant also licensed for use as an adjunct to smoking cessation. The main side-effects are a dry mouth and difficulty sleeping. The drug should not be used if there is a history of epilepsy or eating disorders.

In addition to pharmacological methods, a number of other interventions have been shown to be effective in helping smokers quit:

- Simple advice and/or brief counselling from GPs.
- Group counselling at smoking cessation clinics.
- Mass media campaigns (e.g. No Smoking Day).
- Helplines providing one-to-one telephone support.

Respiratory depressants

If a drug has a depressant action on the central nervous system, large enough doses of it will cause respiratory depression. The most notable of the drugs which cause respiratory depression are the opioid analgesics. Overdose is usually iatrogenic in origin or from illicit drug abuse (heroin). The effects of overdose can be reversed by administration of an opioid-receptor antagonist (e.g. naloxone). Opioid analgesics are contraindicated in respiratory depression and acute alcoholism (alcohol is also a respiratory depressant).

Other drugs that may also cause respiratory depression are barbiturates (when administered at 10–100 times the normal dose), H_1 histamine antagonists and alcohol. Benzodiazepines do not normally cause respiratory depression even at high doses; however, they can do so when administered orally or intravenously to elderly patients or to patients with underlying pulmonary disease.

NON-PHARMACOLOGICAL INTERVENTIONS

Respiratory support

Patients with respiratory disease who are hypoxaemic and/or hypercapnic will often require a form of respiratory support. This support may range from oxygen given briefly via a face mask in a patient with mild hypoxaemia to mechanical ventilation in respiratory failure. The two basic categories of respiratory support are considered below and include:

- Oxygen therapy.
- Assisted ventilation (non-invasive or mechanical).

Oxygen therapy

Oxygen therapy aims to correct hypoxaemia. Progress is monitored, and the amount of oxygen adjusted, according to pulse oximetry and arterial blood gas analysis.

Oxygen can be delivered either by:

- Nasal prongs.
- Face mask.

When delivering an oxygen concentration of > 28%, air must be humidified.

Nasal prongs

These allow the patient to talk and eat whilst receiving oxygen. Air is humidified to avoid discomfort from nasal crusting. Oxygen is delivered at rates of 1–4 L/min, which, when diluted with inspiratory air, equates to oxygen concentrations of 25–30%.

Delivery through nasal prongs is also used in long-term oxygen therapy (LTOT), for example in patients with COPD who have a domiciliary oxygen

Remember that excessive load is a major problem in acute-on-chronic respiratory failure. Taking away some of the work with assisted ventilation will help correct the vicious circle in which lung disease increases work which consumes oxygen which increases work requirement.

A middle-aged, obese man was advised to wear a CPAP mask at night to treat his obstructive sleep apnoea. He gave up on it a few months later because he found it uncomfortable to wear at night and the noise of the pump kept his wife awake.

supply. Because oxygen is flammable, patients must be warned not to smoke when taking an oxygen supply home.

Face masks

These fit over the nose and mouth and are used with higher-flow oxygen (e.g. 6 L/min or an oxygen concentration of 60%). Remember that high concentrations of oxygen should not be given to patients with acute-on-chronic respiratory failure (see p. 93).

Assisted ventilation

In some cases even high-flow oxygen is not sufficient to restore blood gases to adequate levels. A patient with COPD, for example, may maintain near normal blood gases until an infection adds to the workload; some form of ventilatory support is then indicated in order to:

- Offload the respiratory muscles and reduce the work of breathing.
- Improve gas exchange.

Non-invasive ventilation (NIV)

In non-invasive ventilation, respiratory support is given via the patient's upper airway, and intubation is avoided. This method is therefore only suitable if patients can protect their own airway, but has the advantage of reducing the risks of a hospital-acquired infection. The patient breathes spontaneously and the lungs are expanded by a volume of gas delivered, usually at a positive pressure. This decreases the work of the respiratory muscles, particularly the diaphragm.

NIV is particularly effective in patients with acute hypercapnic respiratory failure, particularly in COPD. Lung volumes in these patients do not return to baseline after expiration so that greater pressures are needed to expand the lungs (i.e. there is an intrinsic positive end-expiratory pressure or iPEEP). The posi-

tive pressure of the gas given via the mask therefore reduces the extra work generated by air trapping.

Two basic types of non-invasive ventilation are considered here:

- Continuous positive airway pressure (CPAP).
- Bilevel positive airway pressure (BiPAP).

As the name implies, CPAP delivers a continuous positive air pressure throughout the respiratory cycle and is used to keep the upper airway open in obstructive sleep apnoea. BiPAP is an example of intermittent positive-pressure ventilation (IPPV). BiPAP also reduces the work of breathing but differs in that it senses when inspiration is occurring and delivers a higher pressure during the inspiratory part of the cycle.

Non-invasive ventilation may be used in acute situations or on a long-term basis in patients with COPD; it is also used in weaning from conventional, intubated ventilators.

Mechanical ventilation

True mechanical ventilation links the patient to the ventilator by means of an endotracheal tube (usually inserted via the nose) or, if ventilation is likely to be prolonged, via tracheostomy. An airtight seal is created and gas is delivered either at constant pressure or at PEEP. Indications for mechanical ventilation include:

- Protection of airway in unconscious patients.
- Severe hypoxaemia (e.g. in ARDS).
- Controlling hypercapnia in ventilatory failure (i.e. type 2 respiratory failure) when NIV is inappropriate.

Complications of respiratory support

There are several important complications of respiratory support; most, including those presented by intubation and difficulties in weaning the patient, are outside the scope of this book.

Oxygen toxicity

The use of high-concentration oxygen therapy can have adverse effects on the respiratory system. This is especially evident after prolonged use.

Oxygen intoxication was first recognized by Paul Bert in 1878. He noticed that breathing oxygen at 1 atm for as little as 12 hours can lead to pulmonary congestion (reducing vital capacity), pulmonary oedema, exudation (reducing gaseous exchange) and damage to the pulmonary epithelium.

In the premature infant, administration of high-concentration oxygen can also cause retrolental fibroplasia. Fibrous tissue forms behind the lens and can lead to permanent blindness. This is thought to be caused by vasoconstriction, secondary to a high partial pressure of oxygen. This can be avoided by keeping a low PO_2.

Respiratory distress can occur because of absorption atelectasis.

Absorption atelectasis

Absorption atelectasis is the collapse of an alveolus due to blockage (Fig. 8.7). When breathing 100% O_2, the oxygen in the alveolus is quickly absorbed because there is a huge partial pressure difference between the alveolar gas (about 760 mmHg) and the partial pressure of gases in the venous blood. This results in collapse of the alveolus. It is then difficult to open the collapsed alveoli because of high surface tension effects.

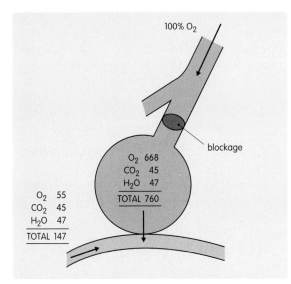

Fig. 8.7 Absorption atelectasis. The sum of the partial pressures (in mmHg) of alveolar gas far exceeds those in the mixed venous blood. Oxygen is taken up rapidly by the blood, causing collapse of the alveoli. (After West 1995, with permission of Lippincott, Williams & Wilkins.)

Absorption atelectasis also occurs in airway occlusion when breathing a normal air mixture. The rate of absorption is much slower as the driving force (the partial pressure difference between venous blood and alveolar gas) is much lower. There is still a partial pressure difference driving diffusion because the fall in oxygen tension from arterial to venous blood is greater than the rise in carbon dioxide tension. Collapse can be avoided by adding even small concentrations of nitrogen. Nitrogen is poorly absorbed because of its poor solubility and therefore remains in the alveoli, delaying or preventing collapse.

Physiotherapy

Physiotherapy is a key part of a respiratory patient's package of care. In addition to managing oxygen therapy as described above, the roles of the physiotherapist include:

Management of respiratory secretions.

Respiratory secretions are cleared by using a combination of small and deep breaths that move secretions up the bronchial tree. These are called active cycle breathing techniques and are used while the patient is lying in a position that encourages drainage of the lung (each lobe has a different position). This is indicated, for example, in cystic fibrosis.

Management of dyspnoea

Techniques, such as sitting forward, can be taught to relieve shortness of breath.

Pulmonary rehabilitation

Many COPD patients are not physically limited by poor respiratory function but rather by being systemically unfit. Pulmonary rehabilitation aims to increase their exercise tolerance through regular group exercises that strengthen upper and lower body muscles. It is combined with educational sessions, e.g. on the link between smoking and COPD.

Surgery

Paradoxically, removal of part of the lung in emphysema can improve lung function. Lung volume reduction surgery is done only in severe emphysema, being one of the last treatment options available.

Presentations of respiratory disease

9

Objectives

By the end of this chapter you should be able to:

- Describe the key differences in presentation between a patient with COPD and one with asthma.
- List important facts that need to be established if a patient complains of coughing up blood.
- Explain the difference between type I and II respiratory failure, in terms of blood gases and symptoms.
- List the three basic mechanisms that contribute to type II respiratory failure.
- Explain why caution must be taken when administering oxygen to a patient with COPD who is in respiratory failure.
- Describe the presentation and management of common respiratory emergencies.

COMMON PRESENTATIONS

The principal symptoms of respiratory disease (breathlessness, cough, sputum, haemoptysis, wheeze and chest pain) are common to many different conditions. Clinical findings often overlap considerably and this can make diagnosis seem difficult. However, a good history focusing on the time course and progression of the illness will often reveal recognizable patterns of symptoms and enable you to narrow down the differential diagnoses. Chapter 10 gives a framework for history taking; the main symptoms of respiratory disease and the key details that you should establish are described below.

It is important to remember that extreme lung disease does not necessarily produce clinical signs (e.g. a silent chest is an ominous sign in severe asthma).

Breathlessness

Breathlessness or dyspnoea is a difficulty or distress in breathing and is a symptom of many different diseases (Fig. 9.1). Breathlessness is a very common reason for referral to a respiratory clinic.

The patient may describe the symptom in a variety of ways. Common terms used are 'puffed', 'can't get enough air' and 'feeling suffocated'. A number of physiological factors (Fig. 9.2) underlie this sensation

and sometimes several mechanisms coexist to cause breathlessness. However, understanding the physiological basis of dyspnoea is of limited help clinically; it is a good history that is vital in diagnosing the underlying disease. Key points to establish include the speed of onset of breathlessness (Figs 9.3–9.5), its progression and variability, exacerbating and relieving factors and response to any treatment. Ask specifically about breathlessness on lying flat (orthonopnoea), which can occur in severe airflow obstruction or cardiac failure.

The severity of the symptom should be assessed by questioning patients on how it affects their daily life (Fig. 9.6).

Fig. 9.1 Causes of breathlessness

physiological	exercise
	high altitude
pathological	respiratory disorders
	cardiac disorders
	obesity
	anaemia
psychological	anxiety (hyperventilation)
pharmacological	drug-induced respiratory disorders
	drug-induced cardiac disorders

(After Munro & Campbell 2000, with permission of Churchill Livingstone.)

Fig. 9.2 Physiology of dyspnoea

Mechanism causing dyspnoea	Responds to:
chemoreceptors	hypercapnia and to lesser extent hypoxaemia
lung receptors (stretch and J receptors)	lung pathology (congestion etc.)
chest wall receptors	awareness by receptors of increased work
sense of effort	awareness by skeletal muscles of increased effort
afferent mismatch	relationship between force generated and lung volume produced; mismatch may lead to dyspnoea

Fig. 9.3 Conditions associated with breathlessness, grouped according to onset

Sudden onset	Onset occuring over hours	Onset occuring over weeks
Pulmonary embolism	Pneumonia	Chronic obstructive pulmonary disease (COPD)
Spontaneous pneumothorax	Exacerbation of asthma	Pleural effusion
Acute pulmonary oedema	Pulmonary oedema	Bronchial carcinoma
Inhalation of foreign body		Pulmonary fibrosis
Acute asthma		Anaemia
Cardiac tamponade		Cardiac failure

Although dyspnoea is a subjective sensation you may be able to see objective evidence of respiratory distress, e.g. use of accessory muscles of inspiration, or obvious tachypnoea. See Chapter 10 for more key signs.

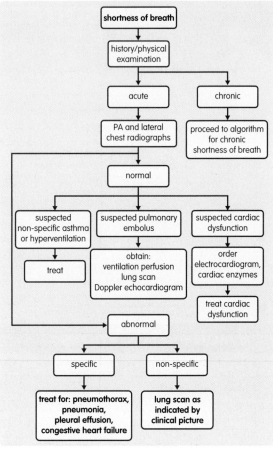

Fig. 9.4 Diagnostic algorithm of breathlessness. (After Greene et al 1998, with permission of Mosby.)

Cough

A cough is the commonest manifestation of lower respiratory tract disease. The cough reflex is a complex centrally mediated defence reflex, resulting from the appropriate chemical or mechanical stimulation of the larynx and the more proximal portion of the tracheobronchial tree. The basic pattern of a cough can be divided into four components:

- Rapid deep inspiration.
- Expiration against a closed glottis.
- Sudden glottal opening.
- Relaxation of expiratory muscles.

A cough may be voluntary but is usually an involuntary response to an irritant such as:

- Infection (URTI/LRTI).
- Cigarette smoke.
- Dusts.
- Dander (e.g. from cats).

Common respiratory diseases causing cough are shown in Figure 9.7. Remember that gastro-oesophageal reflux or ACE inhibitor therapy can cause a patient to cough. Cough can also be due to paralysis of the vocal cords; this 'bovine' cough is low-pitched and occurs when the recurrent laryngeal nerve is compressed, for example by a tumour.

Enquire about the timing of the cough (morning or evening), its chronicity and nature (i.e. productive or unproductive). Answers to these questions should allow you to differentiate between two common causes of cough: asthma and chronic bronchitis (Fig. 9.8).

Sputum

Everybody produces airway secretions. In a healthy non-smoker, approximately 100–150 mL of mucus is produced every day. Normally, this mucus is transported up the airway's ciliary mucus escalator and swallowed. This process is not normally perceived. However, expectorating sputum is always abnormal, and is a sign that excess mucus has been generated. This can result from irritation of the respiratory tract (commonly caused by cigarette smoking or the common cold) or from infection.

Sputum may be classified as:

- Mucoid: clear, grey or white.
- Serous: watery or frothy.
- Mucopurulent: a yellowish tinge.
- Purulent: dark green/yellow.

Fig. 9.5 Diagnostic algorithm of chronic breathlessness. (After Greene et al 1998, with permission of Mosby.)

Fig. 9.6 Key questions in assessing breathlessness

How far can you walk upstairs/uphill without stopping?
How far can you walk on the flat without stopping?
Do you feel breathless when washing or dressing?
Do you feel breathless at rest?

Fig. 9.7 Common respiratory causes of cough

Cause	Nature
asthma	worse at night; dry or productive
COPD	worse in morning; often productive
bronchiectasis	related to posture
post-nasal drip	persistent
tracheitis	painful
croup	harsh
interstitial fibrosis	dry

Fig. 9.8 Patterns of cough in asthma and chronic bronchitis

	Asthma	Chronic bronchitis
timing	worse at night	worse in the morning
chronicity	dry (may be green sputum)	productive
nature	intermittent	persistent
response to treatment	associated wheeze is reversible	associated wheeze is irreversible

179

Always try to inspect the sputum and note its volume, colour, consistency and odour. These details can provide clues as to the underlying pathology (Fig. 9.9). A yellow/green colour usually means infection and is due to myeloperoxidase produced by eosinophils or neutrophils. However, note that sputum in asthma contains high numbers of eosinophils and is often yellow or green without underlying infection.

Most bronchogenic carcinomas do not produce sputum. The exception is alveolar cell carcinoma, which produces copious amounts of mucoid sputum.

You may have to prompt the patient when investigating the volume of sputum. Is enough coughed up to fill a teaspoon/tablespoon/eggcup/sputum pot?

Chronic bronchitis is a particularly important cause of sputum production. This is defined as a cough productive of sputum for most days during at least 3 consecutive months, for more than 2 successive years.

Detailed questioning about cough is needed in patients with chronic bronchitis. Useful questions include:

- Do you cough up sputum/spit/phlegm from your chest on most mornings?
- Would you say you cough up sputum on most days for as much as 3 months a year?
- Do you often need antibiotics from your GP in winter?

Haemoptysis

Haemoptysis is coughing up blood; this needs to be differentiated from other sources of bleeding within the oral cavity and haematemesis (vomiting blood). This distinction is usually obvious from the history. Haemoptysis is not usually a solitary event and so if possible the sputum sample should be inspected.

Haemoptysis is a serious and often alarming symptom that requires immediate investigation (Fig. 9.10). A chest radiograph is mandatory in a patient with haemoptysis, and the symptom should be treated as bronchogenic carcinoma until proved otherwise. Despite appropriate investigations, often no obvious cause can be found and the episode is attributed to a simple bronchial infection.

Important respiratory causes of haemoptysis are:

- Bronchial carcinoma.
- Pulmonary infarction.
- TB.
- Pneumonia (particularly pneumococcal).
- Bronchiectasis.
- Acute/chronic bronchitis.

In investigating the cause of haemoptysis, ask about any preceding events, such as respiratory infection or deep vein thrombosis (DVT) and establish the frequency, volume and whether it is fresh or altered blood. Figure 9.11 gives some characteristic patterns of haemoptysis and possible diagnoses.

Wheeze

Wheezing is a common complaint, complicating many different disease processes. Establish exactly what a patient means by 'wheeze'; used correctly the term describes musical notes heard mainly on expiration and caused by narrowed airways.

Wheezes are classified as either polyphonic (of many different notes) or monophonic (just one note). Polyphonic wheezes are common in widespread airflow obstruction; it is the characteristic wheeze heard in asthmatics. A localized monophonic wheeze suggests that a single airway is partially obstructed; this can also occur in asthma (e.g. by a mucus plug) but may be a sign of narrowing due to a tumour.

The symptom of wheezing is not diagnostic of asthma, although asthma and chronic obstructive pulmonary disease are the commonest causes and they can be difficult to distinguish. You should establish whether the patient wheezes first thing in the morning (common in chronic bronchitis), at night (common in asthma) or on exercising.

Fig. 9.9 Types of sputum

Character	Cause
pink/frothy	pulmonary oedema
yellow/green	infections/eosinophils in asthma
rusty	pneumococcal pneumonia
faol-tasting	anaerobic infection
viscous, difficult to cough up	asthma/infections
large volumes	bronchiectasis
black	cavitating lesions in coal miners
blood-stained	see Figs 9.10 and 9.11

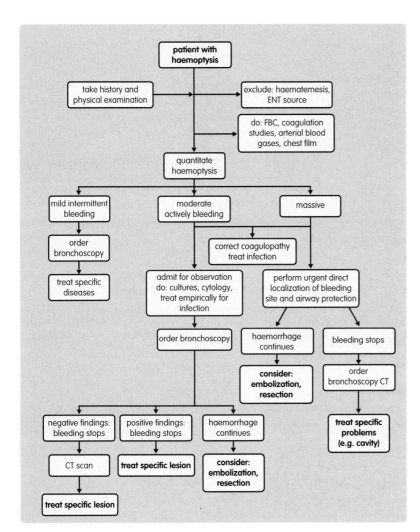

Fig. 9.10 Diagnostic algorithm of haemoptysis. (After Greene, Johnson & Maricic 1993, with permission of Mosby.)

Fig. 9.11 Patterns of haemoptysis	
Pattern	**Possible diagnosis**
recurrent blood-streaked sputum	bronchial carcinoma
frank, becoming progressively darker over 24/48h	infarction
recurrent over years, with purulent sputum	bronchiectasis

Stridor is an audible inspiratory noise and indicates partial obstruction of the upper, larger airways, such as the larynx, trachea and main bronchus. It is very important that you differentiate between a wheeze and stridor because stridor is a serious sign requiring urgent investigation. Causes of obstruction include tumour and inhalation of a foreign body.

Chest pain

Pain can originate from most of the structures in the chest (Fig. 9.12) and can be classified as central or lateral. As with pain anywhere in the body, enquire about site, mode of onset, character, radiation, intensity, precipitating, aggravating and relieving factors and response to any analgesics taken. Make sure you ask specifically about the pain's relationship to breathing, coughing or movement; if it is made worse by these it is likely to be pleural in origin. Pleural pain is sharp and stabbing in character and may be referred to the shoulder tip if the diaphragmatic pleura is involved. It can be very severe and often leads to shallow breathing, avoidance of movement and cough suppression. The commonest causes of pleural pain are pulmonary infarction or infection.

Fig. 9.12 Causes of chest pain

Structure	Possible cause of pain
pleura	pneumothorax, pulmonary infarction
muscle	strain (e.g. from coughing)
bone	rib fracture or tumour
costochondral junctions	Tietze's syndrome
nerves	herpes zoster, Pancoast's syndrome
heart and great vessels	cardiac ischaemia/infarction aortic dissection/aneurysm
oesophagus	spasm, reflux

Respiratory causes of central, or retrosternal, chest pain include bronchitis and acute tracheitis. This pain is often made worse by coughing and may be relieved when the patient coughs up sputum.

Other associated symptoms

In addition to the principal presentations, there are several other symptoms that you should note.

Hoarseness

Ask if the patient's voice has changed at all in recent times, and if so, was there anything that preceded the change, e.g. overuse of the voice, thyroidectomy etc. There may be a simple, benign cause of hoarseness such as:

- Cigarette smoking.
- Acute laryngitis as part of an acute URTI.
- Use of inhaled steroids.

However, there may be a more sinister cause: like the bovine cough noted above, hoarseness may be a sign that a lung tumour is compressing the recurrent laryngeal nerve.

Weight loss

Unintentional weight loss is always an important sign, raising suspicion of carcinoma. Establish how much weight the patient has lost, over what period, and whether there is any loss of appetite. Note, however, that it is common for patients with severe emphysema to lose weight.

Ankle swelling

Patients with chronic obstructive pulmonary disease (COPD) may comment that their ankles swell during acute exacerbations. Ask about this and check for oedema as part of your examination; it is an important sign of cor pulmonale.

ACUTE PRESENTATIONS

Respiratory failure

Respiratory failure is not a presentation seen in isolation but a possible outcome of many different respiratory diseases.

In the initial stages of lung disease, the body may be able to maintain normal blood gases by adapting to increased ventilatory demand. However, if the underlying disease progresses the ventilatory workload may become excessive. The result is a failure to oxygenate the blood or failure to remove carbon dioxide by ventilation. The patient is said to be in respiratory failure, a state which can be diagnosed on the clinical picture and by blood gas analysis. The patient will usually have signs of underlying disease in addition to the clinical features of respiratory failure, which are principally those of hypoxia (Fig. 9.13).

Respiratory failure can be classified into two types, depending on the presence or absence of hypercapnia. It is important to distinguish the two types because this impacts on the therapy given.

Type I respiratory failure

This is the most common type of respiratory failure. The features are:

- Acute hypoxaemia: P_aO_2 low (< 8 kPa).
- P_aCO_2 normal or low.

The patient is hypoxic (and becomes cyanotic, confused and restless) but is normo- or hypocapnic. This can be explained by the patient's response to an initial rise in P_aCO_2. Alveolar ventilation is stimulated and the excess carbon dioxide (and sometimes more than the excess) is excreted.

Almost all acute lung diseases can cause type I respiratory failure. The underlying mechanism for the failure of gas exchange is frequently ventilation : perfusion mismatch. Some common examples are:

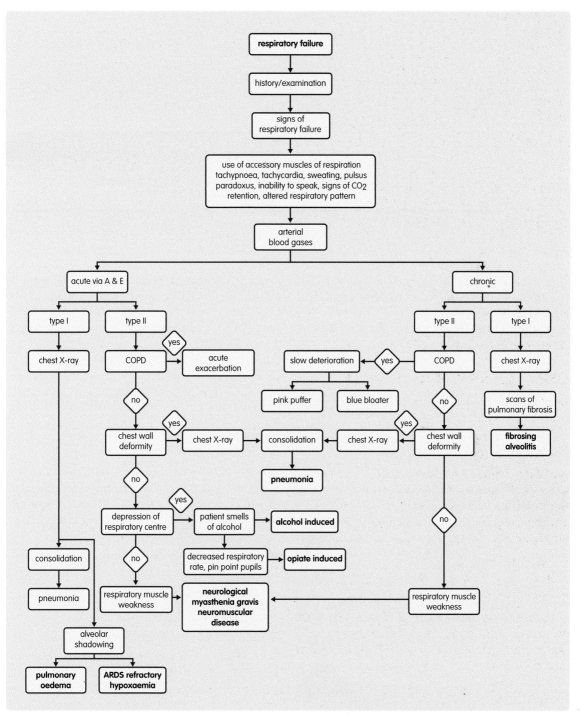

Fig. 9.13 Diagnostic algorithm of respiratory failure. ARDS = adult respiratory distress syndrome. (After Greene, Johnson & Maricic 1993, with permission of Mosby.)

- Severe acute asthma.
- Pneumonia.
- Pulmonary embolism.
- Pulmonary oedema.

Type II respiratory failure

The features of type II respiratory failure are:

- P_aO_2 low (<8 kPa).
- P_aCO_2 high (>6.5 kPa).

The patient is hypoxic and hypercapnic. As the P_aCO_2 rises, the patient will develop additional symptoms and signs including headache, warm peripheries and bounding pulse; with severe hypercapnia a flapping tremor may develop.

Type II respiratory failure is also known as ventilatory failure; the rise in P_aCO_2 is no longer matched by an increase in alveolar ventilation. This can be because:

- Ventilatory drive is insufficient.
- The work of breathing is excessive.
- The lungs are unable to pump air in and out efficiently.

Type II respiratory failure can therefore occur in neuromuscular disorders, CNS depression or when a lung collapses, for example after tension pneumothorax. However, the commonest cause is an acute exacerbation of COPD. Patients with COPD are often hypoxaemic for many years with morning headache being the only sign that P_aCO_2 is slightly raised. An acute exacerbation (e.g. due to respiratory infection) then increases the work of breathing still further, leading to 'acute-on-chronic' respiratory failure.

Management of respiratory failure is discussed in detail in Chapter 6. However, it is important to note here that you should be cautious in giving oxygen to patients with type II respiratory failure. Respiratory drive in these patients has become relatively insensitive to hypercapnia; hypoxaemia plays a more important role in stimulating ventilation. Giving high concentrations of oxygen will therefore suppress ventilatory drive and P_aCO_2 may rise rather than fall.

RESPIRATORY EMERGENCIES

Assessment of patient

Assessment of any emergency is according to the ABC:

A: Airway. Chin lift, head tilt and inspect for obstruction.

B: Breathing.
- Respiratory rate.
- Oxygen saturation.
- Look for symmetrical chest movements and tracheal deviation.
- Listen for stridor or wheeze, auscultate lungs for air entry.
- Peak flow.

C: Circulation.
- Look for cyanosis.
- Heart rate.
- Capillary refill time (should be <2 seconds).
- Blood pressure.

Try to obtain a brief history from the patient; in particular, enquire about allergy, events immediately prior to onset of symptoms, medications (both regular and what has already been tried) and known medical complaints. Additionally, the ability of the patient to talk in sentences will help in assessing severity of dyspnoea.

Arterial blood gases and chest X-rays may be indicated.

The emergency management of common respiratory diseases is discussed below in the format of OSCE style case scenarios.

If the respiratory failure develops quickly, increased P_aCO_2 leads to a rise in pH: respiratory acidosis. If it develops more slowly, there is time for renal compensation and pH may be normal or near-normal. Always look at bicarbonate levels to see if they have risen in compensation.

Whenever you are asked to describe the emergency management of a patient, begin by saying that you would assess and initially manage the patient according to the ABC.

Asthma attack

Case example

John, a 21-year-old, presented to A&E complaining of shortness of breath and wheeze that had been getting progressively worse over the last 8 hours. His symptoms had started after a run. He was not known to be asthmatic but had recently been woken at night by coughing and had suffered from hay fever since childhood. On examination, he was tachycardic, had bilateral high-pitched expiratory wheeze and his peak expiratory flow was 50% of that predicted.

Management of acute asthma

- High-flow oxygen (100%).
- Four to six puffs, each inhaled separately, of a β_2 agonist (salbutamol or terbutaline) from a metered-dose inhaler via a spacer. Repeat every 10–20 min. Give via a nebulizer if life-threatening asthma.
- Prednisolone 40–60 mg orally, or if the patient cannot swallow tablets, parenteral hydrocortisone 400 mg.
- If a poor response to the above, may consider the anticholinergic bronchodilator ipratropium bromide (0.5 mg 4- to 6-hourly via nebulizer) in addition to a β_2-agonist, or a single dose of magnesium sulphate (1.2–2 mg i.v. infusion over 20 minutes).
- If response still poor, could consider the bronchodilator aminophylline i.v. (5 mg/kg loading dose over 20 minutes, then infusion of 0.5–0.7 mg/kg/hour). If the patient already takes regular aminophylline, the loading dose is not required.

Note that asthma attacks can be subdivided according to severity:

- Mild/moderate – patient can talk (complete sentences in one breath), minimal distress and minimal use of accessory muscles. Peak flow 50–75% (moderate) and > 75% (mild) of predicted value.
- Severe – patient cannot complete sentences in one breath, marked distress and use of accessory muscles, peak flow < 50% of predicted value, tachycardia > 110 bpm, tachypnoea > 25 respirations/min.
- Life-threatening – silent chest on auscultation, weak respiratory effort, peak flow < 33% of predicted value, cyanosis, bradycardia, fatigue/exhaustion, confusion/coma.

COPD exacerbation

Case example

Mr Habib, a 59-year old known COPD patient presented to A&E complaining of increased shortness of breath and a change in sputum production (increased volume) compared to normal. He also complained of wheeze, cough and chest tightness, and had been feeling generally unwell and tired over the last few days. Nurses noted that Mr Habib seemed confused.

Management of COPD exacerbation

- Controlled oxygen therapy at 24–28%. In an acute setting, patients are more likely to die from hypoxia than a reduced respiratory drive caused by hypercapnia; therefore give oxygen. However, careful monitoring is still required. Once oxygen saturations are normal (P_aO_2 > 8.0 kPa or S_aO_2 > 90%), check arterial blood gases every 30 min to ensure that there is no carbon dioxide retention and acidosis.
- Bronchodilators – β_2-agonists (salbutamol 5 mg 4-hourly) and anticholinergics (ipratropium 500 µg 6-hourly) via inhaler or nebulizer. Consider i.v. aminophylline.
- Corticosteroids – oral (prednisolone 30–40 mg) or i.v. (hydrocortisone 200 mg).
- Antibiotics if suspicion of chest infection; take sputum and blood for culture before beginning antibiotics.
- Consider ventilatory support – initially non-invasive and then invasive if impending respiratory failure.

Important causes of COPD exacerbations are chest infections and air pollution.

Anaphylaxis

Case example

Mr Lee, a surgical inpatient, was given penicillin by the houseman for a suspected chest infection. Within minutes, he began to feel short of breath, describing a sensation of his throat swelling up, and complained of abdominal pain and itch on the palms of his feet and genitalia. Wheeze, profound swelling of his lips and eyes, rash and severe hypotension were noted. Mr Lee vomited once.

Management of anaphylaxis

- Maintain blood pressure by laying the patient flat and raising the legs.
- Intramuscular adrenaline (epinephrine) (0.5–1.0 mg: 0.5–1.0 mL of adrenaline injection 1 : 1000), repeated at 10-minute intervals depending on the blood pressure.
- 100% oxygen.
- Chlorphenamine (chlorpheniramine) (antihistamine) 10–20 mg intravenously, continued for 24–48 hours.
- Salbutamol can be given intravenously for those patients not responsive to adrenaline.
- Hydrocortisone 200–300 mg intravenously may be given as a second-line drug to reduce further deterioration.
- Intravenous fluids to increase blood pressure.

Common causes of anaphylaxis are food (e.g. peanuts, shellfish), drugs (penicillin, suxamethonium) and insect bites.

Tension pneumothorax

Case example

Mrs Powell, a woman in her early 40s, was brought to A&E after involvement in a car accident. Initial assessment revealed a clear airway but oxygen saturations of only 84%, tracheal deviation to the left, and on the right side of the chest poor chest expansion, a hyperresonant percussion note and poor air entry.

Management of tension pneumothorax (in this case, right sided)

- Place a cannula in the second intercostal space in the midclavicular line. Oxygen saturations

should improve within minutes. Eventually a chest drain will need to be inserted.

Pulmonary embolism

Case example

Mrs Ahmed, a 75-year-old woman, complained of sudden onset of shortness of breath and haemoptysis 10 days following a hysterectomy. Chest X-ray was normal but arterial blood gases showed hypoxia and hypocapnia and D-dimers were raised. ECG showed deep S waves in I, Q waves in III and inverted T waves in III. A ventilation : perfusion scan showed a medium perfusion defect in the left lung.

Management of a pulmonary embolism (PE)

- High-flow oxygen (100%).
- Low-molecular-weight heparin 175 U/kg/24 h subcutaneously (or unfractionated heparin if massive pulmonary embolism). NB: Can be given on suspicion of PE, before imaging has confirmed.
- Oral anticoagulation with warfarin may be started once imaging is obtained. The target INR should be 2.0–3.0 and warfarin should be continued for 4–6 weeks if risk factors for thromboembolic disease were only temporary, 3 months if the PE was idiopathic and 6 months for other causes.
- Thrombolysis (e.g. with streptokinase) is only indicated for massive PE.

History and examination

Objectives

By the end of this chapter you should be able to:

- Describe why the social history is so important in respiratory medicine.
- Describe how features of a patient's past medical history might be relevant.
- Explain why the initial observation of the patient is important.
- Describe the visible effects of long-term steroid use.
- List the causes of tachypnoea.
- List the different patterns of breathing and their significance.
- Describe the common causes of clubbing and how to look for clubbing.
- Describe the significance of unilateral muscle wasting of the hand.
- Describe the relevance of tracheal position in tension pneumothorax.
- Name the common scars seen on the thorax and the possible operations that the patient may have undergone.
- List the surface markings of the lungs for percussion.
- Describe the relationship between added sounds and disease.
- Describe how lung disease alters examination findings.

TAKING A HISTORY

In respiratory medicine your skills in history taking will be tested by both:

- Acute presentations – diagnosis must be quick but may be hindered by the patient's condition.
- Chronic presentations – documenting the key features in an illness that may span many years.

Each situation has its specific challenges and in each a good history should tell you the diagnosis.

This section outlines a generic approach to history taking. In practice, you should tailor your history to the possible diagnoses. In a female patient with a suspected deep vein thrombosis (DVT) you will need to ask about pregnancy, oral contraceptive pill, recent travel or surgery and family history of DVT or PE. Obviously, you will need a different set of questions to establish a diagnosis of asthma.

Initial observations

Before you begin take a few minutes to introduce yourself and to put the patient at ease.

Simple observation at the bedside can often give a good clue to the likely diagnosis:

- Inhalers and oxygen bottles.
- Sputum pots.
- Walking sticks or frames.

How does the patient appear during the interview? Agitated, or distressed? Is there a visible tremor? Is the patient too breathless to speak in full sentences? Is the voice rough or hoarse? Simple observations now will save time later.

Structure of the history

Presenting complaint (PC)

The presenting complaint is a concise statement of the symptoms felt by the patient. Use the patient's own words – this is not a diagnosis. For example, for shortness of breath the patient might use 'out of puff' or 'can't get any air in'.

History of presenting complaint (HPC)

Build up a picture of the presenting complaint, investigating each symptom as described in Chapter 9. You should establish the following details:

- Onset: acute or gradual.
- Pattern: intermittent or continuous.
- Frequency: daily, weekly or monthly.
- Duration: minutes or hours.
- Progression: better or worse than in the past.
- Severity: mild, moderate or severe.
- Character: e.g. is the pain sharp, dull or aching?
- Precipitating and relieving factors: e.g. are any medications used?
- Associated symptoms: e.g. cough, wheeze, haemoptysis, dyspnoea, chest pain, orthopnoea.
- Systemic symptoms: e.g. fever, malaise, anorexia, weight loss.

Has the patient had the problem before? If so, what were the diagnosis, treatment and outcome?

Ask the patient how disabling the problem is and how it affects daily life. In patients with chronic illness, you should establish their exercise tolerance and whether this has declined.

Past medical history (PMH)

Present the PMH in chronological order, listing any hospital admissions, surgical operations and major illnesses.

Take a careful note of anything that might contribute to the presenting complaint; for example:

- Pneumonia – complications include pleural effusion, bronchiectasis.
- 'Wheezy bronchitis' as a child – possibly asthma.
- Severe measles or whooping cough in childhood – may lead to bronchiectasis.
- Previous pulmonary embolism (PE) or deep vein thrombosis (DVT).
- Pregnancy – risk of PE.
- Recent surgery – PE, hospital-acquired or aspiration pneumonia.
- Eczema or hay fever – evidence of atopy.

Has the patient received BCG immunization or experienced tuberculosis contact in the past? Has a chest radiograph ever been taken: it may be useful for comparison.

Note any other factors that might have contributed, for example:

- Recent travel – DVT, legionella.
- Recent life events (e.g. moving house) – stress, house dust.

Drug history (DH)

When taking the drug history, list the patient's current intake of both prescribed and over-the-counter (OTC) drugs, recording dosage, frequency and duration of treatment. Ask the patient what each tablet is for and when it is taken; this gives an indication of patients' understanding of their problems and compliance. Remember that some drugs (e.g. beta-blockers or NSAIDs) can make asthma worse. The oral contraceptive pill is a risk factor for pulmonary embolism. ACE inhibitors prescribed for hypertension can cause cough.

Drug allergies

Ask about any allergies; if the patient mentions an allergy, ask what exactly happened, and how long ago it happened.

Family history (FH)

When noting a family history, it may be easier to draw a pedigree chart. Do any members of the family suffer from a respiratory disorder? A family history of premature emphysema or liver cirrhosis may indicate α_1-antitrypsin deficiency. Is there a family history of pulmonary embolism or deep vein thrombosis. Ask about atopy, asthma, eczema and hay fever. Does anybody in the family smoke?

Social history (SH)

Social history is hugely important in the respiratory system; many respiratory diseases can be caused, or worsened, by social factors such as housing, occupation, hobbies or pets.

Home and social situation

Ask who lives with the patient at home and whether the person is fit and well. Do they have any additional help around the home?

Ask about accommodation:

- Type: house, flat (which floor?) or bed-sit.
- Heating: coal fire, gas fire or central heating.
- Conditions: damp or dry.
- Number of people living in the accommodation.
- Area of town: gives an indication of socioeconomic class.
- Pets: dogs, cats or birds.

Asking about pets is important in a respiratory history. For example, cat dander may precipitate an asthma attack or allergic rhinitis and pet birds are a rare cause of pneumonia.

The smoking history gives clues to correct diagnosis. Most patients with COPD have a 20 or more pack year history. A patient with a diagnosis of COPD and a 10 pack year history may be a misdiagnosed asthmatic.

Fig. 10.1 Occupational causes of lung disease

Disease	Area of work
asbestosis	Vehicle body workers, ship building, demolition
malignant mesothelioma	as above
byssinosis	textile workers
stannosis	tin mining
farmer's lung	farming (exposure to mouldy hay)
coal worker's pneumoconiosis	coal mining
silicosis	mining, quarrying, foundry work etc.
occupational asthma	see Fig. 7.19
berylosis	electronic industries

Ask about the patient's financial situation: is the patient entitled to any state benefits (e.g. social support)? Enquire about diet and exercise.

Smoking and alcohol

A detailed smoking history is essential. You should record:

- Age started.
- Age stopped (if applicable).
- Whether cigarettes, cigars or pipe.
- Average smoked per day.

It may help to convert this information into 'pack years' (where 1 pack year is 20 cigarettes smoked each day for a year).

Ask if the patient drinks alcohol. If yes, convert the weekly intake into units if possible. One glass of wine or one-half pint of beer is equivalent to 1 unit. Remember that some forms of pneumonia (*Staphylococcus aureus* and *Klebsiella*) occur in alcoholics.

Occupation

Present the patient's jobs in chronological order starting from the time the patient left school. Some respiratory conditions have a long latent period between time of exposure and presentation.

Enquire about occupational related disorders (e.g. asbestos exposure and mesothelioma). The length of each job and the job description need to be recorded. Figure 10.1 lists some lung diseases associated with specific occupations. Hobbies may also be relevant.

Once you have finished, check that you have not missed anything and then summarize the key points to add clarity and ease presentation.

EXAMINATION

Overview

As with any examination, it is important that you:

- Introduce yourself if you have not already done so.
- Wash your hands before you begin and when you finish the examination.
- Explain to the patient what you propose to do and ask if this is acceptable.

The structure of the examination is inspection, palpation, percussion and auscultation. For a respiratory examination, patients should be fully exposed to the waist, comfortable, and sitting at 45°, with their hands by their sides.

In clinical examinations, purposefully walk to the end of the bed to observe the patient; this emphasizes that you are observing the patient and also gives you thinking time. Give a running commentary of what you are doing; this needs practice as you will be nervous.

General inspection

The initial observation is vital. If you have not already done so as part of the history, stand at the end of the bed and look at the locker for sputum pots, inhalers and charts. Note any drip stands that are present, venous cannulae, or bandages.

Stand back and note the patient's general appearance. Is the patient:

- Obviously unwell or distressed?
- Alert or confused?
- Thin or overweight?

There are some signs (e.g. use of accessory muscles of inspiration or pallor) that you may notice immediately. Does the patient have a cough and, if so, does it sound productive? Is there any abnormality (e.g. hoarseness) in the voice?

Then run through a systematic general inspection. You should look generally at muscle bulk, noting any cachexia (Fig. 10.2) and then inspect the skin in detail (Fig. 10.3). You may want to inspect the thorax at this point too; these aspects are discussed below.

It is essential that you look closely at how the patient is breathing. In addition to respiratory rate (Fig. 10.4), which is easier to test with the pulse, you should note:

- Signs of dyspnoea (e.g. use of accessory muscles of inspiration such as the sternomastoids, patient 'fixing' upper body by leaning forward, mouth breathing, nasal flaring).

Fig. 10.2 Cachexia

Test performed	Signs observed	Diagnostic inference
observe muscle bulk and general condition of the skin	generalized muscle wasting and lack of nutrition; pallor; dry and wrinkled skin	malignant disease bronchial carcinoma chronic disease renal disease hepatic disease cardiac failure tuberculosis other: anorexia nervosa malnutrition emotional disturbance

Fig. 10.3 Inspection of skin

Test performed	Signs observed	Diagnostic inference
observe the general state of the skin	steroidal skin: shiny excessive bruising thin	prolonged use of corticosteroids: chronic obstructive pulmonary disease asthma fibrosing alveolitis systemic disease (e.g. Crohn's disease)
	generalized dryness and scaling of skin	ichthyosis vulgaris acquired ichthyosis hypothyroidism sarcoidosis
	thin skin	ageing Cushing's syndrome topical or systemic steroid use
observe the colour of the skin	pale skin	pallor anaemia leukaemia shock
	light brown coloured spots on skin	café-au-lait spots neurofibromatosis tuberous sclerosis

Fig. 10.4 Abnormal ventilation rate

Test performed	Signs observed	Diagnostic inference
discretely count the respiratory rate while feeling the patient's pulse	12–20 breaths per minute	normal
	>12 breaths per minute (tachypnoea)	anxiety pain infection pneumothorax pulmonary embolism
	<12 breaths per minute (bradypnoea)	hypothyroidism increased intracranial pressure

Fig. 10.5 Unusual patterns of breathing

Signs observed	Diagnostic inference
hyperventilation with deep sighing respirations (Kussmaul's respiration)	diabetic ketoacidosis aspirin overdose acute massive pulmonary embolism
increased rate and volume of respiration followed by periods of apnoea (Cheyne–Stokes respiration)	terminal disease increased intracranial pressure
prolongation of expiration	airflow limitation
pursed lip breathing	air trapping

- Unusual patterns of breathing (Fig. 10.5).
- Any noises you can hear unaided (e.g. wheeze or stridor).

Hands and limbs

Examination of the hands

The hands can reveal key signs of respiratory disease. Take both the patient's hands and note their temperature. Abnormally warm and cyanosed hands are a sign of CO_2 retention. Check the fingers for nicotine staining. One important sign of respiratory disease is finger clubbing (Figs 10.6 and 10.7). This is a painless, bulbous enlargement of the distal

Fig. 10.6 Clubbing

Test performed	Sign observed	Diagnostic inference

view the nail from the side at eye level; rock the nail from side to side on the nail-bed; look at the nail-bed and nail angle.	increase in the soft tissue of the nail-bed and fingertip, with increased sponginess of the nail-bed	pulmonary causes:
		  tumour (bronchial carcinoma, mesothelioma)
		  chronic pulmonary sepsis (empyema, lung abscess, bronchiectasis, cystic fibrosis)

place nails back to back; a diamond-shaped area is evident between them if clubbing does not exist.	loss of angle between nail and nail-bed	fibrosing alveolitis asbestosis hypertrophic pulmonary osteoarthropathy
	transverse curvature of nail increases	

	in final stages, whole tip of the finger becomes clubbed	cardiac causes:
		  congenital
		  bacterial endocarditis

	clubbing may also affect the toes	other causes:
		  idiopathic causes
		  cirrhosis
		  inflammatory bowel disease

	bones are normal	

fingers; it is accompanied by softening of the nail bed and loss of nail bed angle. Also assess for:

- Muscle wasting (Fig. 10.8).
- Rheumatoid hands (Fig. 10.9).
- Hypertrophic pulmonary osteoarthropathy (HPOA) (Fig. 10.10).
- Hand tremor (Fig. 10.11).

Know the causes of clubbing before any clinical examination. Note that chronic bronchitis does not cause clubbing.

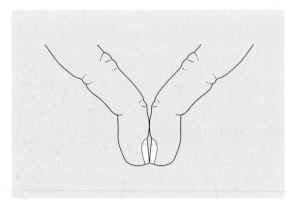

Fig. 10.7 One method of inspecting for clubbing. Normal fingers: note diamond-shaped area.

Examination of the pulse

A normal resting pulse in an adult is 60–100 b.p.m. Bradycardia is defined as a pulse rate of less than 60 b.p.m. and tachycardia of greater than 100. Palpate the radial pulse, wait for a moment and then count for 15 seconds. You can then multiply by four to give a rate per minute. Is the pulse regular and if not how is it irregular? (Fig. 10.12).

In addition to testing pulse volume and character, which are better assessed from the carotid pulse, you should also check for the presence of pulsus paradoxus. In normal individuals the pulse decreases slightly in volume on inspiration and systolic blood pressure falls by 3–5 mmHg. In severe obstructive diseases (e.g. severe asthma) the contractile force of respiratory muscles is so great that there is a marked

Fig. 10.8 Muscle wasting

Test performed	Sign observed	Diagnostic inference

look at the dorsal aspect of the hand for any reduction in muscle bulk
 	
always compare both hands together
	muscle wasting: note the distribution and if it is unilateral or bilateral	localized:
		  unilateral
		  –Pancoast's tumour
		  bilateral
		  –disuse atrophy; rheumatoid arthritis
		
		generalized:
		  diabetes
		  thyrotoxicosis
		  anorexia nervosa

Fig. 10.9 Rheumatoid hands

Test performed	Sign observed	Diagnostic inference

look at the hands for signs of rheumatoid disease	ulnar deviation of fingers
	swan-neck or boutonnière
	  deformity
	Z-deformity of thumb
	subluxation of
	  proximal phalanx
	wasting of small muscles
		rheumatoid disease, which may affect the lung:
		  pulmonary nodules
		  pleural effusion

Fig. 10.10 Hypertrophic pulmonary osteoarthropathy

Test performed	Sign observed	Diagnostic inference

apply pressure to the wrist	tenderness on palpation of the wrist, the pain is over the shafts of the long bones adjacent to the joint
	
	arthralgia and joint swelling
		hypertrophic pulmonary osteoarthropathy, a non-metastatic complication of malignancy – subperiosteal new-bone formation in the long bones of the lower limbs and forearms; clubbing is also present – 90% of cases are associated with bronchogenic carcinoma, especially squamous cell carcinoma
		
		other causes:
		    rheumatoid arthritis
		    systemic sclerosis

Fig. 10.11 Hand tremor

Test performed	Sign observed	Diagnostic inference
ask patient to hold fingers outstretched and spread in front; place a piece of paper on the dorsal aspect of the hands; observe hands at eye level from the side	very fine finger tremor on outstretched fingers; finger tremor is made more obvious by placing a piece of paper on top of the hands	• stimulation of β-receptors by bronchodilator drugs especially nebulized drugs • thyrotoxicosis
ask patient to hold arm outstretched in front; fully extend the wrists; apply pressure to hands; leave patient like this for 30 seconds	flapping tremor (asterixis) against your hands, which is coarse and irregular in nature; maximum activity at wrist and metacarpophalangeal joints	CO_2 retention hepatic failure encephalopathy metabolic diseases subdural haematoma

Fig. 10.12 Abnormal radial pulse

Sign observed	Diagnostic inference
rate <100 beats per minute	normal
rate >100 beats per minute (tachycardia)	pain shock infection thyrotoxicosis sarcoidosis pulmonary embolism drugs e.g. salbutamol iatrogenic causes
full, exaggerated arterial pulsation (bounding pulse)	CO_2 retention thyrotoxicosis fever anaemia hyperkinetic states

fall in systolic pressure on inspiration. A fall of greater than 10 mmHg is pathological. Figure 10.13 shows how to test for this sign.

You will gain marks if your examination looks fluent and professional. It is easy to move smoothly from introducing yourself and shaking the patient's hand to examination of the hands to testing the radial pulse. Then you can discreetly test for respiratory rate without patients realizing and altering their breathing.

Examination of the limbs

Examine the axillary lymph nodes as shown in Figure 10.14. Check the patient's ankles for oedema by applying pressure with fingers and thumb for a few seconds. If there is subcutaneous fluid you may see pitting persisting. Bilateral pitting oedema is seen in many conditions including congestive cardiac failure, liver failure and, important to your respiratory enquiry, cor pulmonale.

Head and neck

Examination of the face

First, observe the face generally. You may notice:

- Signs of superior vena cava obstruction (Fig. 10.15).
- Cushingoid features (Fig. 10.15).

Look at the mouth for signs of:

Fig. 10.13 Pulsus paradoxus

Test performed	Sign observed	Diagnostic inference

measure blood pressure using a sphygmomanometer: cuff pressure is reduced and systolic sound is heard; this initially occurs only in expiration; with further reduction of cuff pressure you can hear systole in inspiration as well; the pressure difference between the initial systolic sound in expiration and when it is present throughout the breathing cycle is what is measured	pulse volume decreases with inspiration, the reverse of normal
	
	large fall in systolic blood pressure during inspiration
		severe asthma
		
		other causes:
		  cardiac tamponade
		  massive pulmonary embolism
		
		fall is exaggerated when venous return to the right heart is impaired

Fig. 10.14 Enlarged axillary lymph nodes

Test performed	Sign observed	Diagnostic inference
method 1: face the patient; place the patient's right arm on your right arm; patient's arm must be relaxed; palpate axilla with left hand; place the patient's left arm on your left arm; palpate left axilla	enlarged lymph node (axillary lymphadenopathy)	localized spread of viral or bacterial infection tuberculosis human immunodeficiency virus (HIV) infection actinomycosis cytomegalovirus (CMV) infection measles
method 2: ask the patient to place hands behind head; palpate axilla by placing your fingers high up in axilla; press tips of fingers against chest wall; move fingers down over ribs		axial lymphadenopathy is often present in breast carcinoma

- Candida infection – white coating on tongue often seen after steroids or antibiotics.
- Central cyanosis (Fig. 10.16).

Then examine the eyes (Figs 10.17 and 10.18) and test for anaemia (Fig. 10.19).

Remember that an anaemic patient may be dangerously desaturated without appearing cyanosed.

Examination of the neck

Examine tracheal position and measure the cricosternal distance (Figs 10.20 and 10.21). Then make sure the patient is at 45° and test the jugular venous pulse (Figs 10.22 and 10.23). Finally, test for cervical lymphadenopathy from behind (Figs 10.24 and 10.25).

Develop a set system of palpating the lymph nodes of the neck (as mentioned above). Sit the patient up and examine from behind with both hands.

Before a clinical examination, learn the lymph nodes of the neck and into which set of nodes different structures drain.

Fig. 10.15 Observation of the face

Test performed	Sign observed	Diagnostic inference

observe the patient's face	oedema
	cyanosis
	puffy eyes
	fixed, engorged neck veins
		superior vena cava obstruction:
		    bronchial carcinoma
		    lymphoma
		    mediastinal goitre
		    fibrosis

	features associated with Cushing's syndrome:
	    moon face
	    plethora
	    acne
	    hirsute
	    oral candidiasis
		long-term administration of steroids
		    ACTH secretion by
		    small-cell
		    bronchial
		    carcinoma

Fig. 10.16 Central cyanosis

Test performed	Sign observed	Diagnostic inference

good natural light is needed
ask the patient to stick tongue out;
look at the mucous membranes of the lips and tongue
	blue discolouration to skin and mucous membrane
	central cyanosis cannot be accurately identified in black and Asian patients
		level of deoxygenated haemoglobin >5 g/dL
		diseases caused by marked ventilation : perfusion mismatch will cause central cyanosis:
		    severe pulmonary fibrosis; chronic bronchitis; right–left heart shunts
		    pneumonia
		    respiratory failure
		    bronchiectasis
		    chronic obstructive pulmonary disease

Before a clinical examination, learn the lymph nodes of the neck and into which set of nodes different structures drain.

Fig. 10.17 Examination of the eyes

Test performed	Sign observed	Diagnostic inference
look at the eyes, noting the position of the eyelid and pupil size; always compare with the other side. if an abnormality is present, check that the pupils are reactive to light	dropping of upper eyelids so that upper part of iris and pupil are covered (ptosis)	third nerve palsy (with dilated pupil) Horner's syndrome (with small reactive pupil); involvement of the sympathetic chain on the posterior chest wall by an apical bronchial carcinoma; T1 wasting and sensory loss also occur. idiopathic (usually in young females) Myasthenia gravis (with bilateral ptosis) Dystrophia Mitochondrial disease (rare)
	small pupil	old age Horner's syndrome Argyll Robertson's pupil: miotic and responsive to accommodation effort, but not to light disease in pons cerebrovascular accident drugs (e.g. opiates)

The thorax

Observation of the thorax

As already noted, it is often easier to inspect the thorax as part of your general inspection. In addition to observing chest wall movement, you should note any lesions, thoracic scars (Fig. 10.26) or radiotherapy tattoos (small green or blue dots used as guidance for radiotherapy). Then observe the shape of the thorax from the front, side and back and look at the curvature of the spine. Chest deformities may be asymptomatic or they may restrict the ventilatory capacity of the lungs. Common chest abnormalities and their clinical significance are shown in Figures 10.27 and 10.28.

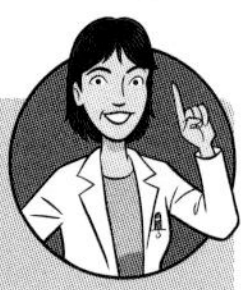

Scoliosis and kyphosis can lead to respiratory failure caused by compressional effects.

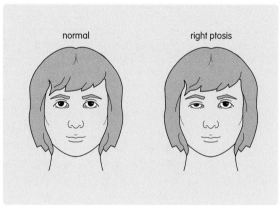

normal   right ptosis

Fig. 10.18 Typical appearance of a patient with ptosis.

Fig. 10.19 Anaemia

Test performed	Sign observed	Diagnostic inference
ask patient to look up, then evert lower lid of eye note the colour of mucous membrane	pale mucous membrane	indication of anaemia; however, anaemia can only be conclusively diagnosed by measuring haemoglobin levels

Fig. 10.20 Tracheal position and crico-sternal distance

Test performed	Sign observed	Diagnostic inference
stand at the front of the patient; pressing gently, place one finger on the trachea judge if the finger slides to one side (tracheal deviation gives an indication of the position of the upper mediastinum; however, the only conclusive method of judging the position is chest radiography)	deviation of the trachea away from the midline	pulled to side of collapse pushed away from mass or fluid contralateral side to tension pneumothorax
measure the distance (in finger breadths) between the sternal notch and cricoid cartilage during a full inspiration	three or four finger breadths	normal
	reduced distance	air flow limitation

Palpation

You should palpate any lumps or depressions you noticed on inspection and test for the symmetry and extent of chest expansion (Fig. 10.29). Testing chest expansion from the posterior is illustrated in Figure 10.30.

Test for the position of the apex beat by moving your hand inwards from the lateral chest until you feel the pulsation. The apex beat should be in the fifth intercostal space at the midclavicular line. The clinical significance of deviations is shown in Figure 10.31.

Test for tactile vocal fremitus as shown in Figure 10.32.

Percussion

The percussion note tells us the consistency of the matter underlying the chest wall, i.e. if it is air, fluid or solid. The correct method of percussion is shown in Figure 10.33 and described in Figure 10.34, which also describes the diagnostic inferences from percussion. Percuss in a logical order, comparing one side with the other and remember to include the axilla (Fig. 10.35). A normal percussion note is described as resonant. In lung pathology the percussion note may be:

When percussing, remember that the upper lobe predominates anteriorly and the lower lobe predominates posteriorly.

- Hyperresonant.
- Dull.
- Stony dull.

Map out any abnormality you find but do not confuse the cardiac borders or liver edge with lung pathology; they will sound dull normally. The note also sounds muffled in a very muscular or obese patient.

Auscultation

Normal breath sounds are described as vesicular and have a rustling quality heard in inspiration and the first part of expiration. Listen to the patient's chest:

- Using the bell of the stethoscope.
- In a logical order comparing the two sides (as for percussion).
- With the patient taking fairly quick breaths through an open mouth.

You should listen for:

- Diminished vesicular breaths (Fig. 10.36).
- Bronchial breathing (Fig. 10.36).
- Added sounds, such as wheezes or stridor (Fig. 10.37), crackles (Fig. 10.38) or pleural rub (Fig. 10.39).

With auscultation always think BAR (B – Breath sounds; A – Added sounds; R – vocal Resonance). Added sounds that disappear when the patient coughs are not significant.

Vocal resonance

The tests for vocal resonance and whispering pectoriloquy are shown in Figures 10.40 and 10.41.

Summary

Once you have finished your examination, sum up the positive findings in a clear and concise manner. Figure 10.42 is a summary of the signs found on examination of the respiratory system as a whole.

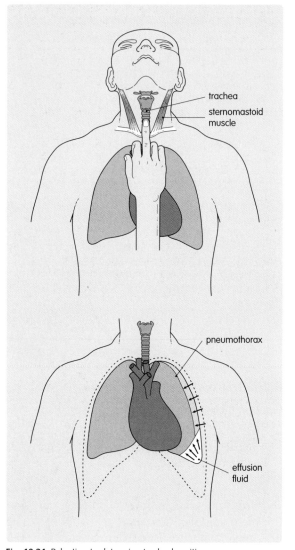

Fig. 10.21 Palpation to determine tracheal position.

Fig. 10.22 Jugular venous pressure

Test performed	Sign observed	Diagnostic inference
patient must be at 45° looking straight ahead; good light is needed; ask patient to rest head comfortably against a pillow, neck slightly flexed; the patient's neck must be relaxed, as it is impossible to assess jugular venous pressure if the sternomastoid muscles are tensed	elevated jugular venous pressure	resting pressure in thorax is raised: • tension pneumothorax • severe hyperinflation is asthma
a normal jugular pulse becomes visible just above the clavicle between the two heads of sternocleidomastoid; jugular venous pressure is difficult to assess and needs much practice; if the jugular pulse is not seen, try the hepatojugular reflex: apply pressure to the liver, increasing venous return to the heart, and so increasing the jugular venous pressure	elevated nonpulsatile jugular venous pressure	superior vena cava obstruction, usually caused by malignant enlargement of the right bronchus
	elevated pulsatile jugular venous pressure	paratracheal lymph nodes cor pulmonale
time against the contralateral pulse and measure the height of the pulse above the heart (giving a measure of pressure); the normal height of the pulse above the atrium is <4 cm	depressed jugular venous pressure	shock dehydration severe infection

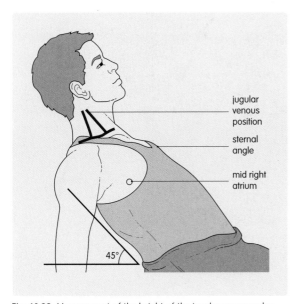

jugular
venous
position

sternal
angle

mid right
atrium

45°

Fig. 10.23 Measurement of the height of the jugular venous pulse.

Fig. 10.24 Cervical lymphadenopathy

Test performed	Sign observed	Diagnostic inference
examine the cervical chain of lymph nodes from behind the patient; it helps if the neck is slightly flexed; most patients extend neck to try and help you	cervical lymphadenopathy	infection carcinoma tuberculosis sarcoidosis
know the nodes which you are feeling	note number of palpable nodes	hard node: calcified soft, matted node: tuberculous
using both hands, start at the mandibular ramus, palpate the submandibular nodes then anterior chain nodes, supraclavicular nodes, and posterior chain nodes in a Z-fashion	describe as for any lump	

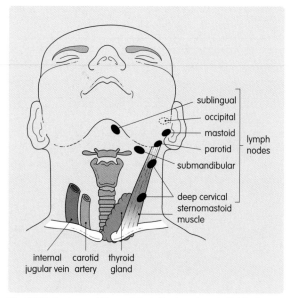

Fig. 10.25 Anatomy of the neck including lymph node distribution.

Fig. 10.26 Thoracic scars

Test performed	Sign observed	Diagnostic inference
look at the thorax for any obvious scars, remembering to look at the front and back of the chest, axilla, and under the breasts	scars present from previous operations	median sternotomy (most open-heart surgery; cardiopulmonary bypass)
		posteriolateral thoracotomy (ligation of posterior descending artery; lung and oesophageal resections)
		lateral thoracotomy (pneumothorax)
		left thoracotomy (closed mitral valvotomy)

Fig. 10.27 Assessing the chest wall and space

Test performed	Sign observed	Diagnostic inference
look at the sternum and its relationship to the ribs	depressed in pectus excavatum (funnel chest)	benign condition requiring no treatment on chest radiograph, the heart may be displaced and appear enlarged
	prominent in pectus carinatum (pigeon chest)	may be secondary to severe childhood asthma
observe the patient from the side; ask patient to fold arms and take a deep inspiration	anteroposterior diameter of chest > lateral diameter (barrel chest)	hyperinflation asthma
ask the patient to stand; stand directly behind the patient and look at the curvature of the spine	increased lateral curvature of the spine (scoliosis)	structural abnormality development abnormality vertebral disc prolapse
next, stand at the side of the patient and again look at the curvature of the spine	increased forward curvature of the spine (kyphosis)	osteoporosis ankylosing spondylitis

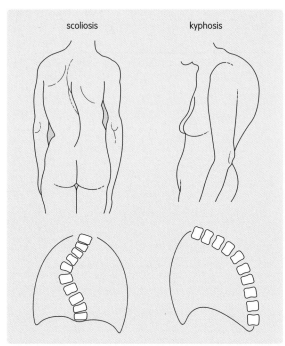

scoliosis   kyphosis

Fig. 10.28 Features of scoliosis and kyphosis.

Fig. 10.29 Chest expansion		
Test performed	**Sign observed**	**Diagnostic inference**
place the flat of both hands on the pectoral region of the chest; ask the patient to take a deep breath, and note any asymmetry	symmetrical rise of hands as chest expands	normal
	asymmetrical rise	unilateral pathology on the depressed side
put fingers of both hands as far around the chest as possible; bring thumbs together in the midline; keep thumbs off chest wall; ask patient to take a deep breath in; note distance between thumbs; examine both front and back	–	–
place a tape measure around the internipple line and measure the difference between inspiration and expiration	>4 cm expansion	normal
	<4 cm expansion	reduced expansion

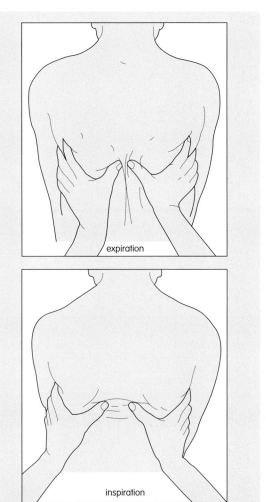

expiration

inspiration

Fig. 10.30 Examining chest expansion from the back. (After Burton, Hodgkin & Ward 1977, with permission of Lippincott-Raven.)

Fig. 10.31 Apex beat	
Sign observed	**Diagnostic inference**
pulsation in fifth intercostal space midclavicular line	normal
deviated pulsation; lower mediastinum displacement	left deviation: cardiomegaly pulmonary fibrosis scoliosis pectus excavatum bronchiectasis right deviation: pneumothorax pleural effusion dextracardia

Fig. 10.32 Tactile vocal fremitus		
Test performed	**Sign observed**	**Diagnostic inference**
place either the ulnar edge or the flat of your hand on the chest wall; ask the patient to repeatedly say '99' or '1, 2, 3'; repeat for front and back, comparing opposite zones	increased resonance	solid areas of lung with open airways consolidation pneumonia tuberculosis extensive fibrosis
the vibrations produced by the manoeuvre are transmitted through the lung substance and felt by the hand; alterations in disease are the same as for vocal resonance	decreased resonance	feeble voice pleural thickening blocked bronchus

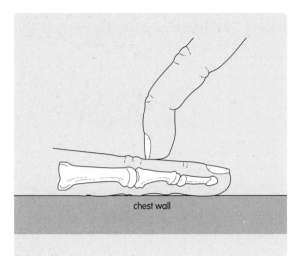

chest wall

Fig. 10.33 Correct method of percussion (see Fig. 10.34 for explanation).

Fig. 10.34 Percussion

Test performed	Sign observed	Diagnostic inference
place your non-dominant hand on the chest wall, palm downwards, with fingers slightly separated; the second phalanx of the middle finger should be in an intercostal space directly over the area to be percussed; strike this finger with the terminal phalanx of the middle finger of the other hand	increased resonance (resonance depends on the thickness of the chest wall and the amount of air in the structures underlying it)	increased air in lung: • emphysema • large bullae • pneumothoraces • asthma
to achieve a good percussion note, the striking finger should be partially flexed and struck at right angles to the other finger; the striking movement must be a flick of the wrist on percussion you will hear a percussion note and feel vibrations	dullness (solid lung tissue does not reflect sound as readily as aerated lung); if a dull area exists, map out its limits by percussing from the resonant to the dull area	consolidation: • fibrosis • collapse • pleural thickening • tuberculosis • extensive carcinoma
percuss from top to bottom including axilla; to check for disease in the lung apices, percuss directly onto the clavicles; do not percuss more heavily than you need and always compare both sides, front and back dullness occurs as you percuss over the liver; note that the right diaphragm is higher than the left diaphragm	stony dullness	fluid present: • pleural effusion

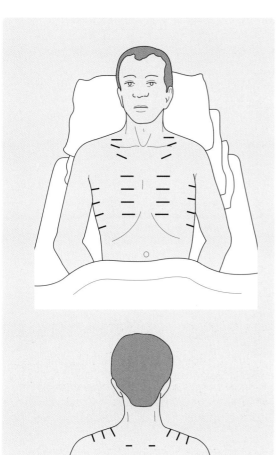

Fig. 10.35 Sites for percussion. (From Munro & Campbell 2000, with permission of Churchill Livingstone.)

Fig. 10.36 Auscultation of the thorax

Sign observed	Diagnostic inference
vesicular breath sounds	breath sounds are produced in the larger airways where flow is turbulent; sounds are transmitted through smaller airways to the chest wall; vesicular breath sounds are normal
	if vesicular breath sounds are reduced or absent: • airway obstruction • asthma • chronic obstructive pulmonary disease • tumour
bronchial breath sounds (described in relation to timing; a gap exists between inspiration and expiration, which are of equal duration; harsh clear breath sounds)	normal, if heard at the tip of the scapula; otherwise caused by: • consolidation • pneumonia • lung abscess
	if inaudible: • severe emphysema • bullae • pneumothorax • pleural effusion

Fig. 10.37 Wheeze and stridor

Sign observed	Diagnostic inference
prolonged musical sound	none: the amount of wheeze is not a good indicator of the degree of airway obstruction
polyphonic sound (many musical notes), mainly in expiration	small airway obstruction: narrowing caused by combination of smooth muscle contraction; inflammation within airways; increased bronchial secretions
monophonic sound	large airway obstruction: a worrying finding, suggesting a single narrowing (e.g. tumour)
loud inspiratory sound	large airway narrowing (larynx, trachea, main bronchi): • laryngotracheobronchitis • epiglottitis • laryngitis

Fig. 10.38 Crackles

Test performed	Sign observed	Diagnostic inference
listen to the patient breathing crackles may be mimicked by rolling hair on your temple between two fingers; timing during the respiratory cycle is of huge significance	non-musical, short, uninterrupted sounds heard during inspiration	crackles represent equalization of intraluminal pressure as collapsed small airways open during inspiration
	early inspiratory crackles	diffuse airflow limitation chronic obstructive pulmonary disease pulmonary oedema
	late inspiratory crackles	conditions that largely involve alveoli: • fibrosis • fibrosing alveolitis • bronchiectasis

Fig. 10.39 Pleural rub

Test performed	Sign observed	Diagnostic inference
listen to the patient breathing	leathery creaking sound associated with each breath inspiratory and expiratory sound that is not shifted by cough; reoccurs at the same time in each respiratory cycle	caused by inflamed surfaces of pleura rubbing together: • pneumonia • pulmonary embolism • emphysema • pleurisy

Fig. 10.40 Vocal resonance

Test performed	Sign observed	Diagnostic inference
auscultatory equivalent to vocal fremitus; place the stethoscope on to the chest and ask the patient to repeatedly say '99' or '1, 2, 3'	normal lung attenuates high-frequency notes; normally, booming low-pitched sounds are heard	as for vocal fremitus

Fig. 10.41 Whispering pectoriloquy

Test performed	Sign observed	Diagnostic inference
place the stethoscope on to the chest and ask the patient to repeatedly whisper '99' or '1, 2, 3'	words are clear and seem to be spoken right into the listener's ears (whispering pectoriloquy)	whispered speech cannot usually be heard over healthy lung; solid lung tissue conducts sound better than normally aerated lung, indicating consolidation, cavitation, tuberculosis, or pneumonia

Fig. 10.42 Summary table of signs found on examination of the respiratory system

	Consolidation	Pneumothorax	Pleural effusion	Lobar collapse	Pleural thickening
Chest radiograph					
Mediastinal shift and trachea	none	none (simple), away (tension)	none or away	towards the affected side	none
Chest wall excursion	normal or decreased on the affected side	normal or decreased on the affected side	decreased on the affected side	decreased	decreased
Percussion note	dull	resonant	stony dull	dull	dull
Breath sounds	increased (bronchial)	decreased	decreased	decreased	decreased
Added sounds	crackles	click (occasional)	rub (occasional)	none	none
Tactile vocal fremitus or vocal resonance	increased	decreased	decreased	decreased	decreased

Investigations and imaging

Objectives

By the end of this chapter you should be able to:

- Summarize the basic haematological tests performed.
- Describe the key information provided by arterial blood gas analysis.
- Describe what tests can be performed on a sputum sample.
- Describe the main use of the histopathology laboratory in diagnosing respiratory disease.
- Describe how to accurately perform a PEFR test.
- List the uses and limitations of the PEFR test.
- Describe tests for airway narrowing.
- Describe the importance of spirometry in differentiating obstructive from restrictive disorders.
- Describe the differences between obstructive and restrictive lung disease.
- Interpret and draw abnormal flow–volume loops.
- Discuss the implications of an abnormal transfer factor test result.
- Describe how airway compliance and resistance can be calculated.
- List indications for exercise testing.
- List indications for ultrasound in respiratory medicine.
- Describe how to read a PA plain film chest radiograph.
- Describe the differences between collapse and consolidation when viewing them on a chest radiograph.
- Describe the silhouette sign and its use.
- Describe an air bronchogram and its use.
- Describe the differences between collapse and consolidation on chest radiographs.
- Describe the uses and limitations of CT and MRI in respiratory imaging.

INTRODUCTION

There are a large number of investigations in respiratory medicine, ranging from basic bedside tests to more invasive procedures such as bronchoscopy. As you read this chapter, you should bear in mind that some of the investigations below are performed only rarely in specialized pulmonary laboratories whilst others are performed by patients at home every day. The investigations that are most commonly performed, and which you should have a thorough knowledge of, include:

- Arterial blood gas analysis.
- Sputum examination.
- Basic tests of pulmonary function.
- Bronchoscopy.
- Chest X-rays.

ROUTINE INVESTIGATIONS

Haematology

In the associated figures, you will find some of the commonly performed haematological tests:

- Full blood count (Fig. 11.1).
- Differential white blood cell count (Fig. 11.2).
- Other haematological tests (Fig. 11.3).

Fig. 11.1 Full blood count

Test	Normal values	Diagnostic inference	
		Increased values	**Decreased values**
haemoglobin (g/dL)	male: 13–18 female: 11.5–16.5	decreased in anaemia (look at MCV for further information); a normal MCV (i.e. normocytic anaemia) is common in chronic disease	
mean cell volume (fl)	76–98	macrocytosis (B12 or folate deficiency etc.)	microcytosis (common in iron deficiency anaemia and thalassaemias)
red blood cells ($\times 10^9$)	male: 4.5–6.5 female: 3.8–5.8	polycythemia; may be secondary to chronic lung disease, smoking, altitude	

Fig. 11.2 Differential white blood cell count

Cell type	Normal values	Diagnostic inference	
		Increased values	**Decreased values**
white blood cell	$4–11 \times 10^9$/L	bacterial infections malignancy pregnancy	viral infections drugs systemic lupus erythematosus overwhelming bacterial infection
neutrophil	$2.5–7.5 \times 10^9$/L 60–70%	bacterial infections malignancy pregnancy	viral infections drugs systemic lupus erythematosus overwhelming bacterial infection
eosinophil	$0.04–0.44 \times 10^9$/L 1–4%	allergic reactions asthma sarcoidosis pneumonia eosinophilic granulomatosus	steroid therapy
monocyte	$0.2–0.8 \times 10^9$/L 5–10%	tuberculosis	chronic infection
lymphocyte	$1.5–4.0 \times 10^9$/L 25–30%	infection cytomegalovirus infection toxoplasmosis tuberculosis	tuberculosis

Fig. 11.3 Other haematological tests

Test performed	Normal values	Diagnostic inference	
		Increased values	**Decreased values**
C-reactive protein (CRP)	normal < 4 mg/L changes more rapidly than erythrocyte sedimentation rate	acute infection, inflammation; same as erythrocyte sedimentation rate	levels often normal in malignancy
anti-streptolysin O (ASO) titre	normal < 200 IU/mL	confirms recent streptococcal infection	

Clinical chemistry

The commonly performed biochemical tests are shown in Figure 11.4.

If malignancy is suspected, you should also perform liver function tests and test alkaline phosphatase as an indicator of metastases. In addition, endocrine tests should be performed for paraneoplastic manifestations.

Tests of blood gases

Arterial blood gas analysis

Blood gas analysis of an arterial blood sample is mandatory in all acute pulmonary conditions. The analysis should always be repeated soon after starting oxygen therapy to assess response to treatment.

A heparinized sample of arterial blood is tested using a standard automated machine, which measures:

- P_aO_2.
- P_aCO_2.
- Oxygen saturation. Blood pH, standard bicarbonate and base excess are either given on the standard readout or can be calculated.

The patient's results are compared with the normal ranges (Fig. 11.5) and assessed in two parts:

- Degree of arterial oxygenation – is the patient hypoxic?
- Acid–base balance disturbances.

Fig. 11.4 Biochemical blood tests

Test performed	Normal values	Diagnostic inference	
		Increased values	Decreased values
potassium	3.5–5.0 mmol/L		adrenocorticotropic hormone (ACTH) secreting tumour β-agonists
angiotensin converting enzyme (ACE)	10–70 U/L	sarcoidosis	
calcium	2.12–2.65 mmol/L	malignancy sarcoidosis squamous cell carcinoma of the lung	
glucose	3.5–5.5 mmol/L	adrenocorticotropic hormone (ACTH) secreting tumour long-term steroid use pancreatic dysfunction	

Fig. 11.5 Arterial blood gases

Test performed	Normal values	Diagnostic inference	
		Increased values	Decreased values
pH	7.35–7.45	alkalosis hyperventilation	acidosis CO_2 retention
P_aO_2	>10.6 kPa		hypoxic
P_aCO_2	4.7–6.0 kPa	respiratory acidosis (if pH decreased)	respiratory alkalosis (if pH increased)
base excess	±2 mmol/L	metabolic alkalosis	metabolic acidosis
standardized bicarbonate	22–25 mmol/L	metabolic alkalosis	metabolic acidosis

Before accurate interpretation of the results, a detailed history of the patient including a detailed drug history is needed.

Pulse oximetry

This is a simple, non-invasive method of monitoring the percentage of haemoglobin that is saturated with oxygen. The patient wears a probe on a finger or ear lobe and this is linked to a unit which displays the readings. The unit can be set to sound an alarm when saturation drops below a certain level (usually 90%). The pulse oximeter works by calculating the absorption of light by haemoglobin, which alters depending on whether it is saturated with oxygen or desaturated. A number of factors may lead to inaccurate oximeter readings. These include:

- Poor peripheral perfusion.
- Carbon monoxide poisoning.
- Skin pigmentation.
- Nail varnish.
- Dirty hands.

Microbiology

Microbiological examination is possible with samples of sputum, bronchial aspirate, pleural aspirate, throat swabs and blood. The aim of examination is to identify bacteria, viruses or fungi.

Tests to request are microscopy, culture and drug sensitivity. The microbiological findings should be interpreted in view of the whole clinical picture.

Bacteriology

Sputum

Testing of sputum for the presence of bacteria is the most common microbiological test performed in respiratory medicine. Obtain the sample, preferably of induced sputum, before antibiotic treatment is started. Collect into a sterile container, inspect the sample, and send to the laboratory.

Request Gram stain, Ziehl–Neelsen stain, and anaerobic cultures. Culture on Lowenstein–Jensen medium to detect tuberculosis. A sputum sample is valuable in diagnosing suspected pneumonia, tuberculosis and aspergillosis, or if the patient presents with an unusual clinical picture.

Failure to isolate an organism from the sputum is not uncommon.

Resistance to commonly used antibiotics is often found in bacteria responsible for respiratory tract infections; therefore, antibiotic sensitivity testing is vital.

Blood culture

A blood culture should always be performed in patients with fever and lower respiratory tract infection. Collect a large volume of blood and divide it equally into two bottles of nutrient media, 20 mL of blood per culture bottle. Collect two or three cultures over 24 hours.

Blood cultures identify systemic bacterial and fungal infections. Results may be positive while sputum culture is negative.

Upper respiratory specimens

Microscopy is generally unhelpful because of the abundant commensals of the upper respiratory tract, which contaminate samples.

Throat specimens can be collected using a Dacron or calcium alginate swab. The tonsils, posterior pharynx and any ulcerated areas are sampled. Avoid contact with tongue and saliva, as this can inhibit identification of group A streptococci.

A sinus specimen is collected with a needle and syringe. The specimen is cultured for aerobic and anaerobic bacteria. Common pathogens of sinuses are *Streptococcus pneumoniae*, *Haemophilus influenzae*, *Mycoplasma catarrhalis*, *Staphylococcus aureus* and anaerobes.

Coxiella burnetii, *Mycoplasma pneumoniae* and *Legionella* are difficult to culture; therefore, results of serology must be used.

Lower respiratory specimens

Techniques used to collect samples include expectoration, cough induction with saline, bronchoscopy, bronchial alveolar lavage, transtracheal aspiration and direct aspiration through the chest wall. Some of these techniques are considered below under the more invasive procedures.

Viral testing

Because of the small size of viral particles, light microscopy provides little information: it is able to visualize viral inclusions and cytopathic effects of viral infection.

Viral serology

Viral serology is the most important group of tests in virology. Serological diagnoses are obtained when viruses are difficult to isolate and grow in cell culture.

Specimens should be collected early in the acute phase because viral shedding for respiratory viruses lasts 3–7 days; however, symptoms commonly persist for longer. A repeated sample should be collected 10 days later.

Specimens should be tested serologically only after the second sample has been received. The laboratory measures antibody type and titre in response to the viral infection: a fourfold increase in titre (rising titre) taken over 10 days is significant.

Viral serology also identifies the virus and its strain or serotype, and is able to evaluate the course of infection.

Cell culture

Specimens for cell cultures are obtained from nasal washings, throat swabs, nasal swabs and sputum. Viruses cannot be cultured without living cells.

Fungal testing

Fungal infections may be serious, especially in the immunocompromised patient, where they can cause systemic infection; invasive fungal infections require blood culture. Repeated specimens from the site need to be taken to rule out contaminants in cultures.

Common fungal infections are *Candida* and *Aspergillus*. Microscopic identification may be difficult for *Aspergillus* because it is common in the environment. Culture is rarely helpful in identifying *Aspergillus*; the *Aspergillus* precipitins test is of more use.

MORE-INVASIVE PROCEDURES

Bronchoscopy

Bronchoscopy allows the visualization of the trachea and larger bronchi and can be used to sample tissues via brushings, lavage or biopsy. Two types of bronchoscope are used:

- Flexible fibreoptic bronchoscope.
- Rigid bronchoscope (under general anaesthetic).

In practice, the flexible bronchoscope is used in most instances. Patients may be lightly sedated to reduce anxiety and suppress the cough mechanism. Topical lidocaine (lignocaine) is used to anaesthetize the pharynx and vocal cords.

The main indications for bronchoscopy are:

- Diagnosis of lung cancer (e.g. after an abnormal chest X-ray or haemoptysis).

- Staging of lung cancer.
- Diagnosis of diffuse lung disease.
- Diagnosis of infections (especially in immunocompromised hosts).

Bronchoalveolar lavage (BAL)

Sterile saline is infused down the flexible bronchoscope and then aspirated. This technique is commonly used to look for evidence of neoplasms or opportunistic infections in immunocompromised patients.

Transbronchial biopsy

Transbronchial biopsy provides samples from outside the airways, e.g. of alveolar tissue. The technique is performed using biopsy forceps attached to a flexible bronchoscope. The bronchoscopist cannot directly visualize the biopsy site and may be assisted by fluoroscopic imaging. Complications include pneumothorax or haemorrhage.

Percutaneous fine needle aspiration

This technique is used to sample peripheral lesions under the guidance of radiography.

Open and thorascopic lung biopsy

In some cases of diffuse lung disease, or where a lesion cannot easily be reached, more extensive lung biopsy is required for diagnosis. Open lung biopsy is performed through a thoracotomy with the patient under general anaesthesia. However, video-assisted thorascopic techniques are increasingly used as a less invasive alternative.

HISTOPATHOLOGY

Histopathology is the investigation and diagnosis of disease from the examination of tissues.

Histopathological examination of biopsy material

The histopathological examination is a vital test in cases of suspected malignancy, allowing a definitive diagnosis to be made. Biopsy material is obtained by the techniques described above, in addition to:

- Pleural biopsy.
- Lymph node biopsy.

Histological features of malignant neoplasms are:
- Loss of cellular differentiation.
- Abundant cells undergoing mitosis, many of which are abnormal.
- High nuclear:cytoplasm ratio.
- Cells or nuclei varying in shape and size.

Other uses of histopathology include diagnosing interstitial lung diseases such as cryptogenic fibrosing alveolitis.

Cytological examination of sputum

Cytological examination is useful in diagnosing bronchial carcinoma and has the advantage of being a non-invasive, quick test; however, it is dependent upon adequate sputum production. Sputum is obtained by:

- Induction–inhalation of nebulized hypertonic saline.
- Transtracheal aspiration.
- Bronchoscopy.
- Bronchial washings.

Exfoliated cells (in the sputum, pleural fluid, bronchial brushings/washings, or fine-needle aspirate of lymph nodes and lesions) are examined, primarily for signs of malignancy.

Pulmonary function tests can seem confusing but there are just three basic questions that most tests aim to answer:
- Are the airways narrowed? (PEFR, FEV_1, FEV_1:FVC, flow–volume loops.)
- Are the lungs a normal size? (TLC, RV and FRC.)
- Is gas uptake normal? (T_LCO and KCO.)
So, as a minimum, make sure you have a good understanding of peak flow monitoring and spirometry and know how you would measure RV, FRC and gas transfer.

INVESTIGATIONS OF PULMONARY FUNCTION

Tests of pulmonary function are used in:

- Diagnosis of lung disease.
- Monitoring disease progression.
- Assessing patient response to treatment.

Tests of ventilation

Ventilation can be impaired in two basic ways:

- The airways become narrowed (obstructive disorders).
- Expansion of the lungs is reduced (restrictive disorders).

These two types of disorder have characteristic patterns of lung function (see Ch. 4) which can be measured using the tests below.

Forced expiration

Peak expiratory flow rate (PEFR) is a simple and cheap test that uses a peak flow meter (Fig. 11.6) to measure the maximum expiratory rate in the first 10 ms of expiration. Peak flow meters can be issued

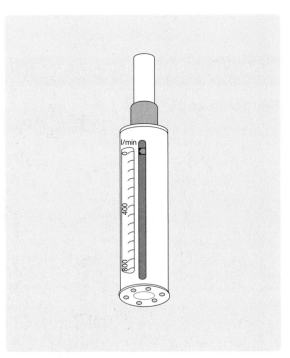

Fig. 11.6 Peak flow meter.

on prescription and used at home by patients to monitor their lung function.

Before measuring PEFR (Fig. 11.7), the practitioner should instruct the patient to:

- Take a full inspiration to maximum lung capacity.
- Seal the lips tightly around the mouthpiece.
- Blow out forcefully into the peak flow meter, which is held horizontally.

The best of three measurements is recorded and plotted on the appropriate graph. At least two recordings per day are required to obtain an accurate pattern. Normal PEFR is 400–650 L/min in healthy adults.

PEFR is reduced in conditions that cause airway obstruction:

- Asthma, where there is wide diurnal variation in PEFR known as 'morning dipping' (Fig. 11.8).
- Chronic obstructive pulmonary disease.
- Upper airway tumours.

Other causes of reduced PEFR include expiratory muscle weakness, inadequate effort and poor technique. PEFR is not a good measure of air flow limitation because it measures only initial expiration; it is best used to monitor progression of disease and response to treatment.

Alex, a 9-year-old boy, was becoming wheezy and short of breath after mild exertion. His GP asked him to keep a peak flow diary, which showed diurnal variation with morning dipping. As this was suggestive of asthma, the GP prescribed bronchodilators which Alex used about three times a week to control his symptoms.

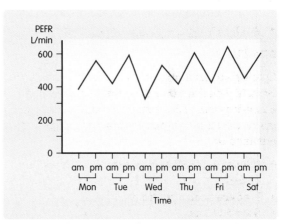

Fig. 11.8 Typical peak expiratory flow rate graph for an asthmatic patient.

Fig. 11.7 Patient performing peak expiratory flow rate test.

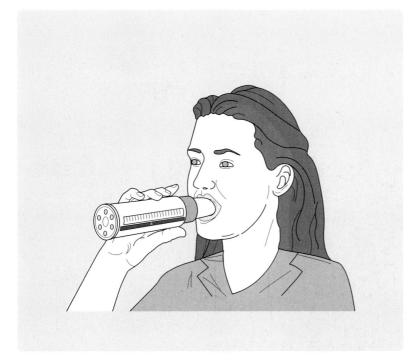

Forced expiratory volume and forced vital capacity

The forced expiratory volume in one second (FEV_1) and the forced vital capacity (FVC) are measured using a spirometer. The spirometer works by converting volumes of inspiration and expiration into a single line trace. The subject is connected by a mouthpiece to a sealed chamber (Fig. 11.9). Each time the subject breathes, the volume inspired or expired is converted into the vertical position of a float. The position of the float is recorded on a rotating drum by means of a pen attachment. Electronic devices are becoming increasingly available.

FEV_1 and FVC

FEV_1 and FVC are related to height, age and sex of the patient.

FEV_1 is the volume of air expelled in the first second of a forced expiration, starting from full inspiration. FVC is a measure of total lung volume exhaled; the patient is asked to exhale with maximal effort after a full inspiration.

FEV_1 : FVC ratio

The FEV_1 : FVC ratio is a more useful measurement than FEV_1 or FVC alone. FEV_1 is 80% of FVC in normal subjects. The FEV_1 : FVC ratio is an excellent measure of airway limitation and allows us to differentiate obstructive from restrictive lung disease.

In restrictive disease:

- Both FEV_1 and FVC are reduced, often in proportion to each other.
- FEV_1 : FVC ratio is normal or increased (> 80%).

Whereas, in obstructive diseases:

- High intrathoracic pressures generated by forced expiration cause premature closure of the airways with trapping of air in the chest.
- FEV_1 is reduced much more than FVC.
- FEV_1 : FVC ratio is reduced (< 80%).

Flow–volume loops

Flow–volume loops are graphs constructed from maximal expiratory and inspiratory manoeuvres performed on a spirometer. The loop is made up of

Patterns of lung function are often tested in exams. Chapter 4 (p. 43) contains more details on patterns of obstructive and restrictive diseases.

Fig. 11.9 Spirometry. The measurement of lung volume by displacement of a float within a sealed chamber is recorded on a paper roll by a pen.

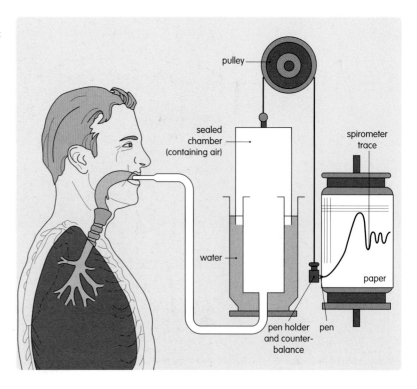

two halves: above the *x*-axis is the flow of air out of the mouth on expiration, and below the *x*-axis, flow into the mouth on inspiration. The loop shape can identify the type and distribution of airway obstruction. After a small amount of gas has been exhaled, flow is limited by:

- Elastic recoil force of the lung.
- Resistance of airways upstream of collapse.

When looking at flow–volume loops, look for a normal-shaped loop (Fig. 11.10A): a triangular expiratory curve created by an initially fast expiration of air, slowing down as total lung capacity is reached, and a semicircular inspiratory curve. Any deviation away from this triangle and semicircle pattern suggests pathology. Additionally read off the FEV_1 (marked by a star) from the *x*-axis. Reduced FEV_1 suggests an obstructive airway disease.

Flow–volume loops are useful in diagnosing upper airway obstruction (Fig. 11.10B), restrictive and obstructive disease.

In restrictive diseases:

- Maximum flow rate is reduced (read from *y*-axis).
- Total volume exhaled is reduced (read from *x*-axis).

- Flow rate is high during latter part of expiration because of increased lung recoil.

In obstructive diseases:

- Flow rate is low in relation to lung volume.
- Expiration ends prematurely because of early airway closure; most easily spotted by a scooped-out appearance after the point of maximum flow rather than the triangular-shaped expiratory curve seen in healthy lungs.

Tests of lung volumes

The amount of gas in the lungs can be thought of as being split into subdivisions (Fig. 4.3, p. 46), with disease processes altering these volumes in specific ways. In measuring tidal volume and vital capacity, we use spirometry; alternative techniques are needed for the other volumes.

Residual volume (RV) and functional residual capacity (FRC)

One important lung volume, residual volume (RV), is not measured in simple spirometry, because gas remains in the lungs at the end of each breath

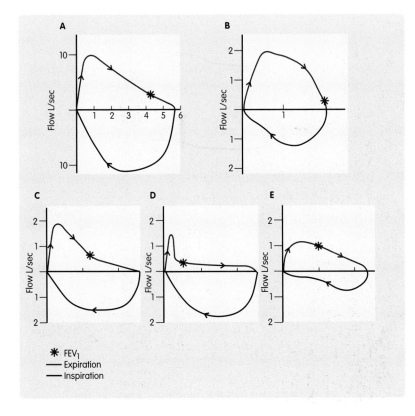

Fig. 11.10 Typical flow–volume loops. (A) Normal. (B) Restrictive defect (phrenic palsy). (C) Volume-dependent obstruction (e.g. asthma). (D) Pressure-dependent obstruction (e.g. severe emphysema). (E) Rigid obstruction (e.g. tracheal stenosis).

✳ FEV_1
— Expiration
— Inspiration

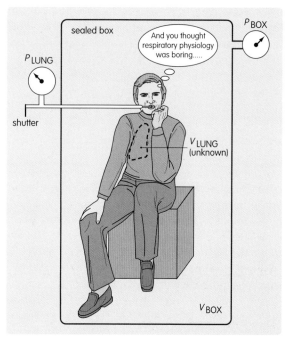

Remember that FRC is the volume of gas remaining in the lung at the end of a quiet expiration. RV is the volume remaining at the end of a maximal expiration. Look back at the subdivisions of lung volumes on page 46 (Fig. 4.3) if you are unsure as to how FRC, RV and TLC relate to each other.

Fig. 11.11 Plethysmography. This assumes pressure at the mouth is the pressure within the lung.

(otherwise the lungs would collapse). Without a measure for RV, we cannot calculate functional residual capacity (FRC) or total lung capacity (TLC).

RV is a useful measure in assessing obstructive disease. In a healthy subject, residual volume is approximately 30% of total lung capacity. In obstructive diseases, the lungs are hyperinflated with 'air trapping' so that RV is greatly increased and the ratio of RV:TLC is also increased. There are three methods of measuring RV: helium dilution, plethysmography and nitrogen washout.

Helium dilution

The patient is connected to a spirometer containing a mixture of 10% helium in air. Helium does not cross the alveolar–capillary membrane into the bloodstream and so after several breaths, the helium concentration in the spirometer and lung becomes equal. Total lung capacity can be calculated from the difference in helium concentration at the start of the test and at equilibrium; then residual volume can be calculated by subtracting vital capacity from total lung capacity.

This method only measures gas that is in communication with the airways.

Body plethysmography

Plethysmography determines changes in lung volume by recording changes in pressure. The patient sits in a large air-tight box and breathes through a mouthpiece (Fig. 11.11). At the end of a normal expiration, a shutter closes the mouthpiece and the patient is asked to make respiratory efforts. As the patient tries to inhale, box pressure increases. Using Boyle's law, lung volume can be calculated.

In contrast to the helium dilution method, body plethysmography measures all intrathoracic gas including cysts, bullae and pneumothoraces, i.e. non-communicating air spaces. This is important in

emphysematous subjects with bullae, in whom helium dilution underestimates residual volume.

Nitrogen washout

Following a normal expiration, the patient breathes 100% oxygen. This 'washes out' the nitrogen in the lungs. The gas exhaled subsequently is collected and its total volume and the concentration of nitrogen are measured. The concentration of nitrogen in the lung before washout is 80%. The concentration of nitrogen left in the lung can be measured by a nitrogen meter at the lips measuring end-expiration gas. Assuming no net change in the amount of nitrogen (it does not participate in gas exchange) it is possible to estimate the FRC.

Anatomical dead space

The volume of anatomical dead space (i.e. areas of the airway not involved in gaseous exchange) is usually about 150 mL, or 2 mL/kg of bodyweight. In a healthy person, the physiological and anatomical dead spaces are nearly equal; however, in patients with alveolar disease and non-functioning alveoli (e.g. in emphysema), physiological dead space may be up to 10 times that of the anatomical dead space.

Fowler's dead space

Fowler's dead space method uses the single-breath nitrogen test to measure anatomical dead space.

The patient makes a single inhalation of 100% O_2. On expiration, the nitrogen concentration rises as the dead space gas (100% O_2) is washed out by alveolar gas (a mixture of nitrogen and oxygen). If there were no mixing of alveolar and dead space gas during expiration there would be a stepwise increase in nitrogen concentration when alveolar gas is exhaled (Fig. 11.12A). In reality, mixing does occur which means that the nitrogen concentration increases slowly, then rises sharply. As pure alveolar gas is expired, nitrogen concentration reaches a plateau (the alveolar plateau). Nitrogen concentration is plotted against expired volume; dead space is the volume at which the two areas under the plot are equal (Fig. 11.12B).

Tests of diffusion

Oxygen and carbon dioxide pass by diffusion between the alveoli and pulmonary capillary blood. The diffusing capacity of carbon monoxide (CO) measures the ability of gas to diffuse from inspired air to capillary blood, and also reflects the uptake of oxygen from the alveolus into the red blood cells. Carbon monoxide is used because:

- It is highly soluble.
- It combines rapidly with haemoglobin.

The single-breath test is the test most commonly used to determine diffusing capacity.

Single-breath test

The patient takes a single breath from residual volume to total lung capacity. The inhaled gas contains 0.28% carbon monoxide and 13.5% helium. The patient is instructed to hold the breath for 10 seconds before expiring. The concentration of helium and carbon monoxide in the final part of the expired gas mixture is measured and the diffusing capacity of carbon monoxide is calculated. You need to know the haemoglobin level before the test.

In practice, the transfer factor is used in preference to the diffusing capacity. In the normal lung, the transfer factor accurately measures the diffusing capacity of the lungs, whereas in diseased lung diffusing capacity also depends on:

- Area and thickness of alveolar membrane.
- Ventilation : perfusion relationship.

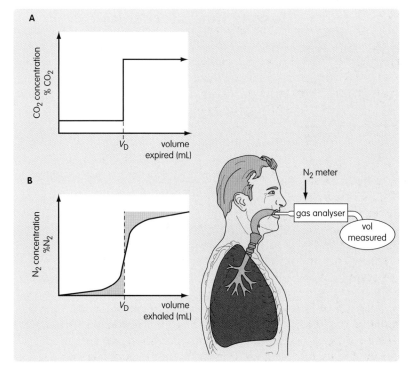

Fig. 11.12 Measurement of anatomical dead space. (A) Using Fowler's method it would be expected that the gas expired from those areas not undergoing gaseous exchange (anatomical dead space) would contain no nitrogen and thus a stepwise change would occur to the nitrogen concentration of expired gas; the volume at which this occurs would be equal to the anatomical dead space volume. (B) On a graph showing the real-world results, a dotted line has been drawn to approximate the step change in nitrogen concentration.

Transfer factor

Transfer factor (T_LCO) is defined as the amount of carbon monoxide transferred per minute, corrected for the concentration gradient of carbon monoxide across the alveolar capillary membrane (Fig. 11.13).

The transfer factor is reduced in conditions where there are:

- Fewer alveolar capillaries.
- Ventilation : perfusion mismatches.
- Reduced accessible lung volumes.

Gas transfer is a relatively sensitive but non-specific test, useful for detecting early disease in lung parenchyma; transfer coefficient is a better test. The transfer coefficient (KCO) is corrected for lung volumes and is useful in distinguishing causes of low T_LCO due to loss of lung volume:

- T_LCO and KCO are low in emphysema and fibrosing alveolitis.
- T_LCO is low, but KCO is normal in pleural effusions and consolidation.

Tests of blood flow

Pulmonary blood flow can be measured by two methods: the Fick method and the indicator dilution technique.

It might help to think of the difference between T_LCO and KCO in terms of a patient who has had a lung removed. Clearly, lung volumes are reduced and therefore so is T_LCO. But KCO corrects for the lost volume, and if the remaining lung is normal, KCO is also completely normal.

Fick method

The amount of oxygen taken up by the blood passing through the lungs is related to the difference in oxygen content between arterial and mixed-venous blood. Oxygen consumption is measured by collecting expired gas in a large spirometer and measuring its oxygen concentration.

Indicator dilution technique

Dye is injected into the venous circulation; the concentration and time of appearance of the dye in the arterial blood are recorded.

Testing patterns of ventilation

Ventilation : perfusion relationships

Ventilation : perfusion relationships are measured by means of isotope scans; these are described in the section on imaging below.

Inequality of ventilation

In diseases such as asthma or COPD the lungs may be unevenly ventilated. Inequality of ventilation is measured using the single-breath nitrogen test, similar to the method for measuring anatomical dead space described above.

Testing lung mechanics

Lung compliance

Compliance is a measure of distensibility. It is defined as the volume change per unit of pressure across the lung. Lung compliance increases in emphysema, as the lung architecture is destroyed. In contrast, pulmonary fibrosis stiffens alveolar walls and decreases compliance (Fig. 11.14).

Lung compliance is measured by introducing a balloon into the oesophagus to estimate intrapleural

Fig. 11.13 Conditions that affect the transfer factor		
	Decreased transfer factor	Increased transfer factor
Pulmonary causes	emphysema; loss of lung tissue; diffuse infiltration	pulmonary haemorrhage
Cardiovascular causes	low cardiac output, pulmonary oedema	thyrotoxicosis
Other causes	anaemia	polycythaemia

Fig. 11.14 Causes of altered lung compliance

Reduced compliance	Increased compliance
pulmonary venous pressure increased	old age
alveolar oedema	emphysema
fibrosis	bronchoalveolar drugs
airway closure	

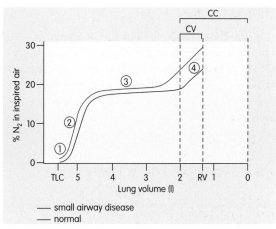

Fig. 11.15 Closing volume. Airways in lower lung zones close at low lung volumes and only those alveoli at the top of the lungs continue to empty. Because concentration of nitrogen in alveoli of upper zones is higher, the slope of the curve abruptly increases (phase 4). Phase 4 begins at larger lung volumes in individuals with even minor degrees of airway obstruction, increasing closing volume. CV = closing volume; CC = closing capacity; TLC = total lung capacity. (Courtesy of The Ciba Collection of Medical Illustrations, illustrated by Frank H Netter, 1979.)

pressure and then the patient is asked to breathe out from total lung capacity into a spirometer. This produces a pressure–volume curve. A lung of high compliance expands to a greater extent than one of low compliance when both are exposed to the same transpulmonary pressure.

Airway resistance

Airway resistance is defined as the pressure difference between the alveolus and mouth required to produce airflow of 1 L/s. Airway resistance is predominantly created by the upper respiratory tract but can be increased by asthma, COPD and endobronchial obstruction (e.g. tumour or foreign body).

Airway resistance can be measured by plethysmography. The patient is instructed to pant, causing pressure within the plethysmograph to increase during inspiration and decrease during expiration. The greater the airway resistance, the greater are the pressure swings in the chest and plethysmograph.

Closing volume

As lung volumes decrease on expiration there is a point at which smaller airways begin to close; this is known as the closing volume of the lungs (Fig. 11.15). Closing volume is usually expressed as a percentage of vital capacity. In young subjects, closing volume is approximately 10% of vital

capacity and increases with age, being approximately 40% of vital capacity at 65 years of age.

In diseases such as asthma or COPD the smaller airways close earlier, i.e. at a higher lung volume. An increase in closing volume against predicted values is a sensitive measure of early lung disease and may even show changes caused by cigarette smoking before the patient is symptomatic.

The test uses the single-breath nitrogen method, as described above.

Exercise testing

Exercise testing is primarily used to:

- Diagnose unexplained breathlessness which is minimal at rest.
- Assess the extent of lung disease, by stressing the system.
- Determine the level of impairment in disability testing.
- Assist in differential diagnosis (e.g. when it is not known whether a patient is limited by cardiac or lung disease).
- Test the effects of therapy on exercise capacity.
- Prescribe a safe and effective exercise regime.

There are a number of established tests, including the shuttle test and a progressive exercise test, which is commonly performed on a cycle ergometer.

In practice, estimates of airway resistance are much more commonly used than plethysmography. PEFR and FEV_1 are both useful estimates of resistance, based on the relationship between resistance and airflow.

Shuttle test

This is a standardized test in which the patient walks up and down a 10-metre course, marked by cones, in a set time interval. The time intervals are indicated by bleeps played from a tape recorder and become progressively shorter. The test is stopped if patients become too breathless or if they cannot reach the cone in the time allowed.

Cycle ergometer progressive exercise test

This is performed in a laboratory and stresses the patient to a predetermined level based on heart rate. A number of tests are made as the patient exercises, including:

* ECG.
* Volume of gas exhaled.
* Concentration of oxygen and carbon dioxide in exhaled gas.

The volume of gas exhaled per minute (V_E L/min), oxygen consumption (VO_2 L/min) and carbon dioxide output (VCO_2 L/min) are then calculated. The test indicates whether exercise tolerance is limited by the cardiovascular or respiratory system and assesses increases in heart rate and ventilation against a known oxygen uptake.

IMAGING OF THE RESPIRATORY SYSTEM

Ultrasound

Ultrasound uses high-frequency sound waves to image internal structures. In respiratory medicine the technique is primarily used in the investigation of pleural effusions and empyemas. Ultrasound can detect an effusion that is not seen on chest X-ray, or localize an effusion before it is drained by thoracentesis.

A variation on this technique, Doppler ultrasound, is a non-invasive method for detecting deep vein thrombosis. It is used in investigating patients with suspected pulmonary thromboembolism. The technique examines blood flow and can detect thrombus in the veins above the popliteal fossa.

Plain radiography

The plain film radiograph is of paramount importance in the evaluation of pulmonary disease. The standard radiographic examinations of the chest are described below.

Posteroanterior erect radiograph (PA chest)

In the PA erect radiograph, X-rays travel from the posterior of the patient to the film, which is held against the front of the patient (Fig. 11.16). The scapula can be rotated out of the way, and accurate assessment of cardiac size is possible. The radiograph is performed in the erect position because:

* Gas passes upwards, making the detection of pneumothorax easier.
* Fluid passes downwards, making pleural effusions easier to diagnose.
* Blood vessels in mediastinum and lung are represented accurately.

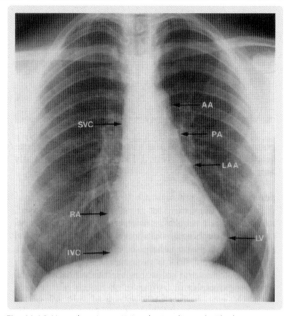

Fig. 11.16 Normal posteroanterior chest radiograph. The lungs are equally transradiant, the pulmonary vascular pattern is symmetrical. AA = aortic arch; SVC = superior vena cava; PA = pulmonary artery; LAA = left atrial appendage; RA = right atrium; LV = left ventricle; IVC = inferior vena cava. (Courtesy of Dr D Sutton and Dr JWR Young.)

Lateral radiograph

Lateral views help to localize lesions seen in PA views; they also give good views of the mediastinum and thoracic vertebrae (Fig. 11.17). Valuable information can be obtained by comparison with older films, if available.

In women of reproductive age, radiography should be performed within 28 days of last menstruation.

Reporting a chest X-ray

Always view chest radiographs on a viewing box and follow a set routine for reporting plain films. If possible, compare with the patient's previous films.

Clinical data

Take down the following details:

> Follow a set pattern for reading chest X-rays – that way you will not miss anything.

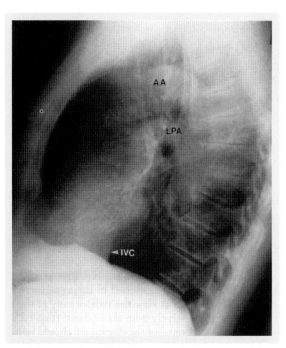

Fig. 11.17 Normal lateral chest radiograph. AA = aortic arch; LPA = left pulmonary artery; IVC = inferior vena cava. (Courtesy of Dr D Sutton and Dr JWR Young.)

- Patient's name.
- Age and sex.
- Clinical problem.
- Date of radiography.

Technical qualities

Note that radiographs contain right- or left-side markers.

With good penetration of X-rays, you should just be able to see the vertebral bodies through the cardiac shadow. In overpenetration, the lung fields appear too black. Conversely, in underpenetration, the lung fields appear too white.

Note the projection (AP, PA or lateral; erect or supine). To deduce whether the patient was straight or rotated, compare the sternal ends of both clavicles.

With adequate inspiration, you should be able to count six ribs anterior to the diaphragm. Make sure that the whole lung field is included.

Heart and mediastinum

When examining the cardiac shadow, observe the position, size and shape of the heart. Are the cardiac borders clearly visible?

Note whether the trachea is central or deviated to either side. Identify blood vessels and each hilum.

Other

Note the following points:

- Diaphragm – visible behind the heart; costophrenic angles acute and sharp.
- Lungs – divide the lungs into zones (upper, middle and lower); compare like with like.
- Bones – ribs, clavicles, sternum, thoracic vertebrae.
- Finally, recheck the apices, behind the heart, and hilar and retrodiaphragmatic regions.

Lateral radiograph

On a lateral radiograph, note the following:

- Diaphragm – right hemidiaphragm seen passing through heart border.
- Lungs – divide lungs into area in front, behind and above the heart.
- Retrosternal space – an anterior mass will cause this space to be white.
- Fissures – horizontal fissure (faint white line that passes from midpoint of hilum to anterior

chest wall); oblique fissure (passes from T4/5 through hilum to the anterior third of the diaphragm).
- Hilum.
- Bones – check vertebral bodies for shape, size and density; check sternum.

Interpreting abnormalities

Once you have completed your overall review of the film, return to any areas of abnormal lucency or opacity and assess them according to:

- Number – single or multiple.
- Position and distribution (lobar, etc.).
- Size, shape and contour.
- Texture (homogeneous, calcified, etc.).

The radiological features of common lung conditions are described below.

Collapse

Atelectasis (collapse) is loss of volume of a lung, lobe or segment for any cause. The most important mechanism is obstruction of a major bronchus by tumour, foreign body or bronchial plug.

PA and lateral radiographs are required. Compare with old films where available. The silhouette sign can help localize the lesion (Fig. 11.18).

The lateral borders of the mediastinum are silhouetted against the air-filled lung that lies underneath. This silhouette is lost if there is consolidation in the underlying lung.

Signs of lobar collapse

Signs of lobar collapse are:

- Decreased lung volume.
- Displacement of pulmonary fissures.
- Compensatory hyperinflation of remaining part of the ipsilateral lung.
- Elevation of hemidiaphragm on ipsilateral side.
- Mediastinal and hilar displacement; trachea pulled to side of collapse.
- Radiopacity (white lung).
- Absence of air bronchogram.

Some signs are specific to lobe involvement.

In upper lobe collapse of the right lung, a PA film is most valuable in making the diagnoses; the collapsed lobe lies adjacent to the mediastinum (Fig. 11.19A).

In the left lung, a lateral film is most valuable in making diagnoses; the lobe collapses superiomedially and anteriorly (Fig. 11.19B).

Lower lobe collapse causes rotation and visualization of the oblique fissure on PA film.

A lateral film is most valuable in diagnosing middle lobe collapse. Thin, wedge-shaped opacity between horizontal and oblique fissures is seen.

Consolidation

Consolidation is seen as an area of white lung and represents fluid or cellular matter where there would normally be air (Figs 11.20 and 11.21). There are many causes of consolidation including:

- Pneumonia.
- Pulmonary oedema.

In contrast to collapse:

- The shadowing is typically heterogeneous (i.e. not uniform).

Fig. 11.18 The silhouette sign

Non-aerated area of lung	Border that is obscured
Right upper lobe	Right border of ascending aorta
Right middle lobe	Right heart border
Right lower lobe	Right diaphragm
Left upper lobe	Aortic knuckle and upper left cardiac border
Lingula of left lung	Left heart border
Left lower lobe	Left diaphragm

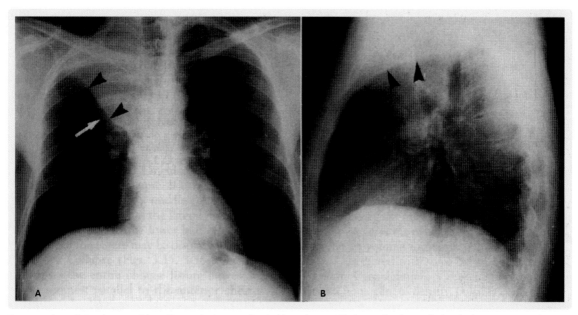

Fig. 11.19 (A and B) Right upper lobe collapse. The horizontal and oblique fissures (black arrowheads) are displaced. There is a mass (white arrow) at the right hilum. (Courtesy of Dr D Sutton and Dr JWR Young.)

Fig. 11.20 Radiological distribution of alveolar processes		
	Bat-wing pattern	
Segmental pattern	**Acute**	**Chronic**
pneumonia	pulmonary oedema	atypical pneumonia
pulmonary infarct	pneumonia	lymphoma
segmental collapse	pulmonary haemorrhage	sarcoidosis
alveolar cell carcinoma		pulmonary alveolar proteinosis
		alveolar cell carcinoma

- The border is ill-defined.
- Fissures retain their normal position.

There are two patterns of distribution:

- Segmental or lobar distribution.
- Bat's-wing distribution.

Peripheral lung fields may be spared (e.g. in pulmonary oedema). Air bronchograms may be seen, because they are delineated by surrounding consolidated lung.

An elderly woman presented to her GP with fever, a productive cough and general malaise. A chest X-ray showed left lower lobe consolidation with air bronchograms. Air bronchograms are mostly seen in infection, when consolidated alveoli are lying adjacent to air-filled small and medium bronchioles. These radiographic features suggested a left lower lobe pneumonia for which she was treated accordingly.

Interstitial patterns

Three types of interstitial pattern exist (linear, nodular and honeycomb), and overlap may occur.

Linear pattern

A linear pattern is seen as a network of fine lines running throughout the lungs. These lines represent

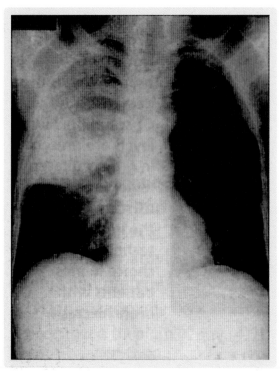

Fig. 11.21 Consolidation of the right upper lobe. (Courtesy of Professor CD Forbes and Dr WF Jackson.)

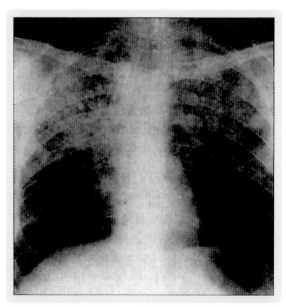

Fig. 11.22 Tuberculosis in a Greek immigrant to the UK. This film shows multiple areas of shadowing, especially in the upper lobes, and several lesions have started to cavitate. (Courtesy of Professor CD Forbes and Dr WF Jackson.)

> Kerley B lines can help to limit the possible diagnoses. They are caused by increased fluid between alveoli, in the interlobular septa. They are seen in pulmonary oedema and malignant lymphatic infiltration.

thickened connective tissue and are termed Kerley A and B lines:

A Upper lobes – long, thin lines.
B Lower lobes – short, thin horizontal lines 1–2 cm in length.

Nodular pattern

This pattern is seen as numerous well-defined small nodules (1–5 mm) evenly distributed throughout the lung. Causes include miliary tuberculosis and chickenpox pneumonia.

Honeycomb pattern

A honeycomb pattern indicates extensive destruction of lung tissue, with lung parenchyma replaced by thin-walled cysts. Pneumothorax may be present.

Normal pulmonary vasculature is absent. Pulmonary fibrosis leads to a honeycomb pattern.

Pulmonary nodules

Solitary nodules

The finding of a solitary pulmonary nodule on a plain chest radiograph is not an uncommon event. The nodule, which is commonly referred to as a coin lesion, is usually well circumscribed, less than 6 cm in diameter, lying within the lung. The rest of the lung appears normal and the patient is often asymptomatic.

A solitary nodule on a chest X-ray may be an artefact or it may be due to:

- Malignant tumour – bronchial carcinoma or secondary deposits.
- Infection – tuberculosis (Fig. 11.22) or pneumonia.
- Benign tumour – hamartoma.

If the patient is older than 35 years of age, then malignancy should be at the top of the list of possible differential diagnoses. If the lesion is static for a long period of time, as determined by reviewing previous radiographs, then it is likely to be a benign lesion. However, a slow-growing nodule in an elderly patient is likely to be malignant.

It is important to take into account clinical history and compare with a past chest radiograph if available. You should be able to distinguish carcinoma from other causes:

- Size of lesion – if lesions is > 4 cm diameter, be suspicious of malignancy.
- Margin – an ill-defined margin suggests malignancy.
- Cavitation indicates infection or malignancy.
- Calcification – unlikely to be malignancy.
- Presence of air bronchogram – sign of consolidation, not malignancy.

Multiple nodules

Metastases are usually seen as well-defined nodules varying in size, which are more common at the periphery of lower lobes (Fig. 11.23); cavitation may be present. Abscesses are cavitated with a thick and irregular wall. Cysts are often large.

Other nodules include:

- Rheumatoid nodules.
- Wegener's granulomatosis.
- Multiple arteriovenous malformations.

Hilar masses

Normal hilar complex includes:

- Proximal pulmonary arteries and bifurcations.
- Bronchus.
- Pulmonary veins.
- Lymph nodes, not seen unless enlarged.

Hilar size varies from person to person, so enlargement is difficult to diagnose (Fig. 11.24). Radiological features of the hilum are:

- Concave lateral margin.
- Equal radiopacity.
- Left hilum lies higher than right.

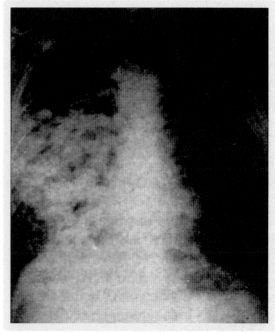

Fig. 11.23 Snowstorm mottling in both lung fields. In this case, the underlying diagnosis was testicular seminoma, with disseminated haematogenous metastases. (Courtesy of Professor CD Forbes and Dr WF Jackson.)

Fig. 11.24 Causes of hilar enlargement

	Bilateral enlargement	
Unilateral enlargement	**Enlarged lymph nodes**	**Enlarged vessels**
bronchial carcinoma	lymphomas	left-to-right cardiac shunts
metastatic malignancy	sarcoidosis	pulmonary arterial hypertension
lymphomas	cystic fibrosis	chronic obstructive pulmonary disease
primary tuberculosis	infectious mononucleosis	left heart failure
sarcoidosis	leukaemia	pulmonary embolism
pulmonary embolus		
pulmonary valve stenosis		

Sarcoidosis commonly presents as bilateral lymphadenopathy.

Tension pneumothorax is seen as a displacement of the mediastinum and trachea to the contralateral side, depressed ipsilateral diaphragm, and increased space between the ribs.

PA films are most valuable in assessing hilar shadow, but you must always consult the lateral film. Technical qualities of the film need to be adequately assessed before conclusions can be made because patient rotation commonly mimics hilar enlargement.

Mediastinal masses

A mediastinal mass typically has a sharp, concave margin, visible due to the silhouette sign. Lateral films may be particularly useful. Mediastinal masses are frequently asymptomatic and are grouped according to their anatomical position (Fig. 11.25). Computerized tomography (CT) is advised where there is a doubt as to the nature of the lesion.

Anterior mediastinal masses

Characteristics of anterior mediastinal masses are:

- Hilar structures still visible.
- Mass merges with the cardiac border.
- A mass passing into the neck is not seen above the clavicles.
- Small anterior mediastinal masses are difficult to see on PA films.

Middle mediastinal masses

- A middle mediastinal mass merges with hila and cardiac border.
- The majority are caused by enlarged lymph nodes.

Posterior mediastinal masses

In posterior mediastinal masses the cardiac border and hila are seen but the posterior aorta is obscured. Vertebral changes may be present.

Pleural lesions

Pneumothorax

Pneumothorax is usually obvious on normal inspiratory PA films. Look carefully at upper zones, because air accumulates first here; you will see an area devoid of lung markings (black lung), with the lung edge outlined by air in the pleural space. Small pneumothoraces can be identified on the expiratory film and may be missed in the supine film.

Tension pneumothorax

Tension pneumothorax is a medical emergency. Review an expiratory film if possible and bear in mind the patient's clinical state. If breathlessness is progressive and you suspect a tension pneumothorax, start treatment without waiting for a chest X-ray.

Pleural effusions

PA erect radiography is performed. Classically, there is a radiopaque mass at the base of the lung and blunting of the costophrenic angle, with the pleural meniscus higher laterally than medially. Large effusions can displace the mediastinum contralaterally.

A horizontal upper border implies that a pneumothorax is also present. An effusion has a more homogeneous texture than consolidation and air bronchograms are absent.

Fig. 11.25 Mediastinal masses

Anterior masses	Middle masses	Posterior masses
retrosternal thyroid	bronchial carcinoma	neurogenic tumour
thymic mass	lymphoma	paravertebral abscess
dermoid cyst	sarcoidosis	oesophageal lesions
lymphomas	primary tuberculosis	aortic aneurysm
aortic aneurysm	bronchogenic cyst	

Mesothelioma

Mesothelioma is a malignant tumour of the pleura, which may present as discrete pleural deposits or as a localized lesion.

On chest X-ray, thickened pleura is seen; in 50% of cases the plural plaques lie on the medial pleura, causing the medial margin to be irregular. Pleural effusions are common, usually containing blood (Fig. 11.26). Rib destruction is uncommon.

Vascular patterns

Normal vascular pattern

Lung markings are vascular in nature. Arteries branch vertically to upper and lower lobes. On erect films, upper lobe vessels are smaller than the lower lobe vessels. It is difficult to see vessels in the peripheral one-third of lung fields.

Pulmonary venous hypertension

On erect films, upper lobe vessels are larger than the lower lobe vessels. Pulmonary venous hypertension is associated with oedema and pleural effusions.

Pulmonary arterial hypertension

Pulmonary arterial hypertension is seen as bilateral hilar enlargement associated with long-standing pulmonary disease.

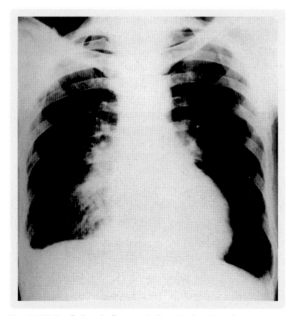

Fig. 11.26 Small pleural effusions. Both costophrenic angles are blunted. (Courtesy of Dr D Sutton and Dr JWR Young.)

Ventilation : perfusion scans

Ventilation : perfusion scans are primarily used to detect pulmonary emboli. The principle is that a pulmonary embolus produces a defect on the perfusion scan (a 'filling defect') which is not matched by a defect on the ventilation scan, i.e. there is an area of the lung that is ventilated but not perfused.

Ventilation scans

Ventilation is detected by inhalation of a gas or aerosol labelled with the radioisotope ^{133}Xe. The patient breathes and rebreathes the gas until it comes into equilibrium with other gases in the lung.

Perfusion scans

Radioactive particles larger than the diameter of the pulmonary capillaries are injected intravenously, where they remain for several hours. ^{99m}Tc-labelled macroaggregated albumin (MAA) is used. A gamma camera is then used to detect the position of the MAA particles. The pattern indicates the distribution of pulmonary blood flow.

Diagnosis of pulmonary embolism

Abnormalities in the perfusion scan are checked against a plain chest X-ray; defects on the perfusion scan are not diagnostic if they correspond to radiographic changes. Scans are classified based on the probability of a pulmonary embolism as:

1. Normal – commonly reported as 'low probability'.
2. High probability.
3. Non-diagnosic.

Non-diagnostic scans include those where patients have obstructive diseases such as asthma or COPD which lead to perfusion and ventilation defects; pulmonary embolus cannot be diagnosed if such a pattern is obtained – other investigations (see below) are then indicated.

Pulmonary angiography

Pulmonary angiography is the gold standard test for diagnosing pulmonary embolus. Indications are:

- When a ventilation : perfusion scan is inconclusive for pulmonary embolus, but the patient is acutely ill.
- Before surgery or thrombolysis for pulmonary embolism.

The test is performed by injection of contrast media through a catheter introduced into the main pulmonary artery using the Seldinger technique. Obstructed vessels or filling defects can be seen clearly and emboli show as filling defects. Despite the accuracy of the test, in practice pulmonary angiography is not often performed because it is invasive and time-consuming. Where ventilation:perfusion scans are inconclusive, and the patient is not acutely ill, it is more common to proceed to lower limb venography or Doppler ultrasound. When angiography is performed, a less invasive test involving computerized tomography (CTPA) is increasingly preferred.

Computerized tomography

Computerized tomography (CT) is the imaging modality of choice for mediastinal and many pulmonary conditions. CT scans provide detailed cross-sectional images of the thorax. The images can be electronically modified to display different tissues (e.g. by using a bone setting compared with a soft-tissue setting).

The patient passes through a rotating gantry which has X-ray tubes on one side and a set of detectors on the other. Information from the detectors is analysed and displayed as a two-dimensional image on visual display units, then recorded.

CT gives a dose of radiation approximately 100 times that of a standard plain film chest radiograph.

Applications of computerized tomography

Detection of pulmonary nodules
CT can evaluate the presence of metastases in a patient with known malignancy; however, it cannot distinguish between benign and malignant masses.

Mediastinal masses
CT is a useful technique in searching for lymph-adenopathy in a person with primary lung carcinoma.

Carcinoma of the lung
CT can evaluate the size of a lung carcinoma, and detect mediastinal extension and staging.

Pleural lesions
CT is effective at detecting small pleural effusions and identifying pleural plaques (Fig. 11.27).

Vascular lesions
Contrast studies allow imaging of vascular lesions (e.g. aortic aneurysms).

High-resolution computerized tomography

High-resolution CT is useful in imaging diffuse lung disease: thinner sections of 1–2 mm show greater lung detail (Fig. 11.28).

Applications of high-resolution computerized tomography
Bronchiectasis. High-resolution CT has replaced bronchography. In dilated bronchi, the technique can show:

- Collapse.
- Scarring.
- Consolidation.

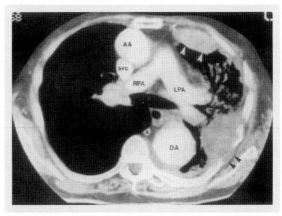

Fig. 11.27 CT scan of a pleural mass. Enhanced CT scan at level of bifurcation of main pulmonary artery. The left lung is surrounded by pleural masses (arrowheads), and the posterior mass is invading the chest wall. The vascular anatomy of the mediastinum is well shown. a = azygos vein (left of descending aorta); RPA = right pulmonary artery; LPA = left pulmonary artery; AA = ascending aorta; SVC = superior vena cava; DA = descending aorta. (Courtesy of Dr D Sutton and Dr JWR Young.)

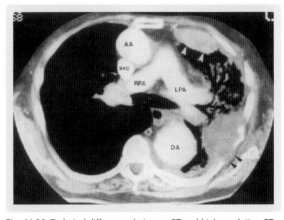

Fig. 11.28 Technical differences between CT and high-resolution CT (HRCT).

Interstitial lung disease. High-resolution CT is more specific than plain film radiography. Disorders that have specific appearances on high-resolution CT include sarcoidosis, occupational lung disease and interstitial pneumonia.

High-resolution CT can be used for biopsy guidance.

Atypical infections. High-resolution CT provides diagnosis earlier than using plain chest radiography and is useful in monitoring disease and response to treatment. It also provides good delineation of disease activity and destruction.

High-resolution CT is used in imaging of patients with AIDS (e.g. PCP).

Diagnosis of lymphangitis carcinomatosa. High-resolution CT can be used in the diagnosis of lymphagitis carcinomatosa.

COPD. High-resolution CT can be used to measure small airways thickening, gas trapping and emphysema.

Magnetic resonance imaging (MRI)

MRI uses the magnetic properties of the hydrogen atom to produce images. MRI gives excellent imaging of soft tissues and the heart, but has limited use in the respiratory system. Flowing blood does not provide a signal for MRI imaging, and vascular structures appear as hollow tubes. MRI imaging can be used to differentiate masses around the aorta or in the hilar regions. It has the advantage of not using ionizing radiation.

SELF-ASSESSMENT

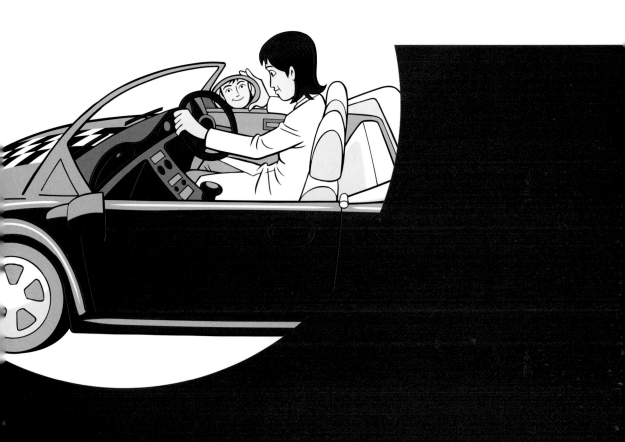

Multiple-choice questions (MCQs)

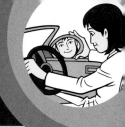

Indicate whether each answer is true or false.

1. **Nasal cavities and air sinuses:**
   a. The maxillary sinus and frontal nasal duct open into the middle meatus.
   b. Consist of three conchae and two air passages opening posteriorly into the choana.
   c. The sphenoethmoidal recess opens between the ethmoid sinus and the middle meatus.
   d. The nasolacrimal duct opens into the inferior meatus.
   e. The upper 2/3 of the nasal cavity is lined by olfactory mucosa.

2. **Bronchioles:**
   a. Contain no smooth muscle in their walls, therefore significantly reduce airway resistance.
   b. Differ from bronchi which contain cartilage in their walls.
   c. Contain Clara cells which secrete highly proteinaceous fluid.
   d. Contribute to more than 50% of resistance to flow in the lower respiratory tract.
   e. Are a major site of gas exchange.

3. **Development of the upper respiratory tract:**
   a. Nerve supply of the branchial arches is derived from the cranial nerves.
   b. The diverticulum lengthens to become the laryngotracheal tube.
   c. The brachial arches are formed by the second week of development.
   d. Defects during development can lead to a fistula.
   e. The fourth and sixth brachial arches are supplied by the branches of the vagus nerve.

4. **Disorders of the larynx:**
   a. Epiglottitis has decreased in incidence due to the pneumococcal vaccine.
   b. Always conduct an ENT examination in acute epiglottitis.
   c. Laryngotracheobronchitis is mainly caused by a viral infection.
   d. Squamous papilloma is common in children.
   e. Medical treatment of squamous papilloma is with gamma interferon.

5. **Cilia:**
   a. They are found on the epithelial surfaces of the mucus-secreting goblet cells.
   b. They play an important role in preventing microorganisms causing infection.
   c. The dynein arms drive ciliary movement.

   d. Kartagener's syndrome is characterized by atrial septal defects.
   e. Energy for ciliary movement comes from microtubule ATPase activity.

6. **Sinuses:**
   a. Sinusitis is common in patients with AIDS.
   b. Sinusitis is common in the maxillary frontal sinuses.
   c. Sinusitis is usually caused by a staphylococcal infection.
   d. In acute sinusitis the cilia beat rapidly to increase secretions.
   e. Acute sinusitis can be treated with oral steroids.

7. **Disorders of the pharynx:**
   a. Obstructive sleep apnoea is common in heart failure patients.
   b. Paradoxical breathing movements are a feature of obstructive sleep apnoea.
   c. Sleep apnoea is diagnostically confirmed with 15 or more apnoea episodes in any hour of sleep.
   d. Nasopharyngeal carcinomas can be associated with Epstein–Barr virus.
   e. The sphenopalatine foramen is always involved in nasopharyngeal angiofibroma.

8. **Development of the lower respiratory tract:**
   a. Gas exchange for respiration can take place in the pseudoglandular period.
   b. The right main bronchus is slightly larger and more vertical than the left main bronchus.
   c. Surfactant is produced by type II pneumocytes in the terminal sac period.
   d. For the first 3 years after birth the alveoli increase in size, not in number.
   e. Squamous epithelium (type I pneumocytes) develops earlier than secretory cells (type II pneumocytes).

9. **Pulmonary circulation:**
   a. In fetal life, the pressure in the pulmonary circulation is greater than in the systemic circulation.
   b. The ductus arteriosus once closed loses its function and becomes the ligamentum teres.
   c. A patent ductus arteriosus (PDA) can be closed by using a prostaglandin agonist.
   d. It is normal to auscultate a murmur in a baby within the first 24 hours of birth.
   e. The bronchial circulation is a subdivision of the pulmonary circulation.

10. Anatomy of the thorax:

a. The upper seven bony ribs articulate anteriorly with the sternum.
b. The external intercostal muscles raise the rib cage and increase the intrathoracic volume.
c. The visceral pleura has an autonomic nerve supply.
d. The neurovascular bundle lies posterior to the subcostal muscles.
e. The parietal pleura has a blood supply from the bronchial arteries.

11. Metabolic functions of the lungs:

a. ACE is produced by the lung epithelial cells in the alveolar ducts.
b. ACE inhibitors (e.g. captopril) inhibit the production of bradykinins.
c. Arachidonic acid is released from membrane phospholipids by the action of phospholipase A_2.
d. All prostaglandins have a vasoconstrictory role.
e. Thromboxanes are synthesized via a cyclo-oygenase-mediated pathway.

12. Ventilation in the healthy lung:

a. Dead space comprises both anatomical and physiological space.
b. Physiological dead space is much greater than anatomical dead space.
c. Minute ventilation is greater than alveolar minute ventilation.
d. Ventilation per unit of lung tissue is higher at the top of the lung.
e. The $\dot{V}/\dot{Q}$ ratio is slightly more than 1.

13. In a normal adult at rest:

a. Alveolar ventilation is about 5 L/min.
b. Pulmonary perfusion is about 5 L/min.
c. P_aO_2 is 4.8–6.0 kPa.
d. Respiratory rate is less than 12 breaths/min.
e. Anatomical dead space is about 300 mL.

14. In quiet breathing:

a. Ventilation is brought about by expansion of the chest, mainly by the intercostal muscles.
b. The abdominal muscles relax during inspiration.
c. The elastic recoil forces of the lung parenchyma are responsible for expiration.
d. Intrapleural pressure is more negative in expiration than in inspiration.
e. The diaphragm is responsible for approximately 75% of the work of ventilation.

15. Airway resistance:

a. Increases with increasing air flow rate.
b. Under laminar flow conditions is directly proportional to radius of the airway to the fourth power.
c. Under laminar flow conditions is described by Poiseuille's law.
d. Increases with increasing lung volume.
e. Can be actively altered.

16. Surfactant:

a. Is secreted by type I pneumocytes.
b. Is not present at birth.
c. Is soluble in water.
d. Decreases lung compliance.
e. Explains hysteresis in pressure–volume curves.

17. Perfusion and diffusion:

a. Carbon monoxide uptake by the lungs is limited by the rate of diffusion.
b. Nitrous oxide uptake by the lungs is limited by the rate of diffusion.
c. In disease-free lungs, oxygen uptake is limited by diffusion.
d. In emphysematous lungs, oxygen uptake is limited by perfusion.
e. It takes 0.75 seconds for oxygen transfer from the alveoli to the bloodstream to plateau.

18. Gas transport in the blood:

a. Once oxygen is bound to the haem group of haemoglobin the ferrous (Fe^{2+}) ion changes to the ferric state (Fe^{3+}).
b. Myoglobin has a greater affinity for oxygen than haemoglobin A.
c. Carbon dioxide and oxygen have similar diffusing capacity in the lung.
d. During exercise an individual will hyperventilate in order to blow off carbon dioxide.
e. Increase in carbon dioxide and decrease in pH enhance dissociation of oxygen from oxyhaemoglobin.

19. The following are true of $\dot{V}_A/\dot{Q}$:

a. Ventilation increases towards the apex of the lung.
b. Perfusion increases towards the base of the lung.
c. $\dot{V}_A/\dot{Q}$ is dependent on lung volume and posture.
d. $\dot{V}_A/\dot{Q}$ is uniform throughout the lung in the healthy patient.
e. Perfusion is increased to those areas of lung which are underventilated.

20. The following statements relate to the pulmonary circulation:

a. The volume of blood is much lower than in the systemic circulation.
b. Alveolar vessels will dilate as the lung expands.
c. Histamine will increase pulmonary vascular resistance.
d. Low P_aO_2 will cause hypoxic vasoconstriction.
e. Hydrostatic pressure can recruit more vessels.

21. The following statements relate to acid–base disturbance:

a. Uncomplicated respiratory acidosis results from an increase in PCO_2.
b. Renal compensation returns the blood gases and pH to normal in respiratory acidosis.

c. Metabolic acidosis may cause respiratory compensation, increasing ventilation and therefore increasing PCO_2.
d. The bicarbonate buffer system is important in the acid–base balance because its pK is very close to physiological pH.
e. Normal physiological pH range is 7.4–7.45.

22. During exercise:

a. Moderate exercise causes an increased P_aCO_2 which drives the ventilatory increase.
b. Oscillations in PCO_2 are similar in amplitude to those at rest due to the fine control achieved by the respiratory system.
c. The build-up of aerobic metabolites in severe exercise leads to an oxygen debt.
d. In moderate exercise ventilation is excessive for metabolic demands and the subject hyperventilates.
e. Exercise may be an important aetiological factor in some asthma.

23. Pulmonary vascular resistance:

a. Is much lower than systemic vascular resistance.
b. Can be further reduced by extension and recruitment of pulmonary capillaries.
c. Is increased during exercise.
d. Is lower than systemic vascular resistance since pulmonary vessels are easily distended.
e. Is higher at the apex of the lung, therefore reducing blood flow to the apex.

24. Central chemoreceptors:

a. Can be found on the ventral surface of the medulla.
b. Respond to hypoxaemia by increasing ventilation.
c. Are sensitive to rapid changes in pH.
d. Have a rapid response to PCO_2.
e. Are responsible for about 10% of the control of ventilation due to short-term changes in PO_2.

25. Peripheral chemoreceptors:

a. Are located in the aortic bodies and carotid sinuses.
b. Are sensitive to hypoxaemia.
c. Have a relatively low blood flow, enabling them to measure small changes in arterial blood gas tensions.
d. Parasympathetic nerves cause vasoconstriction and reduce blood flow to these receptors.
e. Are not sensitive to changes in arterial pH.

26. Ipratropium bromide:

a. Is an antimuscarinic agent.
b. May cause urinary retention.
c. Increases sputum viscosity.
d. Causes bronchodilatation.
e. May affect intraocular pressure.

27. The following drugs are respiratory depressants:

a. Barbiturates.
b. Benzodiazepines.

c. Alcohol.
d. Doxapram.
e. Aminophylline.

28. The following drugs used in the treatment of asthma have an anti-inflammatory action:

a. Glucocorticoids.
b. Salmeterol.
c. Theobromine.
d. Sodium cromoglicate.
e. Terfenadine.

29. Salbutamol:

a. Is an α agonist.
b. May produce a tremor.
c. Is usually administered sublingually.
d. May cause hyperkalaemia with high doses.
e. May cause peripheral vasoconstriction.

30. Pulmonary rehabilitation:

a. When giving oxygen therapy, oxygen only needs to be humidified when given at greater than 28%.
b. CPAP is indicated as a treatment for central sleep apnoea.
c. CPAP is a form of invasive ventilatory support.
d. Lung volume reduction surgery may be used as a last resort in COPD.
e. It improves muscle strength in COPD patients

31. Features of acclimatization include:

a. Polycythaemia.
b. Increased fluid in the interstitium.
c. Hyperventilation.
d. Right shift of the oxyhaemoglobin dissociation curve.
e. An increase in oxidative enzymes.

32. The following relate to respiratory support:

a. Oxygen therapy corrects hypoxaemia in right-to-left shunt.
b. High-dose oxygen is useful in type II respiratory failure.
c. Patients on BiPAP are at risk of aspiration pneumonia.
d. LTOT is only beneficial when used for 19 hours/day.
e. Ventilatory support is usually delivered at a positive pressure.

33. The following relate to long-term oxygen therapy (LTOT) in patients with COPD:

a. It should be given for no more than 8 hours a day, or oxygen toxicity is likely.
b. The newer systems can safely be used in smokers.
c. Oxygen should be given through a mask.
d. It has an effect after 6 months and can then be withdrawn.
e. Arterial saturation should be at least 90%.

34. In emphysema:

a. The distance for diffusion of O_2 is decreased due to destruction of the lung parenchyma.

237

b. Over 10% of cases have α_1-antitrypsin deficiency.
c. The overall surface area for gas exchange is decreased despite the increase in alveolar size.
d. Patients develop stiff fibrotic lungs.
e. Radial traction is increased, therefore reducing airway resistance.

35. Typical features of bronchiectasis are:
a. Cough with small amounts of sputum.
b. Lower lobes are less affected.
c. Empyema.
d. Haemoptysis.
e. Coarse crepitations on auscultation.

36. Referring to α_1-antitrypsin:
a. Deficiency results in increased breakdown of lung parenchyma due to the action of proteolytic enzymes.
b. It is inhibited by aspirin.
c. Deficiency accounts for approximately 2% of cases of emphysema.
d. Deficiency is caused by smoking.
e. Is important in the metabolism of angiotensin II to inactive peptides.

37. In asthma:
a. The peak expiratory flow rate is increased.
b. There is constriction of smooth muscle in bronchioles.
c. There is mucosal oedema in the airways.
d. Mucus secretion is decreased.
e. House dust may be an allergen.

38. Pulmonary embolism:
a. Is usually accompanied by lung infarction.
b. Usually arises from the deep veins of the legs and pelvis.
c. May cause sudden death.
d. Is treated with anticoagulants.
e. Is one of the most frequent causes of postoperative death.

39. Chronic bronchitis:
a. Is associated with hypoplasia of bronchial mucous glands.
b. Is defined as a productive cough for at least 3 months in 2 consecutive years.
c. Is associated with *Haemophilus influenzae* infection.
d. Usually coexists with emphysema.
e. Is associated with cigarette smoking.

40. COPD:
a. Steroids are the mainstay of treatment.
b. Causes some 3000 deaths each year in the UK.
c. May be complicated by pneumothorax.
d. Exacerbations are often caused by *H. influenzae*.
e. Is often caused by a genetic defect.

41. COPD and asthma:
a. TLCO is reduced in both.
b. Both may present with cough.

c. Cough is typically worse in the morning in asthma.
d. Wheeze is only present in asthma.
e. Air trapping is a feature of both disorders.

42. Coal worker's pneumoconiosis:
a. Is caused by asbestos fibres.
b. May cause respiratory failure.
c. Is accompanied by focal emphysema.
d. Has positive association with mesothelioma.
e. May be caused by very low exposure to coal dust.

43. Small-cell carcinoma of the lung:
a. Is usually treated by surgical resection.
b. Shows keratin production on histological examination.
c. Rarely metastasizes.
d. Has a positive association with asbestos exposure.
e. Usually arises in the periphery of the lung.

44. Malignant mesothelioma:
a. Has a positive association with asbestos exposure.
b. Has usually metastasized by the time of presentation.
c. May cause death by respiratory failure.
d. May cause cardiac tamponade.
e. Is an epithelial tumour.

45. Squamous cell carcinoma of the lung:
a. Is associated with cigarette smoking.
b. Shows mucin production on histological examination.
c. May be treated by surgical resection.
d. May produce ectopic hormones.
e. May respond to radiotherapy.

46. Emphysema:
a. Is associated with α_1-antitrypsin deficiency.
b. Is defined as enlargement of air spaces distal to the terminal bronchiole with destruction of the alveolar walls.
c. Causes decreased alveolar surface area.
d. May cause respiratory failure.
e. Is always associated with chronic bronchitis.

47. The following definitions are correct:
a. Haemothorax – collection of blood in the pleural cavity.
b. Pyothorax – collection of lymph in the pleural cavity.
c. Pneumothorax – collection of air in the pleural cavity.
d. Chylothorax – collection of pus in the pleural cavity.
e. Hydrothorax – collection of fluid in the pleural cavity.

48. The following factors have a positive association with the development of lung carcinoma:
a. Coal mining.
b. Haematite mining.
c. Asbestos exposure.

d. Diffuse pulmonary fibrosis.
e. Woodworking with hardwoods.

49. Fibrosing alveolitis:

a. Usually occurs in young people.
b. Is usually caused by inhaled dust.
c. May result in 'honeycomb' lung.
d. Gives an obstructive pattern of deficit on pulmonary function tests.
e. Histologically shows proliferation of type II pneumocytes.

50. Atopic asthma:

a. Is mediated by a type III hypersensitivity reaction.
b. Is associated with hay fever.
c. Is associated with eczema.
d. Is associated with hypoplasia of bronchial wall smooth muscle.
e. May be treated with β_2 agonists.

51. In asthma:

a. Peak expiratory flow rate during an acute attack is usually decreased.
b. The disease results from the destruction of lung parenchyma caused by smoking.
c. An acute attack is characterized by bronchoconstriction which is not usually reversible.
d. Acute asthma can be treated by using ipratropium bromide.
e. Sodium cromoglicate inhibits phosphodiesterase therefore increasing cAMP which leads to bronchodilatation.

52. Acute severe asthma is characterized by:

a. PEFR <33% predicted or best.
b. Pulse of >100 beats/min.
c. Silent chest and cyanosis.
d. Urea >7 mmol/L.
e. Inability to speak in one breath.

53. Cor pulmonale:

a. Is failure of left heart.
b. Is seen in COPD.
c. Is characterized by oedema and raised JVP.
d. Is associated with pulmonary hypertension.
e. Has a good prognosis.

54. Occupational causes of asthma include:

a. Asbestos.
b. Isocyanates.
c. Flour.
d. Seafoods.
e. Dyes.

55. The following relate to sleep apnoea:

a. It is associated with hypertension.
b. Obesity is a risk factor.
c. Women are more often affected than men.
d. It can often be treated conservatively.
e. Patients have an increased risk of road traffic accidents.

56. Lung cancer can metastasize to the:

a. Ovary.
b. Bone.
c. Breast.
d. Prostate.
e. Kidney.

57. Tuberculosis:

a. Is decreasing in developing countries.
b. May be an incidental finding on CXR.
c. Is always asymptomatic in the primary type.
d. May be present with pneumonia.
e. Is not seen in immunized individuals.

58. Interstitial lung diseases:

a. Cause a restrictive pattern of disease.
b. Are sometimes caused by drugs.
c. Invariably cause finger clubbing.
d. May present first with haemoptysis.
e. May coexist with renal disease.

59. Extrinsic allergic alveolitis:

a. Is immunologically mediated.
b. May affect farmers.
c. Causes symptoms related to extent of exposure to antigen.
d. Honeycomb lung may be a feature.
e. There are increased lymphocytes in BAL fluid.

60. Tuberculosis in the immunocompromised:

a. May be caused by MAC.
b. May present with progressive anaemia.
c. Treatment with steroids should be commenced immediately.
d. Is associated with bronchiectasis.
e. May require a pleural biopsy for diagnosis.

61. Prognosis is poor in severe pneumonia when:

a. Urea <7 mmol/L.
b. Respiratory rate <20/min.
c. The patient is confused.
d. The patient is hypertensive.
e. Hypoxaemia is present.

62. Causes of transudate include:

a. Hypothyroidism.
b. Pneumonia.
c. Heart failure.
d. Liver failure.
e. Bronchial carcinoma.

63. Occupational lung diseases:

a. There may be a latency period in non-allergic asthma.
b. Caplan's syndrome is associated with asbestosis.
c. Patients may be eligible for compensation.
d. Can affect workers in animal laboratories.
e. Symptoms may improve at weekends.

64. Surgery is contraindicated in:

a. Lung carcinoma with mediastinal nodes >2 cm diameter.

b. Cystic fibrosis if both lungs are affected.
c. Lung carcinoma if FEV_1 is <0.8 L.
d. Respiratory failure.
e. Most cases of small-cell lung cancer.

65. Features of mycoplasmal pneumonia include:

a. Epidemics typically occur every 10 years.
b. Cold agglutinins are a feature in almost all patients.
c. It is found in water-cooling towers.
d. It is treated effectively with penicillin.
e. Institutional outbreaks amongst the elderly.

66. *Legionella pneumophila*:

a. Is a Gram-positive organism.
b. Causes a pneumonia with a high mortality rate.
c. Antigen may help diagnosis.
d. A vaccine is available.
e. Is ubiquitous in water.

67. Pneumonia may present with:

a. Pleuritic pain.
b. Headache.
c. Haemoptysis.
d. Diarrhoea.
e. Urinary symptoms.

68. Pulmonary embolism:

a. Thrombolysis is indicated in most patients.
b. Heparin is the mainstay of treatment.
c. Anticoagulants should be continued for a week after the event.
d. Can be excluded when a CXR is normal.
e. Is a common finding at autopsy.

69. Small-cell lung cancers:

a. Are treated with chemotherapy with intent to cure.
b. Are the most common type of lung cancer.
c. Have a particularly poor prognosis.
d. Are staged with the TNM classification.
e. Arise from endocrine cells.

70. Bronchial adenocarcinoma:

a. Is more common in women than in men.
b. Is strongly associated with smoking.
c. Stains for keratin histologically.
d. Is often a central tumour.
e. Commonly causes obstructive symptoms.

71. Cavitating lesions in the lung are seen in:

a. Rheumatoid arthritis.
b. TB.
c. COPD.
d. Coal worker's pneumoconiosis.
e. Idiopathic pulmonary haemosiderosis.

72. Features of idiopathic fibrosing alveolitis include:

a. Productive cough.
b. Reduced chest expansion.
c. Wheeze.

d. Weight loss.
e. Pulmonary hypertension.

73. Published guidelines on pulmonary embolism (PE) state:

a. Recent fractures are a lesser risk factor.
b. Obesity is not a proven risk factor.
c. Anticoagulation reduces the risk of fatal recurrent embolism.
d. Serious underlying disease often coexists with PE.
e. Lung scans may be misleading in patients with COPD.

74. Published guidelines on asthma state:

a. Inhaled steroids are always indicated.
b. It is unwise to step down treatment.
c. Avoidance of provoking factors is advised.
d. Bronchodilators may be used twice a day before moving to Step 2.
e. High-dose steroids are contraindicated in children.

75. Sarcoidosis:

a. May be diagnosed using the Schick test.
b. Is characterized histologically by caseous granulomas.
c. Affects the terminal ileum most frequently.
d. May cause interstitial lung fibrosis.
e. May cause hilar lymphadenopathy.

76. Adult respiratory distress syndrome (ARDS):

a. Is associated with inhalation of sulphur dioxide.
b. Is characterized by proliferation of type I pneumocytes.
c. Is characterized by formation of hyaline membranes in the alveoli.
d. Is rarely fatal.
e. Is associated with endotoxic shock.

77. Cystic fibrosis:

a. Is an autosomal dominant genetic condition.
b. Is associated with meconium ileus in infants.
c. May be confirmed by measuring sodium concentration in sweat.
d. Is associated with bronchiectasis.
e. Is associated with infertility in females.

78. Community-acquired pneumonia:

a. Is commonly caused by Gram-negative organisms.
b. Is more common in smokers.
c. May be complicated by empyema.
d. Is more often viral in adults.
e. Has a poorer prognosis if the patient is confused on admission.

79. Carcinoma of the larynx:

a. Is usually of adenocarcinomatous differentiation.
b. Usually affects subjects below 40 years of age.
c. Affects females more commonly than males.
d. Is associated with cigarette smoking.
e. May produce dysphagia.

80. **Wegener's granulomatosis:**

   a. Is a necrotizing vasculitis.
   b. Affects mainly elastic arteries.
   c. Is caused by an antiglomerular basement membrane antibody.
   d. Causes a necrotizing glomerulonephritis.
   e. Causes lung necrosis.

81. **Bronchiectasis:**

   a. Is associated with Kartagener's syndrome.
   b. Usually affects the upper lobes most prominently.
   c. May be complicated by amyloid formation.
   d. Is characterized by bronchial constriction.
   e. May be complicated by metastatic cerebral abscesses.

82. **Causes of a chronic recurrent cough include:**

   a. Asthma.
   b. COPD.
   c. Gastro-oesophageal reflux.
   d. Chronic sinusitis.
   e. ACE inhibitors.

83. **Haemoptysis:**

   a. May be caused by TB.
   b. Is sometimes fatal.
   c. May lead to melaena.
   d. Is commonly sputum streaked with blood in lung cancer.
   e. May be due to acute bronchitis.

84. **Concerning type I respiratory failure:**

   a. $PO_2 < 8\,kPa$.
   b. Tolerance to high arterial oxygen tension develops.
   c. It must be treated effectively with low-dose oxygen.
   d. It differs from type II because it is of pulmonary vascular origin.
   e. It may be caused by spontaneous pneumothorax.

85. **The following relate to respiratory failure:**

   a. It is often caused by ventilation:perfusion mismatching.
   b. The most important investigation is a CXR.
   c. Type I is classically caused by pump failure.
   d. Arterial blood gases may be normal.
   e. Renal compensation frequently occurs in both types.

86. **Features of hypercapnia include**

   a. Flapping tremor.
   b. Peripheral vasoconstriction.
   c. Coma.
   d. Headache
   e. Papilloedema.

87. **Signs of COPD on examination include:**

   a. Pursed lip breathing.
   b. Tracheal tug.
   c. Hoover's sign.

   d. Wheeze.
   e. Hyperinflation.

88. **Finger clubbing is seen in:**

   a. Bronchiectasis.
   b. Asthma.
   c. Chronic bronchitis.
   d. Pulmonary fibrosis.
   e. Cyanotic heart disease.

89. **Signs found on respiratory examination may include:**

   a. Mediastinal shift in a simple pneumothorax.
   b. Hyperresonant lung fields on percussion in pleural effusion.
   c. Decreased vocal resonance in pneumonia.
   d. Decreased chest expansion in lung collapse.
   e. Coarse crackles in pneumonia.

90. **The following relate to lung function tests:**

   a. Transfer factor corrects for lost lung volume.
   b. Normal PEFR is 100–200 in adults.
   c. Closing volume is decreased with air trapping.
   d. Fowler's method measures physiological dead space.
   e. Body plethysmography measures lung compliance.

91. **Features of consolidation on a CXR include:**

   a. Fissures are displaced.
   b. May be in a bat's wing distribution.
   c. Silhouette sign is seen.
   d. Air bronchograms are unlikely to be present.
   e. Peripheral lung fields may be spared.

92. **Diffusing capacity (TLCO):**

   a. Is equivalent to transfer factor.
   b. Corrects for lost lung volume.
   c. Is reduced by exercise.
   d. Is a sensitive test.
   e. Is a specific test.

93. **The following statements relate to lung volumes:**

   a. Functional residual capacity is that amount of air left within the lung following a maximal expiration.
   b. Vital capacity is usually about 4800 mL in the upright 70-kg male subject.
   c. Tidal volume can be measured by spirometry.
   d. Total lung volume is normally increased in fibrosing alveolitis.
   e. The ratio of FEV_1/FVC is usually greater than 80% in asthmatics.

94. **Peak expiratory flow rate:**

   a. Records the volume of a forced expiration in 1 second.
   b. Detects restrictive lung defects.
   c. Is higher in the morning in asthma.
   d. Is dependent on age, gender and height.
   e. Is more accurate than plethysmography in measuring true air flow resistance.

95. Radioisotope lung scanning:

a. With ventilation : perfusion scans can detect pulmonary embolism.
b. Uses microaggregated human albumin to detect ventilation.
c. Is the gold standard test for detecting pulmonary emboli.
d. Is used less often than pulmonary angiograms.
e. Is the basis for the single-breath nitrogen test.

96. Collapse of the lung:

a. Will show the trachea deviated to the opposite side on CXR.
b. Gives an irregular, 'bitty' whiteness on CXR.
c. May occur at birth.
d. May lead to fibrosis.
e. May show a displaced horizontal fissure on CXR.

97. The following relate to bronchoscopy:

a. Rigid bronchoscopy is used more often than fibreoptic.
b. Haemoptysis is a key indication for bronchoscopy.
c. It can be used to sample bronchial secretions.
e. Is used to diagnose mediastinal tumours.
e. In fibreoptic bronchoscopy patients are not sedated.

98. The following are recognized, appropriate investigations:

a. Multiple inert gas procedure for pulmonary embolism.
b. Bronchoscopy in a smoker with a persistent monophonic wheeze.
c. Ultrasound for pleural effusion.
d. Transbronchial biopsy in pulmonary fibrosis.
e. MRI scan in tension pneumothorax.

99. Lung function tests in COPD show:

a. A decrease in gas transfer.
b. A decrease in FEV_1.
c. A decrease in functional residual capacity.
d. An increase in closing volume.
e. An increase in FEV_1 : FVC ratio.

100. Investigations in asthma:

a. Bronchial provocation tests are essential for diagnosis.
b. FEV_1 improves after bronchodilatation.
c. TLCO is decreased.
d. Residual volume may be increased.
e. Skin prick tests are usually negative in extrinsic asthma.

Short-answer questions (SAQs)

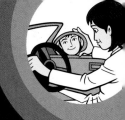

1. What is a surfactant? Describe its functions within the lung.

2. Give the normal values for haemoglobin concentration in the blood. Draw the oxyhaemoglobin dissociation curve, giving arterial and venous PO_2.

3. Define the term venous admixture. If a patient presents with a pulmonary embolus how may the patient's blood gases show a low PO_2 but a normal or lowered PCO_2?

4. Define airway resistance. How is calibre of the airway related to airway resistance under laminar flow conditions and what factors influence smooth muscle tone of the airways?

5. Write short notes on lung carcinoma.

6. Write short notes on bronchial asthma.

7. Write short notes on bronchiectasis.

8. Write short notes on adult respiratory distress syndrome.

9. Write short notes on malignant mesothelioma.

10. Write short notes on cystic fibrosis.

11. Write short notes on pneumonia in the immunocompromised.

12. A 62-year-old woman, with a diagnosis of breast carcinoma, presents to A&E in an anxious state, complaining of shortness of breath and chest pain that is worse on breathing in. She mentions that she has just coughed up a small amount of bright red blood.
    a. What other information should you elicit from the history?
    b. What are the main risk factors for pulmonary embolism?
    c. What investigations should you perform?
    d. How would you manage the patient?

13. A 58-year-old man consults his GP, complaining of increasing shortness of breath. He has been getting progressively more breathless for the last 3 years and now cannot walk upstairs in his home without stopping once or twice. The cough that used to be a feature of the winter months now seems to be present all year round. He has smoked since he was 15 years old and although he has tried to give up several times he has averaged a pack a day over most of this period. His GP sends him for a chest X-ray and some lung function tests.
    a. What lung function tests are indicated and what are they likely to show?
    b. The patient's smoking history equates to how many pack years? What help could his GP give him in his attempts to stop smoking?
    c. How might the patient be treated?
    d. How does smoking cause the symptoms seen in this patient?

14. A 64-year-old chronic smoker presents to A&E with acute dyspnoea and a cough productive of green sputum. On analysis, his blood gases are:

pH	7.22
P_aO_2	4.8
P_aCO_2	8.3
HCO_3^-	35

    a. Is the patient in respiratory failure?
    b. If respiratory failure is present, is it type I or type II?
    c. Comment on his acid–base status.
    d. What treatment would you give the patient?

15. A 33-year-old woman with a known history of asthma presents to A&E with acute shortness of breath. Her asthma has been well controlled with bronchodilators and regular inhaled steroids. The patient woke today with severe breathlessness which has worsened throughout the day. Her inhaled bronchodilators seemed to have little effect on her symptoms. On evaluation she is found to be in respiratory distress, unable to speak in full sentences and with a pulse rate of 110 b.p.m. and using accessory muscles.
    a. What other signs might you notice on examination?
    b. How is acute severe asthma defined?
    c. Comment on the pathogenesis of asthma; why might her bronchodilators not be working?
    d. What treatment would you instigate?

16. A 23-year-old man presents to his GP complaining of breathlessness and wheeze. He has had a non-productive cough for about 4 days. This is worse at night and he been kept awake coughing. On enquiry his family history was notable for eczema and hay fever on his father's side. He has no pets but mentions that his girlfriend has recently acquired a cat.

243

a. What is the likely diagnosis?

b. How might this be confirmed?

c. What are the common precipitants of asthma?

d. What occupations are associated with an increased incidence of asthma?

17. A 65-year-old obese man attends his local GP's surgery after his wife 'insisted that he do something about his snoring'. Although he is not aware of sleeping badly, he awakes unrefreshed and is always tired during the day; he has recently fallen asleep during a meeting at work, which caused much embarrassment. His wife is, however, aware that his sleep is disturbed; she notices that he jolts awake several times each night particularly if he has been to the pub.

a. What tests might the GP perform to diagnose this man's disorder?

b. How might his condition be managed (i) conservatively; (ii) more aggressively?

c. What are the complications of sleep apnoea?

d. Why else might it be important to manage this patient's condition?

18. A 60-year-old man presents to his GP with a 4-month history of a cough which is sometimes tinged with blood. He has also noticed that he has lost about 10 lb in weight over the past 6 months or so. He has smoked heavily for about 40 years and is very worried that his symptoms may be due to 'something sinister'. On examination the patient appeared anxious but there were no signs to confirm his fears. A CXR was normal but flow–volume loop showed a truncated expiratory loop.

a. What are the main causes of haemoptysis?

b. Given the patient's history, what signs would the GP be looking for?

c. What would be an appropriate investigation to perform next?

d. Describe the significance of the flow–volume result? What disorders are likely to generate this pattern?

19. A 78-year-old man is admitted to hospital as an emergency after a home visit from his GP. The patient had a history of recent upper respiratory tract infection, with a sore throat which persisted. Over the course of 2 or 3 days he began to feel increasingly unwell with fever, anorexia and pain in his chest which was worse on coughing. On the day that he was admitted his daughter had visited and found him delirious and confused; she immediately called his GP.

a. What are the core adverse prognostic factors in severe community-acquired pneumonia?

b. What signs might this patient demonstrate on examination?

c. If he went on to develop a complication of pneumonia such as pleural effusion, how might this be treated?

d. Which are the common pathogens in community-acquired pneumonia?

20. A 22-year-old student presented to A&E with breathlessness and chest pain. The breathlessness had come on suddenly whilst he was cycling home from a lecture and the pain was over one side of his chest and worse on breathing and coughing. Examination revealed a tall thin young man with reduced chest expansion. There was hyperresonance to percussion on the right. Breath sounds were diminished and tactile fremitus decreased over the affected side. The trachea was not deviated. On the basis of the clinical findings and a CXR, a diagnosis of spontaneous pneumothorax was made.

a. What is spontaneous pneumothorax and how does it occur?

b. How might a pneumothorax appear on CXR?

c. What procedure might be undertaken in recurrent pneumothoraces?

d. How should a tension pneumothorax be managed?

Extended-matching questions (EMQs)

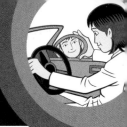

For each scenario described below, choose the *single* most likely option from the list of options.
Each option may be used once, more than once or not at all.

1. Inflammatory disorders of the upper respiratory tract

A. Acute epiglottitis
B. Acute laryngitis
C. Acute pharyngitis
D. Acute sinusitis
E. Chronic laryngitis
F. Chronic sinusitis
G. Infectious rhinitis
H. Laryngotracheobronchitis (croup)
I. Perennial rhinitis
J. Seasonal rhinitis

Instruction: Match the diagnosis to the following clinical scenarios:

1. A 30-year-old man who works in a coal mine comes to the GP complaining of persistent facial pain, headaches and watery rhinorrhoea.
2. A 4-year-old child comes into A&E with a high-grade fever, soft stridor and unable to speak.
3. A 32-year-old comes to the GP complaining of excessive sneezing and watery rhinorrhoea. Further history reveals that he does not get any symptoms affecting the eyes and throat and, recently, his flat mate got a cat.
4. A 2-year-old comes into hospital with a low-grade fever, severe coughing and a hoarse voice. The parents say the symptoms seem worse during the night.
5. A 15-year-old boy complains of excessive sneezing, watery rhinorrhoea and itchy eyes and ears. These symptoms seem to be worse during July and August.

2. Cells and tissues of the lower respiratory tract

A. Alveolar ducts
B. Alveolar macrophages
C. Alveoli
D. Bronchiole
E. Bronchus
F. Respiratory bronchiole
G. Mucosa-associated lymphoid tissue (MALT)
H. Trachea
I. Type I pneumocytes
J. Type II pneumocytes

Instruction: Match the cell or tissue to its description:

1. This structure contains no cartilage and no glands in the submucosa. This part does not have a role in gas exchange.
2. This structure has no contractile element and contains loose submucosa and glands.
3. These cells have flattened nuclei and few mitochondria.
4. These cells have rounded nuclei and are rich in mitochondria. Also, microvilli are present on their exposed surface.
5. These structures have perforations between cells to communicate with adjacent similar structures.

3. Ventilation and gas exchange

A. Expiratory reserve volume
B. Functional residual capacity
C. Inspiratory capacity
D. Residual volume
E. Tidal volume
F. Total lung capacity
G. Vital capacity

Instruction: Match the lung function volume to its description:

1. The volume of air breathed in by a maximal inspiration at the end of normal expiration.
2. The volume of air breathed in and out by a single breath.
3. The volume of air that remains in the lungs at the end of a maximal expiration.
4. The sum of residual volume and vital capacity.
5. The sum of inspiratory reserve volume, tidal volume and expiratory reserve volume.

245

4. Respiratory muscles

A. Diaphragm
B. External intercostals
C. Internal intercostals
D. Levator scapulae
E. Quadratus lumborum
F. Sternocleidomastoids
G. Thoracis transversus

Instruction: Match the respiratory muscle to its description:

1. These muscles are attached to the inferior border of a rib and the superior border of the rib below. They slope downwards and forward. ☐

2. The aorta traverses this muscle at the level of T12. ☐

3. The central part of this domed muscle is tendinous and the outer margin is muscular. ☐

4. Play the greatest role in preventing chest wall recession during quiet inspiration. ☐

5. In addition to the diaphragm and scalene muscles, these muscles raise the ribs anteroposteriorly to produce movement at the manubriosternal joint during forced inspiration. ☐

5. Acid–base balance

A. Compensated respiratory acidosis
B. Compensated respiratory alkalosis
C. Compensated metabolic acidosis
D. Compensated metabolic alkalosis
E. Metabolic acidosis
F. Metabolic alkalosis
G. Respiratory acidosis
H. Respiratory alkalosis
(Normal values: pH 7.35–7.45: PO_2 = 90–110 mmHg; PCO_2 = 34–45 mmHg; $[HCO_3^-]$ 21–27 mmol/L.)

Instruction: Match the acid–base imbalance to the following blood gas results:

1. pH 7.4; PO_2 49 mmHg; PCO_2 26 mmHg; $[HCO_3^-]$ 15 mmol/L. ☐

2. pH 7.4; PO_2 94 mmHg; PCO_2 20 mmHg; $[HCO_3^-]$ 14 mmol/L. ☐

3. pH 7.6; PO_2 94 mmHg; PCO_2 40 mmHg; $[HCO_3^-]$ 35 mmol/L. ☐

4. pH 7.2; PO_2 80 mmHg; PCO_2 55 mmHg; $[HCO_3^-]$ 22 mmol/L. ☐

5. pH 7.2; PO_2 100 mmHg; PCO_2 40 mmHg; $[HCO_3^-]$ 16 mmol/L. ☐

6. Asthma drugs

A. Short-acting β_2 agonist
B. Long-acting β_2 agonist
C. Xanthines
D. Leukotriene antagonist
E. Inhaled corticosteroid
F. Oral corticosteroid

Instruction: Match the drug to its description in the following clinical scenarios:

1. The drug prescribed to an asthmatic adult who uses a reliever (but no other medications) more than once a day. ☐

2. Phosphodiesterases inhibitor which prevents the breakdown of cAMP to cause bronchodilatation, being used in a severe, symptomatic asthmatic adult already on many medications for her asthma. ☐

3. A long-term, severely asthmatic middle-aged woman suffering from side-effects of her medication including osteoporosis, diabetes and recurrent infections. ☐

4. A mild asthmatic complaining that his medication causes oral candidiasis and a hoarse voice. ☐

5. The first medication to try in a newly diagnosed asthmatic. ☐

7. Respiratory drugs

A. Promethazine
B. Codeine phosphate
C. Morphine
D. Bupropion
E. Salmeterol

Instruction: Match the most likely drug to be prescribed to the following clinical scenarios:

1. A middle-aged, non-smoker complaining of a chronic cough. The cough is found to have no underlying cause. ☐

2. An 18-year-old missing days off school and being woken at night because of his asthma. He already takes salbutamol and an inhaled corticosteroid. ☐

3. A terminally ill lung cancer patient with an intractable, dry cough. ☐

4. A smoker requesting a 'boost' to help her with her New Year's resolution to quit smoking. ☐

5. A hay fever sufferer complaining of watery eyes and runny nose. ☐

8. Respiratory investigations

A. Shuttle test
B. Bronchoalveolar lavage
C. Flexible fibreoptic bronchoscopy
D. Peak expiratory flow rate
E. Body plethysmography
F. 6-minute walk test

Instruction: Match the investigation to the following clinical scenarios:

1. A patient whom you suspect to have asthma is asked to keep a diary of peak flow measurements.

2. A camera that is passed through the upper airways to directly visualize pathology and take samples for histology in a lifelong smoker complaining of a new-onset cough with haemoptysis.

3. Saline that is squirted through a bronchoscope and then sucked back up again to collect cells for cytology in a lifelong smoker complaining of new-onset cough with haemoptysis.

4. A sealed box the size of a telephone box, in which the patient whom you suspect of having an interstitial lung disease is asked to sit and perform respiratory manoeuvres. Changes in lung volume are measured.

5. A test of exercise capacity whereby the patient complaining of reduced exercise tolerance is asked to walk up and down between two cones, placed 10 metres apart, in a set period of time. The time in which the patient is allowed to complete the course is progressively reduced.

9. Clinical signs

A. Kyphosis
B. Cushing's syndrome
C. Pectus excavatum
D. Pectus carinatum
E. Horner's syndrome
F. Central cyanosis
G. Peripheral cyanosis
H. Barrel chest

Instruction: Match the clinical sign to the following patients:

1. A forward curvature of the spine in an elderly woman known to have osteoporosis.

2. A hirsute, plethoric, moon-shaped face with acne in a chronic asthmatic.

3. Blue discolouration of tongue and buccal mucous membranes in a patient in acute respiratory distress.

4. A depressed sternum in a young man who has had severe asthma since childhood.

5. A prominent sternum in a young man.

10. Cough

A. Asthma
B. Bronchiectasis
C. Carcinoma of bronchus
D. COPD
E. Cystic fibrosis
F. Gastro-oesophageal reflux disease (GORD)
G. Iatrogenic
H. Inhaled foreign body
I. Pulmonary embolism
J. Tuberculosis

Instruction: Match the most likely diagnosis to the following clinical scenarios:

1. An 3-year-old boy attends hospital having an acute bout of coughing. On auscultation the doctor hears a monophonic inspiratory wheeze.

2. A 12-year-old boy attends hospital after having an acute bout of coughing. On auscultation the doctor hears a polyphonic expiratory wheeze.

3. A 27-year-old man presents with an at least 5-month history of purulent sputum. He has never smoked and he tells you had whooping cough as a child.

4. A 48-year-old woman who is being managed for diabetes and hypertension complains of a constant dry cough.

5. A 60-year-old woman, who smokes 25 cigarettes per day, presents with a 5-week history of cough, malaise and weight loss.

Essay questions

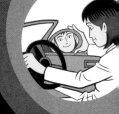

1. Write an account of ventilation and perfusion matching in the normal lung and in disease.

2. Describe the underlying pathology of pulmonary fibrosis and comment on how fibrosis might affect the results of common lung function tests.

3. Write an account of the development of the lower respiratory tract.

4. Describe three ways in which breathing is controlled.

5. Discuss the mechanism of action of steroids and their use in managing respiratory disease.

6. What is meant by the term, paraneoplastic syndrome? Describe how paraneoplastic syndromes might present in lung cancer.

7. What diseases can affect the pleura? With reference to at least two conditions, discuss how pleural disease might present.

8. What is an obstructive disease? Which are the primary tests used to diagnose an obstructive disease?

9. What is ARDS? What are the underlying mechanisms and how does it present?

10. List the three main types of lung cancer and discuss the possible treatments in each.

11. With the aid of a graph, describe lung compliance. How might it be affected by disease?

12. Discuss the drugs used to treat tuberculosis and their side-effects.

13. How does the fetal circulation differ from the adult circulation? Describe one form of congenital defect that can affect the lungs.

14. Describe the mechanism of action of theophylline and list the factors that increase and decrease clearance.

15. What is bronchiectasis and what can cause the disorder? How is it treated?

16. Give a short account of the defence mechanisms of the respiratory system.

17. With the aid of a diagram, describe the paranasal sinuses and comment on the pathology of sinusitis.

18. Discuss the stepwise approach to treating asthma, briefly indicating how each type of drug works.

19. Give an account of the different types of mechanical ventilation, indicating their uses.

20. What are the industrial dust diseases? How do they commonly present?

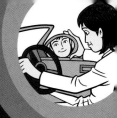

OSCE stations

With these OSCE stations it is a good idea to work with a friend to try to master the station. Use the checklist to give critical feedback to each other. Remember practice makes perfect. Good luck!

Station 1

'This patient has a long history of cough, sputum and shortness of breath. Please conduct a physical examination of the respiratory system. Describe to the examiner what you are doing as you go along.'

Checklist:
- Introduce yourself to the patient and obtain consent.
- General inspection – comment on whether the patient appears comfortable, look for use of accessory muscles, rib cage deformity and count the respiratory rate. Also look around the patient for inhalers, sputum pot, nebulizers, etc.
- Examination of hands – look for clubbing, nicotine staining, peripheral cyanosis and examine for a flap.
- Peripheral and central cyanosis.
- Examination of lymph nodes: cervical, supraclavicular, infraclavicular.
- Closer inspection of chest – skin, veins, hair, chest movement, scars from previous surgery.
- Feel for trachea and apex beat.
- Chest expansion.
- Percussion: technique and areas percussed (both sides).
- Vocal resonance or tactile fremitus tested.
- Auscultation: technique and areas auscultated.

Station 2

'Explain to Derek (who has been recently diagnosed with asthma) how to use a metered-dose inhaler. He will be using a reliever and a preventer inhaler; explain to him the function of each.'

Checklist:
- Introduce yourself to the patient and clearly explain the purpose of the procedure.
- Show the patient the inhaler and how it works.
- Shake container and remove cap of MDI.
- Exhale gently.
- Place mouthpiece in mouth and close lips to get a tight seal.
- Inhale and press canister whilst breathing in.
- Hold breath for 10 seconds.
- Check patient's technique and correct any errors he makes.
- Discuss common problems (e.g. advisable to wash mouth after steroid inhaler use because of the risk of oral thrush).
- Explain to the patient that the reliever is the bronchodilator that relaxes the airways and the preventer is an anti-inflammatory that damps down the airway inflammation.

Remember when explaining information to a patient try to keep it simple and in lay terms.

- Test whether the patient understands and invite any questions.

It is a good idea to know some of the advantages and disadvantages of common inhaler devices used (Fig. OSCE.1). The examiner or the patient may ask you for the alternatives.

Types of devices	Advantages	Disadvantages
metered-dose inhaler (MDI)	compact and lightweight cheap precise and consistent doses quick to use	requires good coordination and technique (may not be suitable for elderly or young children) cold freon effect contains CFCs
MDI + spacer device (± face mask)	no need to coordinate inspiration with depression of canister reduces drug deposition in the mouth eliminates the cold freon effect decreases the incidence of oral thrush	attachments are cumbersome
dry powder inhaler	compact and lightweight easy to use no breath coordination needed does not need a spacer no CFCs	requires a high inspiratory flow to administer the drug some patients dislike not being able to taste drugs
oral tablet	easier to administer drugs doses can be monitored effectively	high doses needed to get the therapeutic effect systemic side-effects
nebulizer	drug is inhaled with normal respiration	noisy not compact and travel friendly expensive requires regular maintenance

Fig. OSCE.1 Advantages and disadvantages of common inhaler devices.

Station 3

'Please measure the peak expiratory rate of this young adult.'

Checklist:
- Introduce yourself and obtain consent.
- Ask if the patient has used a peak flow meter before and explain that you will talk her through it.
- Insert a cardboard mouthpiece into the peak flow meter and push the plastic dial back to 0.
- First demonstrate on yourself – stand up, seal your lips tightly around the mouthpiece, don't cover the sliding scale with your fingers, take as deep a breath as possible and blow as hard and as fast as you can into the mouthpiece with the peak flow meter held horizontally.
- Change mouthpiece.
- Ask the patient to do as you just did, instructing her to do each action as described above. Stress that you will be measuring how hard and fast she is blowing, not the amount she blows out.
- Read the measurement to the nearest L/min. Plot the best of three attempts on a chart to check that it is normal for age, sex and height. If there is no chart, a normal PEFR in a healthy adult is 400–650 L/min.

The examiner may then ask:
'What would be an indication for measuring the peak expiratory flow rate?'

Answers:
- Twice-daily (morning and evening) PEFR monitoring is used to diagnose asthma. Asthmatics have diurnal variation with morning dipping.
- In an acute asthma attack, PEFR measurement is used together with other parameters to assess the severity of the attack.
- Regular monitoring of PEFR can be used to monitor asthma management.

The examiner then shows you a peak flow diary:
'Please comment on the peak flow diary below.'

Name: **Thomas Young**												
Age: **25 years**												
Sex: **Male**												
Date (day/month)	1/6	1/6	2/6	2/6	3/6	3/6	4/6	4/6	5/6	5/6	6/6	6/6
Time	am	pm	am	pm	am	pm	am	pm	am	pm	am	pm
Reliever taken		x		x		x			xx	xx	xx	xx
Preventer taken	x	x	x	x	x	x	x	x	x	x	x	x

PEFR L/min graph (y-axis 200, 400, 600)

Symptoms									x	x	x	x
Notes									Staying at friend's house	Staying at friend's house	Staying at friend's house	Staying at friend's house

Comments:

- This is the peak flow diary of Thomas Young, a 25-year-old man, for 6 days (June 1 to June 6).
- From June 1 to June 4 his peak flow appears within normal limits and stable. During this period he experiences no symptoms and doesn't require his reliever. This indicates that his asthma is well controlled.
- Starting on the morning of June 5 his peak flow begins to fall; he experiences symptoms and begins to take his reliever. This decline in asthma control coincides with a visit to a friend's house, which suggests that something in this new environment is the causative factor. Examples might be a cat, feather pillows or pollen.
- Thomas takes his preventer regularly, suggesting that non-compliance is not the cause of his decline in PEFR.

Station 4

'This is Mr Paterson. He has just been told that he needs a bronchoscopy to investigate a shadow in his lungs seen on chest X-ray. Please explain the procedure to him.'

Checklist:

- Introduce yourself and obtain consent.
- Enquire as to what Mr Paterson understands about the procedure and why it is needed.
- Describe the procedure and its purpose: A bronchoscope is a small camera about the size of a pen that is passed down into your lungs, through your nose to look at the inside of your nose, throat and lungs. It might be possible to see what is causing the shadow on your X-ray, and a small part of your lungs might be snipped away for the cells to be looked at under the microscope.

- Describe preparations and the procedure:
  1. Fast the night before and you may be given a drug before the procedure to empty your stomach.
  2. You will usually be in a sitting-up position on a couch.
  3. A fine needle will be put into your hand, through which will be given medication to make you sleepy.
  4. A small, soft tube will be put into one nostril to give oxygen through.
  5. Local anaesthetic will be sprayed onto the back of your throat – it may make you cough.
  6. The camera will then be passed down your nose.
  7. More anaesthetic may be sprayed as the camera passes your voice box – you may cough again.
  8. The procedure takes 15–20 minutes.
- After the procedure:
  1. If you have had sedation you will not be able to drive, drink alcohol or operate machinery.
  2. It takes about 3 hours for the swallowing reflex to come back.
- Risks:
  1. Nosebleed or a sore throat. These pass in 24 hours.
  2. More serious risks: massive bleeding or a pneumothorax.
- Does that all make sense? Any questions? Any concerns?

MCQ answers

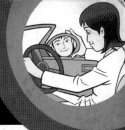

1. a. True The anterior and middle ethmoid sinuses also open into the middle meatus.
    b. False Open anteriorly into the choanae.
    c. False The sphenoethmoidal recess is the opening of the sphenoid sinus.
    d. True
    e. False The upper third is lined by olfactory mucosa.

2. a. False Bronchioles have no cartilage, but they do have smooth muscle. .
    b. True See above.
    c. True Clara cells are present within the bronchiole walls.
    d. False The upper airways contribute about one-half of total resistance.
    e. False Alveoli are the major site of gas exchange.

3. a. True
    b. True
    c. False Formed by the fourth week.
    d. True Can lead to a tracheo-oesophageal fistula.
    e. True Supplied by the superior laryngeal and recurrent laryngeal nerves.

4. a. False Incidence has declined due to the Hib vaccine.
    b. False Never attempt to visualize the throat; always seek help.
    c. True Commonly RSV and parainfluenza virus.
    d. True
    e. False Alpha interferon is the medical treatment.

5. a. False Cilia are found on the type II epithelial cells.
    b. True
    c. True Movement of the dynein arms causes the microtubules to slide across each other.
    d. False Kartagener's syndrome is characterized by dextrocardia.
    e. False Energy is derived from the ATPase activity of the dynein arms.

6. a. True AIDS patients are immunocompromised and therefore are a greater risk for infection.
    b. True
    c. False Sinusitis is caused by *Streptococcus pneumoniae* and *Haemophilus influenzae*.

d. False Cilia stop beating and there is stasis of the secretions.
e. False Acute sinusitis can be treated with topical steroids for symptomatic relief.

7. a. False Central sleep apnoea is common in heart failure patients.
    b. True
    .c. True
    d. True
    e. True

8. a. False Gas exchange is possible in the canalicular period; however, there is small chance of survival.
    b. True
    c. True
    d. False The alveoli increase only in number, not size, for the first 3 years.
    e. True Type I develop at week 24 and type II develop at weeks 24–28.

9. a. True
    b. False It becomes the ligamentum arteriosum.
    c. False Need to use a prostaglandin antagonist – indometacin.
    d. True The murmur is due to the turbulent flow of blood through the ductus arteriosus during its closure.
    e. False The bronchial circulation is a part of the systemic circulation, providing oxygen, nutrients and water to certain parts of the lung.

10. a. False The upper seven ribs articulate with the sternum through their costal cartilages.
    b. True
    c. True Therefore it does not give rise to any sensation of pain.
    d. False The neurovascular bundle lies anterior to the subcostal muscles.
    e. False The blood supply is from the intercostal arteries and branches of the internal thoracic artery.

11. a. False ACE is produced by the vascular endothelial cells.
    b. False ACE inhibitors inhibit the breakdown of bradykinins.
    c. True

d. False   Some prostaglandins also have vasodilatory roles.

e. True

12. a. True   Dead space is the sum of the two.

b. False   In health, physiological dead space is low.

c. True   Due to 'wasted' ventilation.

d. False   Higher at the base.

e. False   Slightly less than 1.

13. a. True   Similar to pulmonary perfusion.

b. True   Ratio of $\dot{V}/\dot{Q}$ is slightly less than 1.

c. False   Normal range for P_aO_2 is > 10.6.

d. False   12–20 breaths/min.

e. False   About 150 mL.

14. a. False   The diaphragm is the main muscle of quiet breathing.

b. True   To allow the abdominal contents to be displaced.

c. True   Elastic recoil drives air out of the lungs.

d. False   Inspiration increases lung volume, making pressure more negative.

e. True

15. a. True   High flows induce turbulence and increase resistance.

b. False   Directly related to the pressure drop between the two ends and the fourth power of the radius.

c. True   Poiseuille's law describes laminar, not turbulent, flow.

d. False   Decreased airway resistance at high volumes.

e. True   For example by mouth breathing.

16. a. False   Secreted by type II pneumocytes.

b. False   After week 32, sufficient surfactant is present.

c. False   Insoluble; it floats on the surface of the alveolar lining fluid.

d. False   Increases compliance by reducing surface tension.

e. True   Allows surface area to vary with volume.

17. a. True

b. False   Nitrous oxide rapidly diffuses into the bloodstream. Instead, transfer is limited by the rise in partial pressure in the blood which reduces the driving force for diffusion. If perfusion of capillaries is high, a low partial pressure is maintained; therefore diffusion gas transfer is limited by rate of blood perfusion.

c. False   Oxygen uptake is perfusion-limited, following a similar pattern to nitrous oxide uptake.

d. False   Oxygen uptake is limited by diffusion because of disease processes in the lung, e.g. increased distance for gaseous diffusion and reduced area of alveolar capillary membrane.

e. False   It takes 0.25 s for oxygen transfer to plateau and 0.75 s for pulmonary capillary blood to be replaced.

18. a. False   The association between oxygen and haemoglobin is not an oxidation; it is an 'oxygenation'.

b. True   Myoglobin accepts the oxygen molecule from oxyhaemoglobin and temporarily stores it for skeletal muscle.

c. False   Carbon dioxide has a 20-fold greater diffusing capacity than oxygen.

d. False   In exercise there is increase in depth of breathing (hyperpnoea) not hyperventilation.

e. True   This is known as the Bohr effect.

19. a. False   Greater at the lung base because of gravity.

b. True   See above.

c. True   Changes in posture alter the ventilation : perfusion ratio.

d. False   Inequalities exist even in health.

e. False   Perfusion is decreased (hypoxic vasoconstriction).

20. a. False   It is only slightly lower.

b. False   Extra-alveolar vessels dilate with increased volume.

c. True   It causes vasoconstriction.

d. False   Low alveolar levels cause vasoconstriction.

e. True   As occurs in exercise.

21. a. True CO_2 is an acidic gas; an uncompensated increase causes acidosis.

b. False   It returns them towards normal but cannot completely correct them.

c. False   Increasing ventilation decreases PCO_2.

d. False   pK is low relative to pH of the blood.

e. False   It is 7.35–7.45.

22. a. False   Reduces P_aCO_2 (CO_2 is blown off).

b. False   Oscillations during exercise stimulate changes in ventilation.

c. False   Anaerobic metabolism takes place, not aerobic.

d. False   It causes hyperpnoea not hyperventilation.

e. True Exercise-induced asthma is a recognized subgroup.

23. a. True Low pressure, low resistance system.
b. True As in exercise.
c. False Resistance is decreased as more capillaries are recruited.
d. True The pulmonary circulation offers lower resistance.
e. True Hydrostatic pressure is lower at the apex.

24. a. True Close to the exits of cranial nerves IX and X.
b. False Respond to hydrogen in concentration.
c. False But response is rapid to PCO_2.
d. True See above.
e. False They are responsible for about 80% of ventilatory drive.

25. a. False They are situated in the carotid and aortic bodies.
b. True The carotid bodies are stimulated by hypoxaemia.
c. False There is a rich supply of blood to the peripheral chemoreceptors.
d. False Parasympathetic nerves cause vasodilatation.
e. False They are sensitive to pH, P_aO_2, P_aCO_2, etc.

26. a. True It is an antimuscarinic bronchodilator.
b. True Other side-effects include dry mouth and constipation.
c. False It reduces mucous secretions.
d. True Hence it is used in COPD.
e. True Acute angle-closure glaucoma has been reported with nebulized ipratropium.

27. a. True Depresses central chemoreceptors.
b. True It is a respiratory depressant.
c. True It is a respiratory depressant.
d. False It is a respiratory stimulant.
e. False It is a respiratory stimulant.

28. a. True Hence their key role in asthma.
b. False A bronchodilator – acts on smooth muscle.
c. False Unlike theophylline.
d. True Acts to stabilize mast cells – mainly used to treat children.
e. True An antihistamine.

29. a. False A β_2 agonist.
b. True Classic fine tremor is seen in inhaled bronchodilators.

c. False Usually inhaled (aerosol or nebulized solution).
d. False May cause hypokalaemia.
e. False May cause peripheral vasodilatation.

30. a. True
b. False CPAP (continuous positive-pressure ventilation) is indicated for obstructive sleep apnoea where it prevents collapse of the upper airways.
c. False CPAP is a form of non-invasive ventilatory support. It is given using a (bulky) facemask.
d. True Paradoxically, taking away diseased emphysematous lung can improve lung function in severe emphysema.
e. True

31. a. True Mitigates the effect of low oxygen saturation.
b. False A feature of pulmonary oedema not acclimatization.
c. True Stimulations of peripheral chemoreceptors by hypoxaemia.
d. True Right shift occurs to aid unloading of O_2.
e. True Oxidative enzymes increase.

32. a. False Blood is not exposed to the O_2.
b. False Hypoxic drive can make high doses dangerous.
c. False BiPAP avoids intubation.
d. False LTOT is beneficial at 15 h/day.
e. True As in positive-pressure ventilation (PPV).

33. a. False 19 h/day is necessary to improve prognosis.
b. False Oxygen should not be prescribed to smokers.
c. False Given through nasal cannulae.
d. False Patients require lifelong therapy.
e. True Minimum recommended saturation.

34. a. True Air spaces are enlarged and their walls destroyed.
b. False Only about 2% have α_1-antitrypsin deficiency.
c. True Due to loss of lung parenchyma.
d. False Compliance is increased.
e. False Radial traction is decreased as supporting architecture is destroyed.

35. a. False Frequently there are copious amounts of sputum.
b. False Dependent lobes more affected due to gravity.
c. True May complicate pneumonia.

d. True   May be long-standing.
e. True   Due to secretions.

36. a. True   Lack of antiprotease causes increased destruction.
b. True   Also inhibited by oxygen radicals released by leucocytes.
c. True   Vast majority of cases are linked to smoking.
d. False   Inherited as an autosomal dominant condition.
e. False   Plays no role in angiotensin conversion.

37. a. False   PEFR is reduced.
b. True   Inflammatory mediators cause bronchoconstriction.
c. True   Due to inflammation.
d. False   Goblet cell hyperplasia increases secretion.
e. True   A common allergen.

38. a. False   Less than 10% of pulmonary emboli cause infarction.
b. True   Hence the risks associated with surgery or fractures to pelvis or lower limb.
c. True   Massive pulmonary embolism may be rapidly fatal.
d. True   Prophylactic measures (TEDS, etc.) are also important.
e. True   Hence prophylactic anticoagulation.

39. a. False   Associated with hyperplasia and hypertrophy.
b. True   Careful history taking is necessary to establish the time frame.
c. True   A frequent cause of exacerbations.
d. True   COPD is chronic bronchitis and emphysema.
e. True   Smoking is the major aetiological factor.

40. a. False   Only of use if reversibility demonstrated by spirometry.
b. False   Causes 30 000 deaths p.a.
c. True   Due to rupture of bullae.
d. True   Common pathogen seen in COPD.
e. False   Genetic defect in only about 2%.

41. a. False   Only reduced in COPD.
b. True   Very common presentation.
c. False   Cough is typically worse at night in asthma but worse in the morning in COPD.
d. False   Wheeze is a feature of both disorders.
e. True   Although, more so in COPD.

42. a. False   Caused by coal dust.
b. True   In advanced disease.

c. True   Due to inflammatory reaction and protease activity.
d. False   Mesothelioma is caused by asbestos exposure.
e. False   Low exposure does not lead to disease.

43. a. False   Usually treated with chemotherapy.
b. False   Squamous cell carcinoma shows keratin.
c. False   Metastases are very common.
d. True   Relative risk rises to 5 with exposure.
e. False   Mostly originates in large bronchi.

44. a. True   Strong association, especially with small fibres.
b. False   Rarely metastasizes.
c. True   Death is usually due to infection, vascular compromise or pulmonary embolism.
d. True   Plus recurrent pleural effusions.
e. False   It is a mesothelial tumour.

45. a. True   Very strong association.
b. False   Adenocarcinomas show mucin production.
c. True   Only treatment of value but tumours are rarely operable.
d. True   For example, PTH production causing hypercalcaemia.
e. True   Used for inoperable tumours.

46. a. True   Panacinar (panlobular) emphysema is associated with α_1-antitrypsin deficiency.
b. True   Enlargement of air spaces is permanent.
c. True   Due to destruction of alveolar walls.
d. True   Either type I or type II respiratory failure.
e. False   Panacinar emphysema is not usually associated with chronic bronchitis.

47. a. True   Common in chest injuries.
b. False   Collection of pus in the pleural cavity.
c. True   May occur spontaneously or after trauma.
d. False   Collection of lymph in the pleural cavity.
e. True   A common feature of congestive heart failure.

48. a. False   No association.
b. True   Associated with occupational exposure to carcinogens.
c. True   Especially crocidolite and amiosite (mesothelioma).
d. True   Relative risk is ×5.
e. False   Associated with nasal carcinoma.

49. a. False   Peak incidence at age 45–65.
b. False   Idiopathic.

c. True   Indicates extensive destruction of tissue.

d. False   Restrictive pattern.

e. True   An increased number of neutrophils is also seen.

50.
a. False   Type I hypersensitivity reaction.

b. True   Hay fever and eczema.

c. True   See above.

d. False   Hypertrophy of smooth muscle.

e. True β_2 agonists ('relievers') cause bronchodilatation

51.
a. True   Due to airway narrowing.

b. False   This describes emphysema rather than asthma.

c. False   Bronchoconstriction is usually reversible.

d. True   Ipratropium bromide is an anticholinergic drug.

e. False   Xanthines work in this way.

52.
a. False   <50%.

b. False   >110 b.p.m.

c. False   Feature of life-threatening asthma.

d. False   Prognostic factor for pneumonia.

e. True   A marker of severe air flow restriction.

53.
a. False   Right heart failure associated with lung disease.

b. True   Chronic lung disease in general is a cause.

c. True   Signs include oedema, cyanosis, tachycardia and raised JVP.

d. True   Pulmonary hypertension leads to right heart failure.

e. False   Prognosis is poor, 50% die within 5 years.

54.
a. False   Cause of asbestosis.

b. True   A common cause.

c. True   Bakers, millers.

d. True   Seafood processors.

e. True   For example textile workers.

55.
a. True   Blood pressure surges during each arousal.

b. True   Plus male sex.

c. False   See above (also common in postmenopausal women).

d. False   Rarely. Patients frequently require CPAP at night.

e. True   Loss of concentration or falling asleep at the wheel.

56.
a. True   All possible sites for metastases.

b. True   All possible sites for metastases.

c. True   All possible sites for metastases.

d. True   All possible sites for metastases.

e. True   All possible sites for metastases.

57.
a. False   Incidence is increasing due to HIV and intercontinental travel.

b. True   In asymptomatic patients.

c. False   Commonly asymptomatic, but sometimes febrile illness.

d. True   Or pleural effusion.

e. False   Although immunization reduces risk by 70%.

58.
a. True   Due to fibrosis.

b. True   For example bleomycin, methotrexate.

c. False   Asbestosis and idiopathic fibrosing alveolitis cause finger clubbing.

d. True   For example in Goodpasture's syndrome.

e. True   See above.

59.
a. True   Immune reaction to antigen.

b. True   As in farmer's lung.

c. True   Concentrated, short exposure causes acute, severe symptoms.

d. True

e. True   Inflammatory marker.

60.
a. True   Opportunistic pathogen.

b. True   A feature of TB caused by MAC.

c. False   Further immunosuppression would probably be fatal.

d. True   Post-infection bronchiectasis.

e. True   TB in any host.

61.
a. False   >7 mmol/L.

b. False   >30 breaths/min.

c. True   A new onset of confusion especially if the patient scores less than 8 on the abbreviated mental test gives the patient a poorer prognosis in severe pneumonia.

d. False   Hypotension (diastolic <60 mmHg).

e. False   May be present in mild pneumonia.

62.
a. True   May also cause pericardial effusions.

b. False   Exudate.

c. True   Left heart failure.

d. True   Cirrhosis.

e. False   Exudate.

63.
a. False   Latency period in allergic form of occupational asthma.

b. False   Caplan's syndrome is coal worker's pneumoconiosis and rheumatoid arthritis.

c. True   In certain diseases (e.g. mesothelioma, asbestosis) within a specified time frame.

d. True   For example in occupational asthma.

e. True   And during holidays.

64. a. False   Size alone is not an indication of metastasis.

b. True   Only indicated in young patients with sufficient respiratory reserve and confined disease.

c. True   Lung function tests are important in assessment.

d. True   Oxygen and/or assisted ventilation to correct hypoxia are more appropriate.

e. True   Has mostly metastasized early.

65. a. False   Epidemics occur about every 3–4 years.

b. False   In 50% of patients.

c. False   Legionella is found in cooling towers.

d. False   No bacterial cell wall so penicillin is ineffective – treated with erythromycin.

e. False   Institutional outbreaks amongst young people.

66. a. False   Gram-negative organism.

b. True   Very severe pneumonia.

c. True   Tests include typical serology.

d. False   No vaccine is available.

e. True   Found in cooling towers and air-conditioning.

67. a. True   In about 60% of patients.

b. True   Frequently in *Chlamydia pneumoniae*.

c. True   In about 15%, classically rusty with *S. pneumoniae*.

d. True   In about 25% of patients.

e. True   Not uncommon.

68. a. False   In those who are haemodynamically unstable.

b. True   Anticoagulation is essential.

c. True   Warfarin should be taken for a minimum of 3 months.

d. False   CXR commonly normal.

e. True   Incidence at autopsy of about 12%.

69. a. False   Not undertaken with intent to cure.

b. False   Non-small-cell is the most common (70%).

c. True   Most aggressive type of lung cancer.

d. False   Staged as limited or extensive.

e. True   From Kulchitsky cells.

70. a. True   Most common in non-smoking elderly women.

b. False   See above.

c. False   Stains for mucin.

d. False   Usually peripheral.

e. False   May be clinically silent.

71. a. True   Cavitating rheumatoid nodules.

b. True   Cavitation may be seen on chest X-ray.

c. False   Does not cause cavitation.

d. True   May rupture producing black sputum.

e. False   Does not cause cavitation.

72. a. False   Typically dry cough.

b. True   As in all restrictive diseases.

c. False   Wheeze is classically absent.

d. True   Often marked.

e. True   Progression over time.

73. a. False   Major risk factor.

b. False   Confirmed as an independent risk factor.

c. True   Anticoagulation usually recommended for 6 weeks to 3 months after PE.

d. True   Malignancy, heart disease, chronic lung disease.

e. True   Due to local variations in ventilation and damaged vascular bed.

74. a. False   Occasional symptoms may be controlled with bronchodilators.

b. False   Treatment may be stepped down at any time.

c. True   Patients are advised to avoid provoking factors such as cat dander.

d. False   If used more than daily, move to Step 2.

e. False   But children requiring high doses should be referred to a specialist.

75. a. False   Kveim test (used in past) or tuberculin test.

b. False   Widespread non-caseating granulomas are present.

c. False   Affects lymphatics and walls of airways and blood vessels.

d. True   In progressive sarcoidosis.

e. True   Classical radiological sign.

76. a. True   Associated with inhalation of toxic gases and smoke.

b. False   Hyperplasia of type 2 pneumocytes.

c. True   Alveolar exudate promotes formation.

d. False   Mortality generally greater than 50%.

e. True   Gram-negative septicaemia.

77. a. False   Autosomal recessive.

b. True   Plus malabsorption and failure to thrive.

c. True   CF sweat test.

d. True   Associated with recurrent infections and bronchiectasis.

e. False   Associated with infertility in males due to immotile sperm.

78.
a. False Hospital acquired pneumonia is mainly Gram-negative.
b. True Due to destruction of cilia.
c. True Or pleural effusion.
d. False More often bacterial.
e. True One of the BTS prognostic factors.

79.
a. False Usually squamous cell carcinoma.
b. False Peak incidence 60–70 years.
c. False $M:F = 5:1$.
d. True Very rare in non-smokers.
e. True Commonly present first with hoarseness.

80.
a. True Rare necrotizing vasculitis.
b. False Affects small arteries and veins.
c. False Aetiology is unknown.
d. True Leading to renal failure.
e. True Mucosal thickening and ulceration.

81.
a. True Rare cause of bronchiectasis.
b. False Dependent lobes are affected.
c. True Kidneys are sometimes affected by amyloid deposits.
d. False Permanent bronchial dilatation.
e. True Complications include pneumonia, pneumothorax, empyema and meningitis.

82.
a. True Common presentation of asthma.
b. True Productive of sputum.
c. True A common cause of cough in non-smoking adults.
d. True From postnasal drip.
e. True A well-known side-effect.

83.
a. True An important cause of haemoptysis.
b. True Massive haemoptysis.
c. True If blood is swallowed.
d. True Frequent and blood streaked.
e. True Simple cause of a sinister sign.

84.
a. True This is the definition of respiratory failure.
b. False Tolerance to increased P_aCO_2 may develop in type II.
c. False High-dose oxygen used in type I.
d. False Differs due to absence of hypercapnia.
e. True Or any disease which causes severe $\dot{V}/\dot{Q}$ mismatch.

85.
a. True Key cause.
b. False Arterial blood gas analysis.
c. False Type II: ventilatory or pump failure.

d. False Defined by a $P_aO_2 < 8\,kPa$.
e. False Renal compensation is common in type II failure (acute-on-chronic).

86.
a. True Flapping tremor is a standard test for CO_2 retention.
b. False Vasodilatation leads to warm peripheries.
c. True In severe cases.
d. True Often headache occurs on waking.
e. True Swelling of the optic disk is sometimes seen.

87.
a. True An attempt to reduce expiratory pressure.
b. True Due to flattened diaphragm (air trapping).
c. True Due to flattened diaphragm (air trapping).
d. True Airways obstruction.
e. True Due to air trapping.

88.
a. True And in other pyogenic lung diseases, e.g. empyema and abscess.
b. False Asthma does not cause clubbing.
c. False Chronic bronchitis never causes clubbing.
d. True In, for example, fibrosing alveolitis.
e. True Due to shunt mechanism.

89.
a. False Tension pneumothorax.
b. False Classically stony dull.
c. False Increased.
d. True Decreased on affected side.
e. True Changed by coughing.

90.
a. False KCO (transfer coefficient) corrects for lost volume.
b. False 400–650 L/min.
c. False Increased with air trapping.
d. False Measures anatomical dead space.
e. False Measures airway resistance.

91.
a. False Displaced in collapse.
b. True Or segmental distribution.
c. False Silhouette of mediastinum is seen against aerated lung.
d. False Bronchi containing air shown against consolidated lung.
e. True Common in pulmonary oedema.

92.
a. True They are synonymous.
b. False KCO corrects for lost volume.
c. False Increased by exercise.
d. True Will highlight even limited disease.
e. False Many causes of reduced TLCO.

93.
a. False At the end of a normal expiration.
b. True Approximately 5 L.

c. True Only RV, FRC and TLC cannot be measured by spirometry.

d. False Lung volume is normally decreased.

e. False Obstructive disorder: <80%.

94. a. False Records the maximum expiratory rate in first 10 ms.

b. False Detects airway resistance (i.e. obstructive defects).

c. False Lower due to morning dipping.

d. True Patient results are assessed against normal values, matched for age, gender and height.

e. False Less accurate but more practical.

95. a. True This is its primary role.

b. False Used to detect perfusion.

c. False Pulmonary angiography is the gold standard.

d. False Less invasive; used more often.

e. False Radioisotopes are not used in this test.

96. a. False Trachea deviated to the affected side.

b. False Homogeneous whiteness is seen.

c. True Congenital atelectasis where lungs fail to expand.

d. True Fibrosis is a recognized complication.

e. True Displaced fissures is a useful sign in differentiating collapse and consolidation.

97. a. False Fibreoptic is used more often (does not require general anaesthetic).

b. True Especially in a smoker.

c. True Bronchial alveolar lavage.

d. False Cannot be reached by bronchoscope.

e. False Light sedation may be used to suppress cough and reduce anxiety.

98. a. False Ventilation : perfusions scans and pulmonary angiography.

b. True Also used in staging lung cancers.

c. True May detect small effusions not seen on CXR.

d. True May require open biopsy.

e. False Medical emergency; aspiration required before investigations.

99. a. True Due to destruction of lung parenchyma.

b. True A measure of airway narrowing.

c. False Increased through air trapping.

d. True Due to air trapping.

e. False Classically reduced in obstructive diseases.

100. a. False Rarely performed; only if diagnosis is in doubt.

b. True Should improve by 15% or more.

c. False No change in TLCO.

d. True Due to air trapping.

e. False Identify allergens (i.e. extrinsic causes).

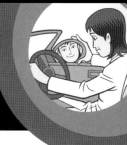

1. Surfactant.

Surfactant is a substance secreted by type II pneumocytes in the alveolus and contains phospholipid (dipalmitoyl phosphatidylcholine, DPC) which reduces the surface tension (ST) of the alveolar lining fluid. It therefore increases lung compliance. Surface tension of surfactant shows hysteresis, i.e. its surface tension is greater on expansion than on compression.

The function of surfactant in the lung is to:

- Reduce the work of breathing ($P \mu T$ – Laplace's law).
- Maintain alveolar stability ($P \mu 1/R$ – Laplace's law).
- Prevent transudation of fluid into the alveoli.

Alveoli vary in size, but because of surfactant the ST of the fluid that lines them is proportional to the surface area and so the $T:R$ ratio remains constant. Thus all the alveoli can be inflated by the same pressure. This prevents collapse of small alveoli and overinflation of large ones.

Surfactant reduces the hydrostatic pressure gradient across the capillary wall (by making tissue pressure less negative), so decreasing the ultrafiltration forces.

2. Normal values for Hb concentration:

Male: 13.5–18.0 g/dL.

Female: 11.5–16.0 g/dL.

See Figure 5.22 Oxyhaemoglobin dissociation curve.

Arterial PO_2 = 100 mmHg (13.3 kPa).

Venous PO_2 = 40 mmHg (5.3 kPa).

3. Venous admixture.

The venous admixture is that blood entering the systemic circulation that has bypassed gas exchange in the lungs. It will not have taken up oxygen or released its carbon dioxide, therefore its levels of PO_2 and PCO_2 are venous levels and for this reason it is termed venous admixture.

In a patient presenting with a pulmonary embolus, some of the pulmonary capillaries of the patient's lung will not be perfused with blood. The blood will not undergo gas exchange. This can be considered as a right-to-left shunt.

This initially causes a rise in arterial PCO_2 and a fall in PO_2. The rise in PCO_2 causes an increase in ventilation.

This allows those areas of lung that are well perfused and ventilated to lower the PCO_2 since a significant proportion (approximately 10%) of CO_2 is dissolved in the blood and is released in the alveoli.

Due to the shape of the oxyhaemoglobin dissociation curve any increase in ventilation doesn't increase O_2 carriage significantly and increases the dissolved O_2 by only a small amount (due to the low solubility of oxygen in the blood).

This non-shunted blood returning to the systemic circulation has a higher PO_2 and a small amount of additional O_2 carriage (in dissolved form) but on mixing with shunted blood this additional dissolved O_2 quickly combines with the unsaturated Hb of the shunted blood and the PO_2 is lowered.

Thus overventilating those areas which are well perfused allows the PCO_2 of arterial blood to be normal or lowered but arterial PO_2 cannot be increased to normal.

4. Airway resistance.

The resistance to flow of a gas within the airways of the lung, i.e. the resistance presented by the airways themselves, is represented by the equation below:

$$\sim 0.5 - 1.5 \, cmH_2O$$

In laminar flow, the flow of a fluid is in streamlines or laminae (parallel to the walls of the tube). The layer closest to the tube wall is believed to be stationary and therefore the resistance to flow is independent of roughness of the tube.

The resistance to flow is dependent on the viscosity of the fluid and the dimensions of the tube.

Poiseuille's law describes the resistance to flow under laminar flow conditions.

$$Resistance = 8\eta l/\pi r^4$$

l = length of tube, r = radius of tube, η = viscosity of fluid.

Thus the resistance to flow is inversely proportional to the radius of the tube to the fourth power.

Factors affecting smooth muscle tone of the airways:

- Nervous factors:
  - Parasympathetic (vagus) → bronchoconstriction. Acetylcholine (Ach) acting on muscarinic receptors. Major importance in control of bronchomotor tone
  - Sympathetic → bronchodilatation. Noradrenaline (norepinephrine) acts via β_2 receptors. Not of major importance in controlling smooth muscle tone in humans, but important in the treatment of asthma.
  - NANC (vagus) → bronchodilatation. It is believed that nitric oxide (NO) is the neurotransmitter responsible. Only effective neural bronchodilator pathway in humans.
- Chemical factors:
  - Constriction caused by:
    Histamine via H_1 receptors
    Prostaglandins
    Leukotrienes

Bradykinin

5-HT via 5-HT$_2$ receptors

Irritants

Cold air

Increased PCO$_2$ via central chemoreceptors

Decreased PO$_2$ via peripheral chemoreceptors

- Dilatation caused by:

Adrenaline (norepinephrine) via β$_2$ receptors

NO

See Figure 4.33.

5. Lung carcinoma:
- Incidence – most common malignant tumour in Britain.
- Age distribution – middle to old age.
- Sex distribution – males > females at present but incidence increasing in females.
- Predisposing factors – cigarette smoking; asbestos exposure; haematite mining; radon and other radioactive gases; chemical exposure: nickel, chromates, mustard gas, arsenic, coal-tar distillates; diffuse pulmonary fibrosis.
- Macroscopic appearances – tumour, usually central (squamous cell, small-cell and large-cell undifferentiated), sometimes peripheral (mainly adenocarcinoma).
- Microscopic appearances – squamous cell, small-cell, adenocarcinoma, large-cell undifferentiated.
- Spread – direct to pleural membranes, lymphatics to hilar lymph nodes includes subcarinal node, blood to anywhere in systemic circulation if erodes into a pulmonary vein, transcoelomic across pleural cavities.
- Prognosis – related to type (worse with small-cell) and stage (some squamous cell and adenocarcinomas may be surgically resectable) but overall 5-year survival rate 4–7%.

6. Bronchial asthma:
- Definition – reversible airways obstruction due to increased irritability of bronchial tree.
- Types – atopic, non-atopic, aspirin-induced, occupation, allergic bronchopulmonary aspergillosis.
- Mechanisms – type I, type II, type III, or mixture of hypersensitivity reactions. Immediate early response due to mast cell degranulation and release of histamine and leukotrienes. The late asthmatic response is due to recruitment and activation of inflammatory cells within the airway and the release of cytokines and other mediators.
- Consequences – bronchial obstruction with distal overinflation, mucus plugging of bronchi, mucous gland hypertrophy, bronchial wall smooth muscle hypertrophy, inflammation extending into bronchioles, possible centrilobular emphysema.
- Treatment – β$_2$ adrenoceptor agonists (short and long acting), corticosteroids, sodium cromoglicate and aminophylline.

7. Bronchiectasis:
- Definition – permanent dilatation of bronchi and bronchioles.
- Causes – bronchial obstruction and severe inflammation, e.g. measles, cystic fibrosis, chronic bronchitis, immotile cilia syndromes.
- Features – dilatation of bronchi and bronchioles, destruction of alveolar walls, pulmonary fibrosis.
- Complications – pneumonia, empyema, septicaemia, meningitis, metastatic abscesses, amyloid formation.
- Treatment – symptomatically, treat active infections, surgical resection of localized areas of bronchiectasis.

8. ARDS:
- Definition – diffuse alveolar damage with hyaline membrane formation.
- Causes – shock (haemorrhagic, cardiogenic, septic, anaphylactic, endotoxic), trauma (direct lung trauma, multisystem trauma), viral or bacterial pneumonia, gas inhalation (nitrogen dioxide, sulphur dioxide, chlorine), narcotic abuse, ionizing radiation, gastric aspiration, disseminated intravascular coagulation, oxygen toxicity.
- Pathogenesis – diffuse alveolar damage ± oxygen toxicity.
- Histological appearances – hyaline membranes, oedema, red cells, proliferation type II pneumocytes.
- Prognosis – 50% mortality rate.

9. Malignant mesothelioma:
- Definition – malignant tumour derived from mesothelial cells.
- Site – usually pleural, sometimes peritoneal.
- Causes – asbestos especially blue asbestos, long latent period (20–30 years).
- Macroscopic appearances – malignant tumour, often spindle-celled, distinguished from diffuse adenocarcinoma.
- Spread – locally through pleural cavities, distant spread less common.
- Prognosis – poor, may remain localized for years but universally fatal.

10. Cystic fibrosis:
- Definition – autosomal recessive genetic condition affecting production of exocrine secretions.
- Pathogenesis – deletion in cystic fibrosis transmembrane conductance regulator leading to unresponsiveness to cAMP control and defective transport of chloride ions and water across epithelial cell membranes.
- Diagnosis – genetic or sweat test (increased sodium concentration).
- Features – meconium ileus in infants, failure to thrive, recurrent lung infections, bronchiectasis, chronic pancreatitis, malabsorption, male infertility.

11. Pneumonia in the immunocompromised:

- Causes of immunosuppression – human immunodeficiency virus–acquired immune deficiency syndrome (AIDS), severe combined immunodeficiency (SCID), intensive chemotherapy and/or radiotherapy for disseminated malignancy.
- *Pneumocystis carinii* pneumonia – common in AIDS, a fungus, diffuse radiographic shadowing.
- Cytomegalovirus – common in AIDS, reactivation of dormant infection or acquisition through blood products, owl's eye nuclei.
- Aspergillus – any immunodeficiency state, fungus, diagnosis from bronchial washings.
- Cryptococcus – fungus, diagnosis by serology or direct examination of bronchial washings.
- Varicella zoster virus.
- Lymphoma – neoplastic but can give a pneumonic pattern on radiography.
- Kaposi's sarcoma – neoplastic but can give a pneumonic pattern on radiography.

12. a. Any other symptoms (e.g. syncope, calf swelling)? Was haemoptysis a solitary event? Explore risk factors: recent surgery, etc. Is there a family history of DVT or PE? Is she a smoker?

  b. Malignancy (as seen here), recent surgery, fractures, recent stroke/MI; pregnancy; immobility; clotting disorders.

  c. CXR, $\dot{V}/\dot{Q}$ scan – depending on results and her status possibly Doppler/CTPA.

  d. Anticoagulation – heparin and then overlap with warfarin. Warfarin to be continued for at least 3 months. Measure INR to assess response – aim for INR of 2–3. Also other prophylaxis, e.g. TED stockings.

13. a. Spirometry is the most useful test here; likely to demonstrate decrease in FEV_1 and reduction in FEV_1/FVC. Also test of bronchodilator response. Exercise testing would assess level of disability. Progressive exercise test likely to show decreased uptake of oxygen against predicted; shuttle test should also show reduced exercise capacity.

  b. Approx. 40 pack years. This would be consistent with a diagnosis of COPD (patients normally > 20 pack years). GP could give him information (advice, Quitline, contact details for support groups, etc.) and drugs, e.g. nicotine replacement patches.

  c. As per BTS guidelines. Strongly encouraged to stop smoking to reduce further damage. Encouraged to exercise. Drug treatment in mild cases: short-acting β_2 agonists or ipratropium p.r.n. Corticosteroids if subject has concomitant asthma.

  d. Cough and sputum due to chronic bronchitis: cilia have been damaged by smoke which also causes inflammation, hypertrophy of mucous glands, etc. Elastic tissue of lung parenchyma is destroyed as granulocytes release large amounts of protease. Loss of compliance causes early airway collapse and air trapping.

14. a. The patient is hypoxaemic with $P_aO_2 < 8\,\text{kPa}$ – i.e. respiratory failure.

  b. Type II respiratory failure as the patient is hypercapnic with $P_aCO_2 > 6.5\,\text{kPa}$. He is hypoventilating and the CO_2 in the blood cannot be blown off in the lungs. (Type I respiratory failure is defined as a $P_aCO_2 < 6.5\,\text{kPa}$. This is a ventilation:perfusion mismatch.)

  c. pH is below the normal range, i.e. there is an acidosis. This can be explained by rise in CO_2 – it is a respiratory acidosis. Looking at bicarbonate levels (and using the Henderson–Hasselbalch equation) we see that $[HCO_3^-]$ has risen in order to compensate for the rise in CO_2; renal compensation has occurred in order to bring pH towards normal. This is typical of the acute-on-chronic situation where long-standing disease allows the renal system time to compensate, but an acute exacerbation (e.g. infection) tips the patient into respiratory failure.

  d. Treat underlying cause of respiratory failure (i.e. antibiotics for infection). Give nebulized bronchodilators. Give oxygen, but in type II respiratory failure limit the concentration to 24% at first, using a controlled-flow mask. Tolerance to high levels of PCO_2 may have built up over a long period of time in this patient, reducing the central chemoreceptor drive. Hypoxic drive (low PO_2) from the peripheral chemoreceptors then becomes vital. This is significant clinically because if these patients are given high levels of oxygen, this raises the PO_2, reducing the drive for ventilation. The patient may therefore stop breathing and die. If, despite treatment, P_aCO_2 continues to rise, or a safe P_aO_2 cannot be achieved, consider mechanical ventilation.

15. a. On inspection: cyanosis, hyperinflated lungs, tachypnoea (possibly > 25).

  On palpation: pulsus paradoxus.

  On percussion: hyperinflation (hyperresonant lungs).

  On auscultation: polyphonic wheeze.

  b. See BTS guidelines: pulse > 110; respiratory rate > 25; inability to complete sentences; PEFR < 50% predicted/best.

  c. Mention proinflammatory components, preformed and rapidly generated mediators. Early and late phases; cytokines, etc., promotion of inflammatory response is underway and bronchodilators will do little to mitigate airway narrowing.

  d. Test blood gases. Immediate treatment with high-dose oxygen, nebulized salbutamol. Hydrocortisone i.v. or prednisolone p.o. Then assess.

16. a. Extrinsic asthma – probably triggered by cat dander (evidence of atopy in family). IgE-specific antibodies produced, leading to inflammatory cascade and airway hyperresponsiveness.

  b. Could be confirmed by skin prick test to cat dander showing weal.

c. Cold air, exercise, stress, allergens (pollen, animal fur/dander, house dust mites), drugs (NSAIDs, β-blockers), infection.

d. Many different occupations (see Fig. 10.1); includes animal laboratory workers, shellfish processors, spray painters, health professionals (latex or drugs). Establish whether symptoms are better at weekends/holidays.

17. a. Pulse oximetry, video recordings or referral to sleep laboratory for full testing (full monitoring during sleep). Fifteen apnoeas/hypoapnoeas during 1 hour of sleep is diagnostic.

b. Weight loss, avoidance of alcohol and tobacco. Or more likely, CPAP via nasal mask during sleep. In very rare cases (where anatomy of jaw is abnormal) surgery to relieve obstruction.

c. Consequences for him and his wife: reduced quality of life, daytime sleepiness, morning headache, decreased libido, depression is common. Also blood pressure surges during arousal, may lead to hypertension. Serious complications: pulmonary hypertension and type II respiratory failure.

d. Also much higher risk of RTA due to lapses of concentration or falling asleep at the wheel.

18. a. Bronchial carcinoma, TB, PE. Haemoptysis over years can sometimes occur in bronchiectasis.

b. Cachexia, finger clubbing, HPOA, lymphadenopathy. Signs of SVC syndrome, etc. Chest may be normal on examination, or signs of obstruction (e.g. monophonic wheeze).

c. Given history and abnormal test, flexible fibreoptic bronchoscopy would be next investigation.

d. Flow–volume loop showed truncated expiratory limb, indicating there is an intrathoracic obstruction.

19. a. Adverse prognostic factors: new mental confusion; urea >7 mmol/L; tachypnoea >30 breaths/min; hypotension – diastolic <60 mmHg.

b. Fever, confusion, cyanosis, hypotension, tachycardia, tachypnoea. Chest examination: may be signs of consolidation (dull to percussion, decreased expansion, increased vocal resonance, crackles/bronchial breathing), pleural rub.

c. If effusion is large and patient is symptomatic, drainage is indicated. Drain slowly (<2 L/h). If bacteriology shows aspirate is infected – empyema – then further antibiotics. A loculated empyema may require intrapleural streptokinase. If persists, surgery is indicated.

d. CAP: *Streptococcus pneumoniae* most common, also *Haemophilus influenzae* and *Mycoplasma pneumoniae*.

20. a. Not traumatic; may be primary spontaneous (no underlying disease) or secondary to pre-existing disease such as COPD. Primary spontaneous is common in tall, thin young men due to rupture of subpleural blebs at apices.

b. May be able to see reflection of pleura; lung collapsed towards heart border; in tension pneumothorax the trachea is deviated from the affected side (NB: a medical emergency – CXR should not be performed, treatment should be started immediately.)

c. Recurrent pneumothoraces: pleurodesis is indicated. Irritating agent is introduced into pleural space so that inflammatory reaction causes adhesion of parietal and visceral pleura.

d. Air removed with large-bore syringe partially filled with saline (in second intercostal space midclavicular line). Air is allowed to bubble through the syringe.

EMQ answers

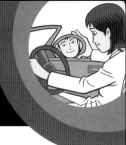

1. Inflammatory disorders of the upper respiratory tract

1. F   Chronic sinusitis.
2. A   Acute epiglottitis.
3. I   Perennial rhinitis.
4. H   Laryngotracheobronchitis (croup).
5. J   Seasonal rhinitis.

2. Cells and tissues of the lower respiratory tract

1. D   Bronchiole.
2. H   Trachea.
3. I   Type I pneumocytes.
4. J   Type II pneumocytes.
5. C   Alveoli.

3. Ventilation and gas exchange

1. C   Inspiratory capacity.
2. E   Tidal volume.
3. D   Residual volume.
4. F   Total lung capacity.
5. G   Vital capacity.

4. Respiratory muscles

1. B   External intercostals.
2. A   Diaphragm.
3. A   Diaphragm.
4. C   Internal intercostals.
5. F   Sternocleidomastoids.

5. Acid–base balance

1. A   Compensated respiratory alkalosis.
2. C   Compensated metabolic acidosis.
3. F   Metabolic alkalosis.
4. G   Respiratory acidosis.
5. E   Metabolic acidosis.

6. Asthma drugs

1. E   Inhaled corticosteroids.
2. C   Xanthines.
3. F   Oral corticosteroids.
4. E   Inhaled corticosteroids.
5. A   Short-acting β_2 agonist.

7. Respiratory drugs

1. B   Codeine phosphate is a specific antitussive therapy suitable for a chronic idiopathic cough.
2. E   Salmeterol.
3. C   Morphine may be used in terminally ill patients where issues of addiction are irrelevant. It also provides the strong pain relief, which is usually needed.
4. D   Bupropion.
5. A   Promethazine.

8. Respiratory investigations

1. D   Peak expiratory flow rate.
2. C   Flexible fibreoptic bronchoscopy.
3. B   Bronchoalveolar lavage.
4. E   Body plethysmography.
5. A   Shuttle test.

9. Clinical signs

1. A   Kyphosis, if severe may cause respiratory compromise.
2. B   Cushing's syndrome, a side-effect of high-dose steroids (may be required in severe asthma).
3. F   Central cyanosis.
4. C   Pectus excavatum – chronic respiratory difficulties while the skeleton is still forming in childhood may cause this deformity.
5. D   Pectus carinatum – often a congenital abnormality.

10. Cough

1. H Inhaled foreign body.

2. A Asthma.

3. B Bronchiectasis, severe whooping cough in childhood, predisposes to bronchiectasis in later life.

4. G Iatrogenic; the likely cause is ACE inhibitors.

5. C Carcinoma of bronchus.

Index